Difficult Conditions in Laparoscopic Urologic Surgery

Ahmed M. Al-Kandari • Inderbir S. Gill

(Editors)

Difficult Conditions in Laparoscopic Urologic Surgery

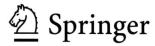 Springer

Editors

Ahmed M. Al-Kandari
Department of Surgery (Urology)
Faculty of Medicine,
Kuwait University, Jabriyah
Kuwait

Inderbir S. Gill
Department of Urology
University of Southern California,
Los Angeles, CA
USA

ISBN 978-1-84882-104-0   e-ISBN 978-1-84882-105-7
DOI 10.1007/978-1-84882-105-7
Springer London Dordrecht Heidelberg New York

British Library Cataloguing in Publication Data
A catalogue record for this book is available from the British Library

Cover design: eStudioCalamar, Figueres/Berlin

Printed on acid-free paper

Springer is part of Springer Science+Business Media (www.springer.com)

Preface

Laparoscopic surgery has changed the way that many surgical conditions are managed. Urologists are among the specialists who pioneered the field of laparoscopy and continued to improve and explore more technical methods that have led to successful procedures, with excellent functional outcome and minimal morbidity. The collaborative efforts that we, the editors, have had together from the live transmission of a laparoscopic conference by Dr. Gill from the United States to operating together on multiple visits have resulted in this book.

When I suggested this book idea to Dr. Gill two years ago, he supported it immediately since he and I felt the need to educate junior and even senior urologists about the safest ways to do laparoscopic urologic surgery. Laparoscopic urologic procedures have recently duplicated most open surgical procedures in an efficient and accurate way with the least morbidity, confirming that it is minimally invasive surgery. This has led more urologists and patients to request laparoscopic surgery to deal with their conditions. Subsequently, we felt an essential need to educate junior urologists, like residents and fellows, as well as urologists interested in learning and performing laparoscopic urologic procedures.

This book is unique in that it will review common, useful information about certain laparoscopic procedures, including technique and instruments, and then discuss common difficulties faced during each operation. We also discuss the uncommon and occasionally even anecdotal cases and the safest ways to deal with them.

We are honored to have a group of world experts in laparoscopic urologic surgery valuably contribute to our book. This book is medium sized and includes a good number of illustrative pictures, drawings, and images that aim to make reading it informative, educational, and interesting. This book is good preoperative refresher reading that will remind the surgeon regarding important steps and possible difficulties.

We hope that this book will continue to accumulate experiences of difficult conditions in laparoscopic surgery and add to the literature in a more instructive way in the future.

Ahmed M. Al-Kandari
Inderbir S. Gill

Contents

Contributors

Amr M. Abdel-Hakim, MBBcH MSc Urol MD Urol
Department of Urology,
Cairo University, Cairo,
Egypt

Mahmoud A. Abdel-Hakim, MD Dr. med. PhD FEBU
Department of Urology, Cairo University,
Sahafeen, Cairo, Egypt

Angus G. Alexander, MBBCh FCS (SA) Cert. Paeds. Surg. (UCT)
Department of Pediatric Urology,
The Hospital for Sick Children,
Toronto, ON, Canada

Ahmed M. Al-Kandari, BM BCh FRCS(C)
Department of Surgery (Urology),
Faculty of Medicine, Kuwait University,
Jabriyah, Kuwait

Alireza Aminsharifi, MD
Department of Urology,
Shiraz University of Medical Sciences,
Shiraz, Fars, Iran

Juan C. Astigueta Pérez, MD
Department of Urology,
Instituto Regional de Enfermedades
Neoplasicas Norte, Trujillo, La Libertad,
Peru

Mohamed A. Atalla, MD
The Arthur Smith Institute for Urology,
Hofstra University Medical School,
North Shore LIJ Health System,
New Hyde Park, New York, USA

Andre Berger, MD
Department of Urology,
University of Southern California,
Los Angeles, CA, USA

Ricardo Brandina, MD
Department of Urology,
University of Southern California,
Los Angeles, CA, USA

David Canes, MD
Department of Urology,
Lahey Clinic Hospital, Burlington,
MA, USA

Sanket Chauhan, MD
Department of Urologic Surgery,
Global Robotics Institute,
Florida Hospital-Celebration Health,
Celebration, FL, USA

Mahesh R. Desai, MS FRCS(Edin) FRCS(Eng)
Department of Urology,
Muljibhai Patel Urological Hospital,
Nadlad, Gujarat,
India

Philip J. Dorsey, Jr., MD MPH
Department of Urology,
Tulane University School of Medicine,
New Orleans, Louisiana, USA

**Ahmed S. El-Feel, MD Dr. med.
PhD FEBU**
Department of Urology, Cairo University,
Dokki, Cairo, Egypt

Ahmed R. El-Nahas, MD
Department of Urology,
Urology and Nephrology Center,
Mansoura, Dakahlia, Egypt

Walid A. Farhat, MD FRCS C
Department of Surgery,
Sickkids Hospital, University of Toronto,
Toronto, Ontario, Canada

Golena Fernández Moncaleano, MD
Department of Urology,
Fundación Universitaria de Ciencias de la
Salud–Hospital de San José (University
Foundation of Health Science–Saint
Joseph Hospital), Bogotá, Columbia

**Arvind P. Gapule, MS(Surgery)
DNB(Genitourinary surgery) MNAMS**
Division of Laparoscopic Surgery,
Department of Urology,
Muljibhai Patel Urological Hospital,
Nadlad, Gujarat, India

Ahmed E. Ghazi, MD, MSc FEBU
Department of Urology,
Krankenhaus der Elisabethinen Linz,
Linz, Austria

Camilo Andrés Giedelman Cuevas, MD
Department of Urology,
Centro de Cirugía Robotica y de Invasion
Minima, Instituto Medico La Floresta,
Caracas, Venezuela

Inderbir S. Gill, MD
Department of Urology,
University of Southern California,
Los Angeles, CA, USA

Raj K. Goel, MD
Department of Urology,
University of Western Ontario Schulich
School of Medicine, Windsor, ON,
Canada

Khurshid A. Guru, MD
Department of Urology,
Roswell Park Cancer Institute,
Buffalo, NY, USA

Ahmed M. Harraz, MD
Department of Urology,
Urology and Nephrology Center,
Mansoura, Dakahlia, Egypt

Hamdy M. Ibrahim, MD
Department of Urology,
Fayoum University, Fayoum, Egypt

Günter Janetschek, MD
Department of Urology,
Medical University of Salzburg,
Salzburg, Austria

Jihad H. Kaouk, MD
Center for Laparoscopic and Robotic
Surgery, Cleveland, OH, USA

Louis R. Kavoussi, MD
The Arthur Smith Institute for Urology,
Hostra University Medical School,
North Shore LIJ Health System,
New Hyde Park, NY, USA

Rakesh V. Khanna, MD
Glickman Urological and Kidney Institute,
Cleveland Clinic, Cleveland,
OH, USA

Ahmed M. Mansour, MD MRCS
Department of Urology,
Roswell Park Cancer Institute,
Buffalo, NY, USA

Shashikant Mishra, MD
Department of Urology,
Muljibhai Patel Urological Hospital,
Nadlad, Gujarat, India

Akbar Nouralizadeh, MD
Department of Urology,
Shahid Labbafinejad Hospital, Urology
and Nephrology Research Center, Shahid
Beheshti University of Medical Sciences,
Tehran, Iran

Kenneth Palmer, MD
Department of Urologic Surgery,
Global Robotics Institute,
Florida Hospital-Celebration Health,
Celebration, FL, USA

Manoj B. Patel, MD
Department of Urologic Surgery,
Global Robotics Institute,
Florida Hospital-Celebration Health,
Celebration, FL, USA

Vipul R. Patel MD
Department of Urologic Surgery,
Global Robotics Institute,
Florida Hospital-Celebration Health,
Celebration, FL, USA

Amr M. Sayed, MD
Department of Anesthesia, Intensive Care
Medicine and Pain Management,
Ain Shams University, Cairo, Egypt

Hani S. Shaaban, MD MSc
Department of Surgery, Adan Hospital,
Reqqa, Ahmadi, Kuwait

Shrenik Shah, MCh
Department of Urology,
Civil Hospital and B J Medical College,
Ahmedabad, India

Ahmed A. Shokeir, MD PhD FEBU
Department of Urology,
Urology and Nephrology Center,
Mansoura, Egypt

Nasser Simforoosh, MD
Department of Urology,
Shahid Labbafinejad Hospital,
Urology and Nephrology Research Center,
Shahid Beheshti University of Medical
Sciences, Tehran, Iran

Rene J. Sotelo Noguera, MD
Department of Urology,
Centro de Cirugía Robotica y de Invasion
Minima, Instituto Médico la Floresta,
Caracas, Venezuela

Robert J. Stein, MD
Center for Laparoscopic and Robotic
Surgery, Glickman Urological and Kidney
Institute, Cleveland Clinic, Cleveland,
OH, USA

**Gerald Y. Tan, MB ChB (Edinburgh)
MRCS (Edinburgh) M Med (Surgery)
FAMS (Urology) FICS**
Department of Urology, Tan Tock Seng
Hospital, Singapore

Ashutosh K. Tewari, MD MCh
Ronald P. Lynch Professor of Urologic
Oncology and Director, Lefrak Institute of
Robotic Surgery Brady Foundation,
Department of Urology Weill Medical
College of Cornell University, New York
Presbyterian Hospital, New York, USA

Wesley M. White, MD
Division of Urologic Surgery,
The University of Tennessee Medical
Center, Knoxville, TN, USA

Eboni J. Woodard, MD
The Arthur Institute for Urology,
Hofstra University Medical School,
North Shore LIJ Health System,
New Hyde Park, NY, USA

Introduction

Ahmed M. Al-Kandari and Inderbir S. Gill

Minimally invasive therapy is evolving as a newly accepted modality for different surgical specialties. This is due to improvements in equipment and techniques of different procedures. Urology has been at the forefront of developing these minimally invasive surgical procedures.

Laparoscopic urologic procedures are now the result of decades of improvements, starting with inspection, ablation, and reconstruction, and moving towards robotic-assisted and single-port techniques. The learning curve for each procedure is an important aspect of improvement and mastering.

It is essential that beginners in laparoscopic urologic procedures know all the steps and laparoscopic anatomy for common, straightforward cases. They should master these procedures before doing more difficult ones. In each laparoscopic urologic procedure, there are some difficult steps that the surgeon must be aware of and understand how to deal with in order to accomplish the procedure safely.

In this book, the editors aim to collect the experience of worldwide experts in laparoscopic urologic procedures. The format of the chapters is easy-to-read, with an introduction and description of the difficulties, and then examples illustrated with pictures. The solutions that the authors have used to overcome difficulties are also discussed. Finally, a conclusion summarizes the chapter. The purpose of this book is to serve as a practical guide for residents, fellows, and urologists at the beginning of their experience in laparoscopy. It may also be useful to experienced laparoscopic urologists who wish to learn more about what their colleagues from different institutions and different countries are doing.

It is the editors' hope that the illustrations, in addition to the website with samples of video materials, will be a great help in fully understanding the material included in this book.

In this introductory chapter, we provide comments to supplement the information provided in other chapters in order to enhance the book's insights.

A.M. Al-Kandari (✉)
Department of Surgery (Urology), Faculty of Medicine, Kuwait University, Jabriyah, Kuwait
e-mail: drakandari@hotmail.com

A.M. Al-Kandari and I.S. Gill (eds.), *Difficult Conditions in Laparoscopic Urologic Surgery*,
DOI: 10.1007/978-1-84882-105-7_1, © Springer-Verlag London Limited 2011

Chapter 3: Difficulties in Anesthesia for Urologic Laparoscopy

- The urologist willing to start or advance in their laparoscopic procedure should develop a good relationship with the anesthetist. Communication with the anesthetist during lengthy laparoscopic surgery is important, especially during the initial learning curve.
- Careful preoperative general medical evaluation, especially for patients with pre-existing medical problems, is essential for a successful and safe post laparoscopic outcome.
- Careful patient positioning and padding of pressure areas are important to avoid post-operative position-related complications.

Chapter 4: Difficulties in Urologic Laparoscopic Instrumentation

- Detailed knowledge of all the necessary laparoscopic instruments should be completely mastered by the surgeon and the surgical team to prevent avoidable instrument problems.
- Access-related problems can be safely avoided with thorough surgical anatomical knowledge and specific preparation for each case.
- Particular care is required when obtaining laparoscopic access in obese, thin, and pediatric cases.
- Good laparoscopic access should allow for easy visualization and reach of the target organs with ergonomic instrument handling.

Chapters 7–8: Laparoscopic Radical Nephrectomy

- Preoperative preparation of vascular anatomy and a tumor in relation to adjacent structures is a helpful method to avoid difficulties.
- The use of all possible helpful equipment and respect for oncological principles is essential for safe surgery.

Chapter 9: Difficulties in Laparoscopic Live Donor Nephrectomy

- Preoperative planning with computed tomography (CT) angiography is essential for safe surgery.
- The editors prefer the transperitoneal access, which provides more operative room.
- Hem-o-lok® (Teleflex Medical, Research Triangle Park, NC) clipping for the artery is safe and the editors use the endovascular stapler for the vein after complete kidney mobilization.
- Careful dissection of the ureter with the gonadal vessels is important to avoid ischemic damage to the ureter.

Chapter 12: Difficulties in Laparoscopic Adrenalectomy

- Both retroperitoneal and transperitoneal accesses are used; one must choose their preference according to experience and comfort level with the approach.

- In the transperitoneal approach, full mobilization of the spleen on the left side and the liver on the right side are important and helpful movements that will expose the adrenal efficiently.
- Thermal energy instruments are helpful tools for adrenal dissection and mobilization.

Chapter 14: Difficulties in Laparoscopic Simple Prostatectomy

- This technique is definitely less invasive than open prostatectomy.
- Intraperitoneal, extraperitoneal, and transvesical techniques can be used in this procedure.
- Traction on the middle lobe with traction suture is helpful in facilitating the enucleation.
- The use of thermal energy devices, such as ultrasonic devices, can be helpful in minimizing oozing when enucleating the adenoma.

Chapter 16: Difficulties in Robotic Radical Prostatectomy

- The the transperitoneal approach is preferred because it provides a larger working space.
- The editors prefer the descending approach, in which seminal vesicles and vas are dissected first.
- Managing the dorsal vein complex can be done with suture as well as an endovascular stapler.
- Avoiding thermal sources in nerve sparing cases is essential for better potency outcomes.
- Currently more robotic-assisted radical prostatectomies are done in the USA, which suggests that they may replace standard laparoscopy.

Chapter 19: Difficulties in Laparoscopic Retroperitoneal Lymph Node Dissection

- This technique should be performed by experienced laparoscopic surgeons.
- This technique is far less invasive than open surgery, and the patient should be offered this option when an experienced surgeon is available.

Chapter 21: Difficulties in Laparoscopic Pyeloplasty

- The editors prefer transperitoneal access, which allows more operative room to suture, although the retroperitoneal route is quite acceptable if the surgeon feels comfortable with it.
- In thin individuals and on the left side, the transmesocolic approach is very helpful.
- Careful dissection of the ureteropelvic junction (UPJ) and handling of the important crossing vessels are essential.
- Traction suture on the pelvis can be a helpful trick for good exposure.
- Delicate handling of the UPJ is important while suturing to avoid ischemic injury due to tissue crushing.

- Pre- or intra-operative ureteral stenting is equally acceptable and depends on the surgeon's experience.

Chapter 22: Difficulties in Laparoscopic Surgery for Urinary Stones

- Most stone interventions utilize shockwave lithotripsy, percutaneous nephrolithotomy or ureteroscopy, and to lesser extent laparoscopy, and, rarely, in some centers, open surgery.
- Complete stone removal with careful dissection of the ureter or renal pelvis and accurate incision are important technical issues in laparoscopic stone surgery to minimize postoperative difficulties and morbidities.

Chapter 27: Difficulties in Laparoscopic Pediatric Urologic Surgery

- It is important to know that not all laparoscopic surgeons will deal with pediatric cases. However, if one decides to take on pediatric cases, then knowledge of the detailed technical steps and instruments is crucial.
- Inserting trocars in children should be carefully assessed to avoid trocar-related injuries since children have small organ anatomy with shorter distances in comparison to adults.

Chapter 30: Difficulties in Laparoscopic Training, Mentoring, and Medico-Legal Issues

- If a surgeon is keen to learn laparoscopy and has the required skills, then it is not too late.
- Various worldwide courses of laparoscopy are very helpful in learning about laparoscopy, from beginner to advanced levels.
- Visiting experts or inviting them to your institution and assisting them while performing laparoscopic procedures can help one to learn important steps.

These are just a few comments about some of the aspects of laparoscopic urologic procedures that the editors wanted to share with readers. It is our hope that, by adding them, readers will find the book more informative and helpful.

Difficulties in Laparoscopic Access

2

Hamdy M. Ibrahim, Hani S. Shaaban, Ahmed M. Al-Kandari, and Inderbir S. Gill

Introduction

Laparoscopic surgery has developed rapidly over the last few years, and many surgical procedures formerly carried out through large abdominal incisions are now performed laparoscopically. Reduction of the trauma of access by avoidance of large wounds has been the driving force for such development.[1] However, the insertion of needles and trocars necessary for the pneumoperitoneum and the performance of the procedure are not without risk.[2] The technical modifications imposed by surgical laparoscopy are obvious (e.g., number and size of trocars, location of insertion sites, specimen retrieval), and therefore morbidity may be substantially modified. Complications such as retroperitoneal vascular injury, intestinal perforation, wound herniation, wound infection, abdominal wall hematoma, and trocar site mestastasis have been reported.[3]

Laparoscopy currently plays a key role in urological surgery. Its applications are expanding with experience and evolving data confirming equivalent long-term outcome. Although significant port-site complications are uncommon, their occurrence impacts significantly on perioperative morbidity and rate of recovery. The incidence of such complications is inversely related to surgeon experience. Ports now utilize bladeless tips to reduce the incidence of vascular and visceral injuries, and subsequently port-site herniation. Metastases occurring at the port site are preventable by adhering to certain measures. Whether performing standard or robot-assisted laparoscopy, port-site creation and maintenance is critical in ensuring minimal invasiveness in laparoscopic urological surgery. Although patient factors can be optimized perioperatively and port design continues to improve, it is clear that adequate training is central in the prevention, early recognition, and treatment of complications related to laparoscopic access.[4] Despite numerous recent technical advances in minimally invasive surgical technique, the potential exists for serious morbidity during initial laparoscopic access. Laparoscopic access entry injuries are reported at rates of 0.05–0.3%. Such injuries likely occur more frequently than reported and carry a mortality rate as high as 13%.[5,6] Studies have shown that no trocar design, including safety shields

H.M. Ibrahim (✉)
Department of Urology, Fayoum University, Fayoum, Egypt
e-mail: hamdyibrahim4@yahoo.com

A.M. Al-Kandari and I.S. Gill (eds.), *Difficult Conditions in Laparoscopic Urologic Surgery*,
DOI: 10.1007/978-1-84882-105-7_2, © Springer-Verlag London Limited 2011

and direct-view trocars, can completely prevent serious injuries.[6-8] Safe access depends on adhering to well-recognized principles of trocar insertion, knowledge of abdominal anatomy, and recognition of the hazards imposed by previous surgery.[9]

Anatomical Considerations

Abdominal wall anatomy should receive special attention prior to laparoscopy because many laparoscopic complications result from trocar placement.

Abdominal Scars

Previous surgery is associated with a greater than 20% risk of adhesions of bowel or omentum to the anterior abdominal wall. Of special concern are incisional scars immediately adjacent to the umbilicus because bowel adherent underneath the umbilicus may be at risk for injury, regardless of the technique used. In addition to location, the width and depth of the scar should be evaluated because a wide or retracted scar may be associated with an increased risk of intra-abdominal adhesion formation, although no data are available to support this observation. If the dome of the bladder is involved, there is increased risk of bladder injury at the time of suprapubic trocar placement.[10]

Abdominal Wall Thickness

Although abdominal thickness correlates with patient weight, short stature or truncal obesity may increase abdominal wall thickness out of proportion to patient weight. Routine evaluation of the abdominal wall prior to laparoscopy is important because the success of trocar insertion may depend on altering the technique based on abdominal wall thickness.[11]

Umbilicus

The umbilicus should be examined for signs of umbilical hernia. Techniques for trocar insertion should be adjusted, and closure of the defect should be considered. In the absence of incarcerated bowel, the skin over the hernia can be carefully incised and the peritoneal cavity entered using an open technique.

Abdominal Wall Vessels

The anterior abdominal wall contains two sets of bilateral vessels: the superficial and the inferior (deep) epigastric vessels. These arteries originate from the femoral and external iliac arteries, respectively, and are accompanied by a large vein in most cases. Immediately above the symphysis pubis, they are both located an average of 5.5 cm from the midline and course either laterally or cephalad. In order to avoid injuring these vessels during lateral trocar placement, the superficial vessels should be visualized by transillumination and the inferior vessels should be laparoscopically visualized whenever possible.[12]

Port Design

Port design has also improved significantly since the beginning of urological laparoscopy. Initially pyramidal cutting trocars were the mainstay. Trocars with shielded blades were then developed and are still the preferred port type in many centers. More recently, non-bladed trocars are increasingly being used as a growing number of studies suggest reduced complication rates. These ports spread muscle and fascia rather than incise it and theoretically allow spontaneous re-approximation after trocar removal. A randomized prospective multicenter trial comparing radially expanding trocars to standard cutting trocars, in gastrointestinal surgery, has shown significantly reduced wound complications in the radial expansion group.[13,14]

Two primary entry systems are available in laparoscopy: the first-generation conventional entry method where the push-through spike principle is applied, and the second-generation entry method where the Archimedes spin principle is employed.

Conventional entry, irrespective of make or model of instrument, requires two components, a central trocar with a sharp cutting, or pointed, distal end and an encasing cannula. Surgeons palm the access instrument with the dominant hand and apply considerable penetration force (PF), generated through the dominant upper arm muscles, axially at port site, to push the spike across different tissue layers towards the intended body cavity. Several versions, modifications, and models have attempted to render this entry system less hazardous while maintaining the spike and cannula design.

The second-generation entry method uses the spin principle, where the entry instrument comprises a threaded cannula only, which ends in a notched blunt tip. No central trocar is required as a laparoscope is mounted into the cannula during insertion and removal. No axial PF is applied; tissue layers part radially and the visually guided cannula pulls tissue up along its outside thread using Archimedes' principle.[15]

Conventional primary port insertion requires application of considerable axial PF to the push through the trocar cannula access unit. The anterior abdominal wall dents towards the viscera; entry is blind and uncontrolled with the probability of overshoot. The compilation of these potentially dangerous performance shaping factors (PSFs) during primary port insertion renders access less forgiving and sets the stage for inadvertent injury.

Second-generation entry systems cushion human error through system redesign and avoid integration of identified PSF. Error recognition is likely when mishaps occur and error recovery is possible before the situation evolves and harms the patient. When specific PSFs of conventional entry are eliminated during primary entry, port placement becomes less hazardous. Interactive and real-time visual entry avoids application of axial force at port site, requires no sharp or pointed trocars, and allows for controlled port placement.[16]

Port Insertion Techniques

Laparoscopic approaches to the urological organs and the prostate can be performed using the retroperitoneal or transperitoneal approach. Each approach has distinct advantages and disadvantages. Laparoscopic radical nephrectomy and adrenalectomy have been performed most commonly via the transperitoneal approach. In general, the retroperitoneal approach is used less frequently because the working space is smaller, landmarks are less easily identified, and the operative strategy requires a steeper learning curve. However, the retroperitoneal location of the kidney and adrenal allows a more direct approach without the need to mobilize or retract the viscera. In addition, it provides greater direct access to the vasculature and drainage systems of the urological organs.[17]

The Transperitoneal Approach

There are three main options for initial port insertion: closed access using the Verres needle, open Hasson technique, or use of an optical port. The site of insertion depends on the procedure and whether the site is approached trans- or retroperitoneally. To avoid the epigastric vessels, the site is generally located lateral to the rectus abdominus or just below the tip of the 12th rib, respectively, in upper renal tract laparoscopy. In pelvic laparoscopy, the site is para- or infraumbilical, according to the type of approach.

Closed Access

Using the Veress Needle

This procedure involves blind insertion of the Veress needle to create a pneumoperitoneum. The needle design allows tactile feedback as it passes through various layers of the abdominal wall. Intra-abdominal pressure is initially set at 15–20 mm Hg for primary port insertion, which is done via inserting a separate port-site system. In upper-tract laparoscopy with the patient in the flank position, the needle can be inserted in the iliac fossa or upper quadrant.[18]

  The insertion site should always be away from previous surgical scars to reduce the risk of visceral injury. The Veress needle is placed in the midclavicular line at the level of the umbilicus in patients without previous open abdominal surgery, while in those with previous open surgery the needle is placed in the ipsilateral abdominal quadrant farthest from the previous incision. After placing the Veress needle into the peritoneal cavity, insufflation to 15 mmHg pneumoperitoneum is established. Certain safety steps are used to confirm entry into the peritoneal cavity, including absence of gas or blood at aspiration of a syringe through the Veress needle, injection of 5 cc saline that cannot be aspirated, low initial intraperitoneal pressure, and no rapid increase in intraperitoneal pressure at the commencement of insufflation. If any of these steps are not satisfactory, the Veress needle is removed and reinserted. No more than three attempts are made with the Veress needle. If still unsuccessful, open trocar placement or a nonbladed visualizing trocar entry technique is used for direct vision into the peritoneal cavity. Radially expandable sheaths are the most commonly used trocars.[19,20]

Open Access

Using the Hasson Technique

The open procedure is carried out as follows: A 1.5-cm semicircular incision in the inferior border of the umbilicus is made and the subcutaneous tissue dissected. The fascia is then grasped with two Kocher clamps and lifted to separate these layers from the underlying viscera. The fascia and peritoneum are incised with scissors to gain access to the peritoneal cavity. The fascial defect is secured by passing two single stitches on both sides of the incision, aiming to avoid any gas leak. Afterward, the Hasson's blunt tip trocar is inserted and attached to both sutures. Subsequently, the insufflator is connected to the trocar and pneumoperitoneum is established.[21]

Using the Bailez Technique

A variation of the Hasson technique for laparoscopic access has been developed in children. Access to the peritoneal cavity is obtained using the following approach: a semicircumferential incision is made in the inferior part of the umbilicus and the umbilical skin lifted and dissection carried out underneath to expose the area of the umbilical scar where the peritoneum and the skin meet. On separating the skin from the peritoneum, the abdominal cavity is opened without an incision. The opening is sometimes enlarged with a hemostat to allow the introduction of a blunt nonarmed 5- or 10-mm trocar into the peritoneal cavity without forceful manipulation (Fig. 2.1). The rest of the procedure is accomplished as usual. At the end of the procedure, the opening is closed with a polydioxanone figure-of-8 stitch and the skin reapproximated with 5-0 polyglactin subcuticular sutures.[22]

The open technique using a peritoneal cut-down and trocar insertion under direct visualization is associated with fewer problems than blind insertion of the Veress needle and primary trocar. Nevertheless, the Hasson technique, believed to be safer than blind insertion of the Veress needle, also carries the risk of potential complications. Hasson's experience with open laparoscopic access demonstrates complications related to primary access in 0.5% of patients.[23] In an effort to decrease the complications associated with the introduction of the first trocar, many variations of the Hasson technique have been proposed. Suggested alternatives include modifications to the traditional open approach, as well as techniques using a blunt tip trocar, a visualizing trocar, and a finger to gain initial access to the peritoneal cavity.[8,24,25] Others have suggested using an alternative site of entry for laparoscopy in patients with previous abdominal surgery.[26] The incision made in the Hasson technique is done infraumbilically where a considerable amount of subcutaneous fat can

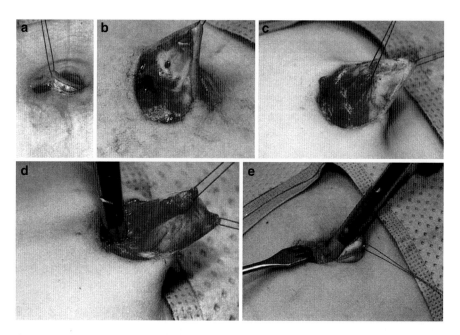

Fig. 2.1 (**a**) A semicircumferential incision is made in the inferior part of the umbilicus. (**b**) Umbilical skin lifted and dissection carried out underneath to expose the area of the umbilical scar. (**c**) Figure illustrating where the peritoneum and the skin meet. (**d**) The opening is sometimes enlarged with a hemostat. (**e**) The introduction of a blunt nonarmed 5 mm trocar

be encountered, while the technique described herein takes advantage of the fact that at the umbilicus the skin and peritoneum are in contact with each other without interposed fat. Therefore, this approach is believed to be advantageous for obese patients.[22]

Optical Access

Optical access trocars have been developed as an alternative method of peritoneal entry. The theoretical advantage of these trocars is that each layer can be identified prior to transection. Two visual entry systems are available: one system retains the conventional trocar and cannula push-through design, where the visual trocar transects abdominal myofascial layers by applying axial PF generated by the surgeon's dominant upper body muscles, while the second visual cannula system applies radial PF generated by the surgeon's much weaker dominant wrist muscles to part the abdominal myofascial layers.

The First Disposable Visual Entry System

This system retains a push-through trocar and cannula design where the spike principle recruits considerable PF thrust, denting tissues towards viscera. After pneumoperitoneum is established with the Veress needle, the pressure is increased to 20 mm Hg. A Visiport™ (Covidien, Mansfield, MA), a disposable device consists of an optical obturator with a blunt, clear window at its distal tip and a recessed knife blade. Following the skin incision and blunt dissection into the fascia, the trocar connected to a 0° laparoscope is inserted. Under constant visualization, it is moved into the abdomen by activating the retracted blade at the instrument tip. The subcutaneous fatty tissue, anterior fascia of the rectus muscles, rectus muscles, posterior fascia of the rectus muscles, transversalis fascia, and peritoneum are traversed with slight rotating movements and moderate pressure. The trigger is activated when passing through fascia and peritoneum. The trocar advances by dilating the tissue planes and the correct position in the abdomen of the instrument can be recognized easily. After the peritoneal cavity is entered and pneumoperitoneum is started, the handpiece of the optical access trocar is removed and the 0° laparoscope is replaced with a 30° endoscope. All secondary trocars are placed under direct vision.[27]

The Second Reusable Visual Entry System

The Endoscopic Threaded Imaging Port (EndoTIP™) (Karl Storz, Tuttlingen, Germany), is a reusable visual entry cannula that may be used as a primary and ancillary port and may be used to perform intra- or retroperitoneal operations. It consists of a stainless steel proximal valve and distal hollow cannula section. A single thread winds diagonally on the cannula's outer surface, which ends distally in a blunt notched tip. EndoTIP™ is available in different lengths and diameters for different surgical applications. The reusable retaining ring, or Telescope Stopper (TS), keeps the mounted telescope from sliding out of focus during insertion. This system has no trocar and is a hollow threaded cannula with a blunt distal tip to engage abdominal tissue layers. It uses the Archimedes spin principle to tent tissue away from viscera, while relaying clear real-time monitor images of the port site. In addition, the outer thread avoids overshoot and renders port insertion and removal incremental and less forceful.[28] Despite visualization of tissue layers, these ports cannot prevent serious injuries as outlined by the review of the Food and Drug Administration's database by Sharp et al.[29]

The Retroperitoneal Approach

The retroperitoneoscopic approach to the kidney and adrenal has been described in detail previously.[30,31] Briefly, patients are given gentle bowel preparation and are positioned on the operative table in the full 90° flank position with the table flexed and the kidney rest elevated. The technique used is a three-port approach. A 1.5-cm incision is made at the tip of the 12th rib and the retroperitoneum is entered. A trocar-mounted 800-cc balloon is used to create a working space outside and posterior to Gerota's fascia. A 10-mm 30° laparoscope is used to visualize proper dilation through the balloon. Following balloon deflation, a 10-mm blunt port is inserted and CO_2 pneumoretroperitoneum is established under high flow at a patient pressure of 15 mm Hg.[17]

Two ancillary ports are then placed, of which the size depends on the indications; they may be 5 or 12 mm. One port is placed at the junction of the paraspinal muscles and the 12th rib, while the other is placed in the midaxillary line 2 cm above the anterior superior iliac crest. The psoas muscle is identified, the intermediate stratum of the transversalis fascia is divided, and the kidney and adrenal are retracted anteromedial. Mobilization remains completely posterior to the kidney and/or adrenal until vascular control is complete. Further steps involving ablative techniques, radical or partial nephrectomy, ureterectomy, or adrenalectomy have been previously described.[17,32]

Laparoscopic Access Difficulties

Factors that cause difficulties in laparoscopic entry to the peritoneal cavity or the retroperitoneal space are mainly related to patient factors and to some extent to surgeon factors.

Patient Factors

Obesity

Obesity is an ever-increasing problem. A thick layer of adipose subcutaneous tissue limits access, especially in the insertion of the initial camera port. The angle of insertion is more critical as this adipose layer limits free rotational movement of working ports. Patients who are grossly obese are at a significantly greater risk of complications when undergoing laparoscopic surgery. It is generally recommended that an open (Hasson) technique should be performed for primary entry in patients who are morbidly obese, although even this technique may be difficult. If a Veress needle approach is used in the patient who is morbidly obese, it is important to make the vertical incision as deep as possible in the base of the umbilicus, since this is the area where skin, deep fascia, and parietal peritoneum of the anterior abdominal wall will meet. In this area, there is little opportunity for the parietal peritoneum to tent away from the Veress needle and allow preperitoneal insufflation and surgical emphysema. If the needle is inserted vertically, the mean distance from the lower margin of the umbilicus to the peritoneum is 6 cm (±3 cm). This allows placement of a standard length needle even in extremely obese women. Insertion at 45°, even from within the umbilicus, means that the needle has to traverse distances of 11–16 cm, which is too long for a standard Veress needle.[33,34]

Ports need to be placed closer to the operation site, or longer ports and instruments must be used. The potential risk of misplacement of ports with associated injury is also higher for those choosing initial Verres needle insufflation. Open Hasson access requires a larger skin incision to see in the obese patient, and the overall operation time is generally prolonged. If the surgeon realizes intraoperatively that he or she is far away or aiming with difficult angle to the target organ, then new ports should be inserted, which will make the procedure more efficient and close the previous ports.

Very thin patients are also potentially at risk of trocar-related injury, mainly with the primary port, as adjacent organs and major vessels are much closer to the abdominal wall. Great care, therefore, must be taken when performing first entry and a Hasson approach or insertion at Palmer's point is preferable in this situation.[11,35] Care and caution are essential when doing laparoscopy in children where open access may be advised and even continuous monitoring of all the laparoscopic instruments is essential to avoid inadvertent injury during the surgery.

Previous Surgery in the Area of Interest

Previous surgery can influence laparoscopy in many ways. It may cause difficulty in placing a Verres needle because of abdominal wall adhesions and limitations in proper insufflation. In retroperitoneal laparoscopy, a previous significant breach of the retroperitoneum increases the potential for significant adhesions and limitations in creating a sufficient working space.[36]

The rate of adhesion formation at the umbilicus may be up to 50% following midline laparotomy and 23% following low transverse incision.[37] The umbilicus may not, therefore, be the most appropriate site for primary trocar insertion following previous abdominal surgery. The most usual alternative site is in the left upper quadrant, where adhesions rarely form, although even this may be inappropriate if there has been previous surgery in this area or splenomegaly. The preferred point of entry is 3 cm below the left costal margin in the mid-clavicular line (Palmer's point). A small incision is made and a sharp Veress needle inserted vertically. A check for correct placement using the pressure/flow test is performed. CO_2 is then insufflated to 20 mmHg pressure and a 2–5 mm endoscope is used to inspect the undersurface of the anterior abdominal wall in the area beneath the umbilicus. If this is free of adhesions, the trocar and cannula can be inserted under direct laparoscopic vision. If there are many adhesions present, it is possible to dissect these free via secondary ports in the lower left abdomen or an alternative entry site can be selected visually.[35]

If the initial intraperitoneal pressure is high (>10 mm Hg) and there is no rapid increase in intraperitoneal pressure at the commencement of insufflation, the Veress needle is removed and reinserted. No more than three attempts are made with the Veress needle. If still unsuccessful, open trocar placement or a nonbladed visualizing trocar entry technique is used for direct vision into the peritoneal cavity.[20]

Anatomical Variations

Patients with a large degree of hydronephrosis or giant hydronephrosis that crosses the midline and causes significant anatomic distortion are at risk of injury to the intra-abdominal organs. Open (Hasson) access into the peritoneum is performed to avoid injury to the already displaced abdominal contents.[38] Prelaparoscopic deflation of the hydronephrotic kidney with intraoperative or preoperative nephrostomy tube insertion may also be performed. Variation in the course and size of parietal vessels attributable to inferior vena caval obstruction or portal hypertension are also susceptible to provoking unexpected injuries to parietal vessels.[39]

Surgeon Factors

It is well established that both the retroperitoneal and transperitoneal approaches have distinct advantages and disadvantages with regard to urological laparoscopic surgery. In practical terms, the selection of one approach over the other depends on an individual surgeon's experience and training.[40] Surgeon experience is paramount in getting a safe, versatile access and in reducing the rate of port-site and other complications. With experience comes skill at accurate port placement, preventing inadvertent injury as well as maximizing surgical ergonomics, and, therefore, reducing fatigue.[31]

Conclusion

Gaining safe and accurate access is the first and most important step in achieving a safe and efficient laparoscopic surgery. Detailed knowledge of the organ anatomy and prior surgical history with availability of all the important surgical tools is an important requirement to do safe laparoscopy.

Caution is vital in laparoscopic access and especially in children and thin or obese patients, and also in patients with previous surgeries. Open access is always an alternative for safe laparoscopy in difficult case scenarios.

References

1. Cuschieri A. Minimal access surgery and the future of interventional laparoscopy. *Am J Surg*. 1991;161:404-407.
2. Fitzgibbons RJ, Salerno GM, Filipi CJ. Open laparoscopy. In: Zucker KA, ed. *Surgical Laparoscopy*. St. Louis, MO: Quality Medical Publishing; 1991:87-97.
3. Mayol J, Garcia-Agular J, Ortiz-Oshiro E, De-Diego Carmona JA, Fernandez-Represa JA. Risks of the minimal access approach for laparoscopic surgery: multivariate analysis of morbidity related to umbilical trocar insertion. *World J Surg*. 1997;21:529-533.
4. Pemberton JR, Tolley DA, Van Velthoven RF. Prevention and management of complications in urological laparoscopic port site placement. *Eur Urol*. 2006;50:958-968.
5. Chandler JG, Corson SL, Way LW. Three spectra of laparoscopic entry access injuries. *J Am Coll Surg*. 2001;192:478-490.
6. Bhoyrul S, Vierra MA, Nezhat CR, Krummel TM, Way LW. Trocar injuries in laparoscopic surgery. *J Am Coll Surg*. 2001;192:677-683.
7. Schäfer M, Lauper M, Krähenbühl L. Trocar and Veress needle injuries during laparoscopy. *Surg Endosc*. 2001;15:275-280.
8. Catarci M, Carlini M, Gentileschi P, Santoro E. Major and minor injuries during the creation of pneumoperitoneum. A multicenter study in 12,919 cases. *Surg Endosc*. 2001;15:566-569.
9. Antevil JL, Bhoyrul S, Brunson ME, Vierra MA, Swadia ND. Safe and rapid laparoscopic access – a new approach. *World J Surg*. 2005;29:800-803.
10. Godfrey C, Wahle GR, Schilder JM, Rothenberg JM, Hurd WW. Occult bladder injury during laparoscopy: report of two cases. *J Laparoendosc Adv Surg Tech A*. 1999;9:341-345.
11. Hurd WW, Bude RO, DeLancey JO, Gauvin JM, Aisen AM. Abdominal wall characterization with magnetic resonance imaging and computed tomography. The effect of obesity on the laparoscopic approach. *J Reprod Med*. 1991;36:473-476.
12. Hurd WW, Amesse LS, Gruber JS, Horowitz GM, Cha GM, Hurteau JA. Visualization of the bladder and epigastric vessels prior to trocar placement in diagnostic and operative laparoscopy. *Fertil Steril*. 2003;80:209-212.

13. Shafer DM, Khajanchee Y, Wong J, Swanström LL. Comparison of five different abdominal access trocar systems: analysis of insertion force, removal force and defect size. *Surg Innov.* 2006;13(3):183-189.

14. Leibl BJ, Schmedt CG, Schwarz J, Kraft K, Bittner R. Laparoscopic surgery complications associated with trocar tip design: review of literature and own results. *J Laparoendosc Adv Surg Tech A.* 1999;9:135-140.

15. Corson SL, Chandler JG, Way LW. Survey of laparoscopic entry injuries provoking litigation. *J Am Assoc Gynecol Laparosc.* 2001;8:341-347.

16. Ternamian AM. A trocarless, reusable, visual-access cannula for safer laparoscopy; an update. *J Am Assoc Gynecol Laparosc.* 1998;5(2):197-201.

17. Viterbo R, Greenberg RE, Al-Saleem T, Uzzo RG. Prior abdominal surgery and radiation do not complicate the retroperitoneoscopic approach to the kidney or adrenal gland. *J Urol.* 2005;174:446-450.

18. Aron M, Desai MM, Rubenstein M, Gill I. Laparoscopic instrumentation. In: de la Rosette J, Gill I, eds. *Laparoscopic Urologic Surgery in Malignancies.* Berlin, Germany: Springer; 2005:271-285.

19. Marcovich R, Del Terzo MA, Wolf JS Jr. Comparison of transperitoneal laparoscopic access techniques: Optiview visualizing trocar and Veress needle. *J Endourol.* 2000;14:175-179.

20. Seifman BD, Dunn RL, Wolf JR. Transperitoneal laparoscopy into the previously operated abdomen: effect on operative time, length of stay and complications. *J Urol.* 2003;169: 36-40.

21. Fitzgibbons RJ, Salerno GM, Filipi CJ. Open laparoscopy. In: Zucker KA, ed. *Surgical Laparoscopy.* St. Louis, MO: Quality Medical Publishing; 1991:87-97.

22. Franc-Guimond J, Kryger J, González R. Experience with the Bailez technique for laparoscopic access in children. *J Urol.* 2003;170:936-938.

23. Hasson HM, Rotman C, Rana N, Kumari NA. Open laparoscopy: 29-year experience. *Obstet Gynecol.* 2000;96:763-766.

24. String A, Berber E, Foroutani A, Macho JR, Pearl JM, Siperstein AE. Use of the optical access trocar for safe and rapid entry in various laparoscopic procedures. *Surg Endosc.* 2001;15: 570-573.

25. Grundsell H, Larsson G. A modified laparoscopic entry technique using a finger. *Obstet Gynecol.* 1982;59:509-510.

26. Gersin KS, Heniford BT, Arca MJ, Ponsky JL. Alternative site entry for laparoscopy in patients with previous abdominal surgery. *J Laparoendosc Adv Surg Tech A.* 1998;8:125-130.

27. Thomas MA, Rha KH, Ong AM, et al. Optical access trocar injuries in urological laparoscopic surgery. *J Urol.* 2003;170:61-63.

28. Ternamian AM. Laparoscopy without trocars. *Surg Endosc.* 1997;11:815-818.

29. Sharp HT, Dodson MK, Draper ML, Watts DA, Doucette RC, Hurd WW. Complications associated with optical-access laparoscopic trocars. *Obstet Gynecol.* 2002;99:553-555.

30. Gill IS. Laparoscopic radical nephrectomy for cancer. *Urol Clin North Am.* 2000;27: 707-719.

31. Fahlenkamp D, Rassweiler J, Fornara P, Frede T, Loening SA. Complications of laparoscopic procedures in urology: experience with 2, 407 procedures at 4 German centers. *J Urol.* 1999;162:765-771.

32. Sung GT, Gill IS. Anatomic landmarks and time management during retroperitoneoscopic radical nephrectomy. *J Endourol.* 2002;16:165-169.

33. Holtz G. Insufflation of the obese patient. In: Diamond MP, Corfman RS, DeCherney AH, eds. *Complication of Laparoscopy and Hysteroscopy.* 2nd ed. Oxford, United Kingdom: Blackwell Science; 1997:22-25.

34. Hurd WH, Bude RO, DeLancey JO, Gauvin JM, Aisen AM. Abdominal wall characteristics with magnetic resonance imaging and computed tomography. The effect of obesity on the laparoscopic approach. *J Reprod Med.* 1991;36:473-476.

35. Royal College of Obstetricians and Gynaecologists. Preventive entry-related gynaecological laparoscopic injuries. Green-top Guideline 49. http://www.rcog.org.uk/files/rcog-corp/uploaded-files/GT49PreventingLaparoscopicInjury2008.pdf. Published January 5, 2008. Accessed April 24, 2010.

36. Parsons JK, Jarrett TJ, Chow GK, Kavoussi LR. The effect of previous abdominal surgery on urological laparoscopy. *J Urol.* 2002;168:2387-2390.

37. Audebert AJ, Gomel V. Role of microlaparoscopy in the diagnosis of peritoneal and visceral adhesions and in the prevention of bowel injury associated with blind trocar insertion. *Fertil Steril.* 2000;73:631-635.

38. Ibrahim HM, Al-Kandari AM, Taqi A, et al. Etiology and management of adult giant hydronephrosis. *Arab J Urol.* 2008;6(2):21-25.

39. Guleria K, Manjusha, Suneja A. Near fatal haemoperitoneum of rare origin following laparoscopic sterilization. *J Postgrad Med.* 2001;47:143.

40. Gill IS. Laparoscopic radical nephrectomy for cancer. *Urol Clin North Am.* 2000;27:707-719.

Difficulties in Anesthesia for Urologic Laparoscopy

3

Amr M. Sayed

Laparoscopic techniques have rapidly increased in popularity because of multiple advantages: smaller incisions compared with traditional open techniques, reduction in the postoperative pain, lower postoperative pulmonary complications, lower incidence of postoperative ileus, and early ambulation. All of these aspects carry substantial medico-economic advantages.[1]

Urologic laparoscopy techniques are minimally invasive and have rapidly gained acceptance.[2] Laparoscopic procedures performed in urology include diagnostic procedures for evaluating undescended testis, orchiopexy, varicocelectomy, bladder suspension, pelvic lymphadenectomy, nephrectomy, partial nephrectomy, nephroureterectomy, adrenalectomy, prostatectomy, and cystectomy. The physiological consequences of laparoscopy are related to the combined effects of elevated intraperitoneal pressure following carbon dioxide (CO_2) insufflation to create a pneumoperitoneum, effects of systemic absorption of carbon dioxide, and alteration of patient position.[3] The lengthy operative duration, unsuspected visceral injury, and the difficulty in evaluating the amount of blood loss are additional factors that contribute in the complexity of anesthetic practice for laparoscopic surgery. Understanding of the pathophysiologic consequences of elevated intra-abdominal pressure (IAP) is crucial for the anesthesiologist in order to prevent or adequately respond to changes in the perioperative period.[4]

Pulmonary Changes in Laparoscopy

Pneumoperitoneum is created by insufflation of carbon dioxide (CO_2) – which is currently the routine gas used for laparoscopy – results in ventilatory and respiratory changes. Changes in pulmonary function during abdominal insufflation include reduction in lung volumes, decrease in pulmonary compliance, and increase in peak airway pressure.[5]

Reduction in functional residual capacity (FRC) and lung compliance associated with supine positioning and induction of anesthesia would be aggravated by CO_2 insufflation and cephalad shift of the diaphragm during head-down tilt.[6]

A.M. Sayed
Department of Anesthesia, Intensive Care Medicine and Pain Management, Ain Shams University, Cairo, Egypt
e-mail: amrafatah@hotmail.com

A.M. Al-Kandari and I.S. Gill (eds.), *Difficult Conditions in Laparoscopic Urologic Surgery*, DOI: 10.1007/978-1-84882-105-7_3, © Springer-Verlag London Limited 2011

Table 3.1 Pulmonary changes associated with laparoscopy (Adapted from Schellpfeffer and Crino[42])

Increased	Decreased	No significant change
Peak inspiratory pressure	Vital capacity	PaO_2 (in healthy patients)
Intrathoracic pressure	Functional residual capacity (FRC)	
Respiratory resistance	Respiratory compliance	
$PaCO_2$		

Hypoxemia because of reduction in FRC is uncommon in healthy patients during laparoscopy. However, reduction in FRC may result in significant hypoxemia because of ventilation-perfusion mismatch and intrapulmonary shunting in obese patients or in patients with preexisting pulmonary diseases such as those in the American Society of Anesthesiologists (ASA) classes III and IV (Table 3.1).[7]

Carbon dioxide is the gas of choice for laparoscopic surgery. It does not support combustion as nitrous oxide (N_2O), and therefore can be used safely with diathermy. Compared with helium, the high blood solubility of CO_2 and its capability for pulmonary excretion reduces the risk of gas embolism. CO_2 insufflation into the peritoneal cavity increases arterial carbon dioxide tension ($PaCO_2$), which is anesthetically managed by increasing minute ventilation. Absorption of carbon dioxide depends on vascularity and the surface area, making absorption greater in pelvic extraperitoneal laparoscopic procedures than abdominal intraperitoneal ones. Mullet and colleagues examined end-tidal CO_2 ($EtCO_2$) and pulmonary CO_2 elimination during CO_2 insufflation for laparoscopic cholecystectomy and pelviscopy. CO_2 absorption reached a plateau within 10 min after initiation of intraperitoneal insufflation, but continued to increase slowly throughout extraperitoneal insufflation. The resulting rise in $PaCO_2$ is unpredictable, particularly in patients with severe pulmonary disease (Fig. 3.1).[8]

Fig. 3.1 Change in total respiratory compliance during pneumoperitoneum for laparoscopic procedure. The intra-abdominal pressure was 14 mm Hg, and the head-up tilt was 10°. The airway pressure (Paw) versus volume (V) curves and data were obtained from the screen of a Datex Ultima monitoring device. Curves are generated before insufflation (A) and 30 min after insufflation (B). Values are given for tidal volume (TV, in mL); peak airway pressure (Ppeak, in cm H_2O); plateau airway pressure (Pplat, in cm H_2O); total respiratory compliance (C, in mL/cm H_2O); and end-tidal carbon dioxide tension (PETCO$_2$, in mmHg) (Adapted from Joris[4])

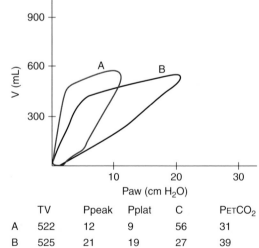

	TV	Ppeak	Pplat	C	PETCO$_2$
A	522	12	9	56	31
B	525	21	19	27	39

Cardiovascular Changes in Laparoscopy

The hemodynamic response to peritoneal insufflation depends on the interaction between many factors including the degree of IAP achieved,[9] patient positioning,[10] neurohumoral response,[11] cardiorespiratory status of the patients and the intravascular volume status.[6] Principally, the physiologic responses include an elevation in systemic vascular resistance (SVR), mean arterial blood pressure (MAP), and myocardial filling pressures, accompanied by an initial fall in cardiac index (CI), with little change in heart rate. The rise in the IAP that occurs with pneumoperitoneum compresses vessels of the venous system, causing initially an increase in the venous return, which is then followed by a sustained decrease.[12] The decrease in cardiac output is a multifactorial phenomena, related to the decline in venous return[13] followed by a reduction in left ventricular end-diastolic volume when measured using transesophageal echocardiography (TEE) (Fig. 3.2).[14]

The compression of the arterial vasculature increases afterload and hence the SVR.[15] Using flow-directed pulmonary artery catheters in healthy patients, Joris and colleagues[16] observed a significant (35–40%) reduction in CI with induction of anesthesia, which was further decreased to 50% of baseline following peritoneal insufflation. Branche and colleagues observed a similar phasic hemodynamic response to pneumoperitoneum.[12] These hemodynamic changes would carry a detrimental effect on patients with depressed ejection fractions. Pulmonary edema, perioperative myocardial ischemia, and arrhythmias could manifest during lengthy laparoscopic surgery. Ishizaki et al. reported that $IAP \leq 12$ mm Hg had minimal hemodynamic effects, and recommend this pressure value to avoid cardiovascular compromise during CO_2 insufflation (Table 3.2).[10]

Neurohumoral Response

Vasopressin and catecholamines are mediators activating the sympathetic nervous system. Joris and colleagues observed a marked increase in plasma vasopressin immediately after peritoneal insufflation in healthy patients and the profile of vasopressin release paralleled the time course of changes in SVR.[16]

Patient Positioning

The patient's positioning may have significant effects on the hemodynamic consequences of pneumoperitoneum. By using transesophageal echo (TEE), Cunningham and colleagues reported a significant reduction in left ventricular end-diastolic area on assumption of the reverse Trendelenburg position, indicating reduced venous return. Left ventricular ejection fraction was maintained throughout in otherwise healthy patients. However, such changes in left ventricular loading conditions might have adverse consequences in patients with cardiovascular disease.[11]

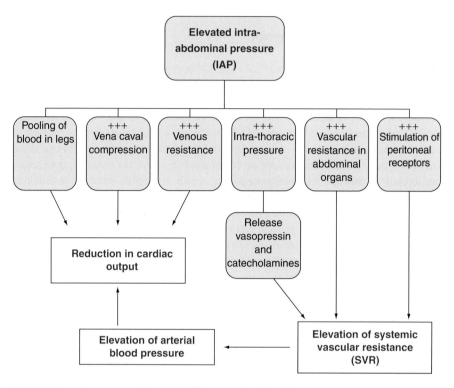

Fig. 3.2 Schematic representation of the different mechanisms leading to decreased cardiac output during pneumoperitoneum for laparoscopy (Adapted from Joris[4])

Table 3.2 Hemodynamic changes during laparoscopy (Adapted from Schellpfeffer and Crino[42])

Increased	Decreased	No change
SVR MAP CVP	CO (initially, then increases) Venous return (at IAP > 10)	Heart rate (may increase due to hypercapnia or catecholamine release)
PAOP		
Left ventricular wall stress		
Venous return (at IAP < 10)		

SVR systemic vascular resistance, MAP mean arterial pressure, CVP central venous pressure, PAOP pulmonary artery occlusion pressure, IAP intra-abdominal pressure

Miscellaneous Changes

Renal System

The renal system is affected by the mechanical compressive effects of pneumoperitoneum that accounts for almost 50% reduction in glomerular filtration rate, renal plasma flow, and urine output during laparoscopic interventions.[17] Urine output increases significantly following pneumoperitoneum deflation. Oliguria has been associated with prolonged duration of pneumoperitoneum during laparoscopic nephrectomy.[18] A possible mechanism for intraoperative oliguria during laparoscopic surgery is an increase in stress hormone levels, such as antidiuretic hormone (ADH).[19] Thus, oliguria during prolonged laparoscopic procedures does not reflect depletion in the intravascular volume.

Cerebral Circulation

Cerebral blood flow velocity and intracranial pressure both increase during CO_2 pneumoperitoneum, with implications for patients with intracranial mass lesions.[20]

Splanchnic Circulation

The splanchnic circulation flow is reduced, but it is counterbalanced by the splanchnic vasodilating effects of carbon dioxide. The effects of pneumoperitoneum on the splanchnic circulation are not clinically significant.[20]

Intra-operative Complications Throughout Laparoscopic Urologic Procedures

Various complications may possibly occur in laparoscopic procedures:
- *Pulmonary* complications include pneumothorax, pneumomediastinum, hypoxemia, hypercapnia, and pulmonary aspiration.
- *Cardiovascular* involvement could be in the form of dysrhythmias, hypotension, hypertension, venous gas embolus, and venous thrombosis.
- *Miscellaneous* complications include vascular injury, visceral perforation, oliguria, hypothermia, peripheral nerve injury, and surgical emphysema.[21]

Anesthesia for Patients Undergoing Urologic Laparoscopic Surgery

The number of patients presenting for laparoscopic surgery is increasing, with a great percentage of them having cardiac, respiratory, or renal dysfunctions and other system affections. The changes that occur during abdominal insufflation prior to laparoscopic surgery and the hemodynamic consequences that take place turn these situations into great challenges anesthetically. The challenging aspect is that preoperative dysfunctions will still exist after the operation, needing further postoperative care; furthermore perioperative myocardial ischemia, infarction, and arrhythmias are the most common cause of morbidities following anesthesia and surgery for cardiac patients undergoing noncardiac surgery. In patients with severe pulmonary dysfunction, prolonged postoperative mechanical ventilation could delay the discharge of the patient from the operating room and may prolong the intensive care unit (ICU) stay. Elevated blood urea nitrogen (BUN), serum creatinine, history of renal dysfunction, left ventricular dysfunction, advanced age, jaundice, and diabetes mellitus are predictive of postoperative renal dysfunction.

Challenges in Cardiac Patients Undergoing Laparoscopic Surgery

The role of anesthetist in the preoperative period is divided into three stages: (1) the patient's risk assessment, (2) evaluation of functional capacity, and (3) determination of surgical risk; this is to help in patient selection for surgery and optimization of medical status.

Risk Assessment

In 2007, the American College of Cardiology and the American Heart Association (ACC/AHA) produced updated guidelines for perioperative evaluation for noncardiac surgery. These guidelines differentiate clinical predictors of increased perioperative cardiac risk into three categories (major, intermediate, and minor). For patients with major clinical risk predictors, their elective nonurgent surgical procedures, whether open or laparoscopic, should be postponed till they undergo preoperative evaluation and treatment, if needed (Table 3.3).

Functional Capacity

The patient's exercise tolerance is assessed by history and is expressed as metabolic equivalents (1 MET=3.5 mL O_2/kg/min) on a scale defined by the Duke Activity Status Index that estimate patient's maximal oxygen consumption capacity. METs greater than 10 are classified as excellent, 7–10 METs are good, 4–7 METs moderate, and, lastly, METs less than 4 is a poor functional capacity. Activities that require more than 4 METs include moderate cycling, climbing two flights of stairs, and jogging.

Surgical Risk Factors

The type of surgery and the resultant degree of hemodynamic stress influences the risk to the patient. Some procedures previously counted as high risk are now categorized as intermediate risk, owing to improved perioperative management. The risks of not performing

Table 3.3 Active cardiac conditions (major clinical risk predictors) for which patients should undergo evaluation and treatment before noncardiac surgery (class I, level of evidence: B) (Adapted from Fleisher et al.[22])

Medical disorder

Unstable coronary syndrome
   Unstable severe angina (CSS class III or IV)
   Recent M.I. (recent MI as more than 7 days and less than or equal to 30 days)

Decompensated heart failure (HF)   NYHA class IV worsening or new onset HF

Significant arrhythmias
   Mobitz II
   Third degree A-V block
   Symptomatic ventricular arrhythmias
   Supraventricular tachyarrhythmias (SVTs)
   Atrial fibrillation (A.F.) with uncontrolled ventricular rate

Severe valvular lesions   Severe stenotic lesions

the surgery should be taken into account, and the experience and skill of the surgeon and anesthetist. Endoscopic and laparoscopic procedure ranges from low risk to intermediate risk surgery where reported cardiac risk generally less than 1%.[22]

Preoperative Therapy

For patients undergoing laparoscopic urologic procedures, most cardiac medications should be continued preoperatively. There is evidence that continuation of angiotensin-converting enzyme (ACE) inhibitors may increase the incidence of hypotension and some physicians have recommended withholding them for 24 h preoperatively.

In goal-directed optimization, patients with high risk factors should be admitted preoperatively to a high-dependency or intensive care unit for invasive monitoring (including pulmonary artery catheter), manipulation of fluid, and inotropic therapy in order to achieve the optimal cardiac index, oxygen delivery, and consumption. Patients receiving antiplatelets present a challenge in management. Dual-antiplatelet therapy using aspirin and clopidogrel carries a 0.4–1.0% increased absolute risk of major bleeding compared with aspirin alone.[23] Increased blood loss in patients taking aspirin has been reported in noncardiac surgery, including general surgical, gynecologic, urologic operations, and in dermatologic surgery. Merritt and Bhatt concluded that monotherapy with aspirin need not be routinely discontinued for elective noncardiac surgery.[24] Burger et al. reviewed the surgical literature with regard to the risks of stopping low-dose aspirin versus the risks of bleeding and found that, in the majority of surgeries, low-dose aspirin may result in increased frequency of procedural bleeding (relative risk 1.5), but not an increase in the severity of bleeding complications or perioperative mortality due to bleeding complications.[25]

Intraoperative Monitoring

Standard intraoperative monitoring is recommended for all patients undergoing minimal-access procedures. There may be hemodynamic consequences to the rise in the intra-abdominal pressure during laparoscopic interventions; invasive monitoring by arterial and pulmonary artery catheters may be useful in patients at high risk, especially if they have had a recent myocardial infarction with cardiac failure, provided that the anesthetist has the experience to insert them and interpret the data. The pulmonary artery catheter is most useful in monitoring volume status and cardiac performance, such as cardiac output/index, mixed venous oxygen saturation, systemic and pulmonary vascular resistances. Transesophageal echocardiography may be used to assess volume status and valvular disease and is the best way to detect ischemia early (segmental wall motion abnormalities), but requires expertise to interpret.[26] $EtCO_2$ is most commonly used as a noninvasive indicator of $PaCO_2$ in assessing the adequacy of ventilation during laparoscopic procedures. Temperature should be monitored throughout laparoscopic surgery.

Intraoperative Management

The oxygen supply/demand ratio must be maintained to avoid ischemia in coronary artery disease patients. During pneumoperitoneum, the rise of the systemic vascular resistance would impair oxygen supply/demand ratio. The maintenance of arterial blood pressure and reduction of heart rate should reduce the risk of ischemia.[26]

Anesthetic Agents

In laparoscopic surgery, general anesthesia is the technique of choice, owing to the lengthy procedure and the diaphragmatic cephalad migration. The choice of anesthetic agents does not significantly affect the risks of perioperative complications, provided that hypertension, tachycardia, and hypotension are avoided. Anesthetic agent choice should be governed by the experience and skill of the anesthetist and their familiarity with the techniques and drugs. Etomidate has the fewest cardiovascular effects, but most people are more familiar with thiopentone or propofol, both of which should be titrated carefully to effect. Pretreatment with a dose of opioid (fentanyl and sufentanil, 1.5–5 and 0.25–1 µg/kg, respectively) reduces the required dose of induction agent and attenuates the hemodynamic response to intubation. Remifentanil is a new, potent, ultra-short-acting opioid, in a dose 0.05–2 µg/kg/min has great ability to produce hemodynamic stability and suppress the stress response. Concerns were previously raised that isoflurane might cause a "coronary steal" situation, but these have subsided. The concerns regarding the use of N_2O during laparoscopy, as it might lead to bowel distension and postoperative nausea and vomiting, has been a controversial issue. Clinically there is no significant difference in bowel distension and postoperative nausea and vomiting when N_2O-oxygen was compared to air-oxygen and no conclusive evidence suggesting N_2O cannot be used during laparoscopy.[27] The rise in the SVR that accompanies peritoneal insufflation leads to afterload elevation and increase in the left ventricular workload, adding more stress to the coronary circulation disrupting the oxygen supply/demand ratio. At this stage a vasodilator agent is of value in reducing the elevated SVR; inhalational anesthestic agents, especially isoflurane and sevoflurane, are the agents of choice, as the hemodynamic profile of sevoflurane resembles that of isoflurane.[28] In cardiac patients, sevoflurane had a cardiovascular outcome data equivalent to that of isoflurane.[29] When intravenous vasodilator agent is warranted, hydralazine is recommended for perioperative hypertension in a dose of 5–20 mg in a titrated intravenous (IV) boluses every 15–20 min until the desired blood pressure is reached. Fenoldopam mesylate is a selectively D_1-dopamine receptor agonist with moderate affinity for α(alpha)$_2$-adrenoceptors (infusion rates studied in clinical trials range from 0.01 to 1.6 µg/kg/min) reduces systolic and diastolic blood pressure in patients with malignant hypertension. It offers advantages in the acute resolution of severe hypertension compared to sodium nitroprusside, particularly in patient with preexisting renal impairment.[30] Esmolol is an ultra-short-acting selective β(beta)$_1$-antagonist that reduces heart rate and to a lesser extent blood pressure. Successfully used to prevent tachycardia and hypertension in response to perioperative stimuli such as intubation, surgical stimulation, and emergence from general anesthesia, esmolol is given by infusion in a dose 50–300 µg/kg/min. Labetalol α(alpha)- and β(beta)-blocker for treatment of hypertension can be used as a bolus; the initial dose is 0.1–0.25 mg/kg IV over 2 min, then repeated every 10 min to a total of 300 mg. When used as a continuous infusion, it is usually started at 2 mg/min and titrated to effect.[31] Owing to their systemic vasodilatory effects, intravenous isradipine and nicardipine have been shown to be effective in the treatment of postoperative hypertension in cardiac surgical patients, with minimal side effects.[32]

Challenges in Patients with Pulmonary Disease Undergoing Laparoscopic Surgery

Six risk factors predispose patients to postoperative pulmonary complications:

- Preexisting pulmonary disease
- Thoracic or upper abdominal surgery
- Smoking
- Obesity
- Age (>60 years)
- Prolonged general anesthesia (>3 h)

Chronic obstructive pulmonary disease (COPD) is the most common pulmonary disorder encountered in anesthetic practice. During preoperative assessment using a pulmonary function test, patients with a forced expiratory volume in the first second (FEV_1) less than 50% of predicted (1.2–1.5 L) usually have dyspnea on exertion, whereas those with an FEV_1 less than 25% (< 1 L for men) typically have dyspnea with minimal activity. The latter patients often exhibit CO_2 retention and pulmonary hypertension. Many patients have concomitant cardiac disease and should also receive a careful cardiovascular evaluation. Laparoscopic procedures commonly lead to elevation of $PaCO_2$; mechanical ventilation should be adjusted through manipulation of tidal volume and respiratory rate to achieve normocapnia and avoid hypercarpia. The use of arterial blood gas sampling and capnogram are helpful monitoring devices is such situations.[33]

Challenges in Patients with Perioperative Renal Dysfunction and Renal Failure

Preoperative preparation is of benefit for patients with renal disease undergoing urologic laparoscopic procedures. Hemodynamic instability is common, especially on a lengthy laparoscopic extensive surgery such as laparoscopic nephrectomy. From the standpoint of renal dysfunction, there may be a varying degree of decreased ability to concentrate urine, decreased ability to regulate extracellular fluid and sodium, impaired handling of acid loads, hyperkalemia, and impaired excretion of medications as in end stage renal disease (ESRD). Renal impairment is confounded by anemia, uremic platelet dysfunction, arrhythmias, pericardial effusions, myocardial dysfunction, chronic hypertension, neuropathies, malnutrition, and susceptibility to infection. If a contrast study is definitely indicated, the patient should be well hydrated and the contrast dose limited to the minimum needed, plus the addition of N-acetylcysteine, which acts as a nephroprotective agent to prevent contrast-induced nephropathy.[34]

Preoperatively patients must be euvolemic, normotensive, normonatremic, and normokalemic. Patients should not be acidotic or severely anemic, or without significant platelet dysfunction as this would carry deleterious bleeding consequences in a laparoscopic urologic procedure. Dialysis usually corrects uremic platelet dysfunction and is best performed within the 24 h before surgery, though 1-deamino-8-d-arginine vasopressin (DDAVP) may also be administered to correct platelet dysfunction.

Patients with ESRD who have left ventricular dysfunction undergoing laparoscopic urologic procedures would need invasive monitoring in the form of invasive blood pressure, pulmonary artery catheter (PAC) to measure pulmonary capillary wedge pressure (PCWP) and left ventricular functions. A sterile technique should be strictly followed when inserting any catheters to reduce risk of infection. Hyperkalemia should be considered in patients with ESRD who develop ventricular arrhythmias or cardiac arrest. Rapid administration of calcium chloride temporizes the cardiac effects of hyperkalemia until further measures (administration of glucose and insulin, hyperventilation, administration of sodium bicarbonate and potassium-binding resins, and dialysis) can be taken to shift potassium intracellularly and to decrease total body potassium.[35]

Contraindications for Laparoscopic Procedures

Relative contraindications for laparoscopy include increased intracranial pressure, patients with ventriculoperitoneal or peritoneojugular shunts, hypovolemia, congestive heart failure or severe cardiopulmonary disease, and coagulopathy. Morbid obesity, pregnancy, and prior abdominal surgery were previously considered contraindications to laparoscopic surgery; however, with improved surgical techniques and technology, most patients with these conditions can safely undergo laparoscopic surgery.[36]

Postoperative Pain Management in Laparoscopic Urologic Surgeries

Pain is a form of stress and produces an elevation in stress hormones and catecholamines. Good pain management results in shorter hospital stay, reduced morbidities (especially in patients with less physiologic reserve, such as those in the intensive care unit), and better immune function, less catabolism and endocrinal derangements, and fewer thrombo-embolic complications. Recent studies have shown the value of preemptive analgesia in some surgical situations. The blockade of the pathways involved in pain transmission before surgical stimulation may decrease the patient's postoperative pain. Balanced (multimodal) analgesia is the term applied for using two or more analgesic agents that act by different mechanisms to achieve a superior analgesic effect without increasing adverse events compared with increased doses of single agents. For example, epidural opioids can be administered in combination with epidural local anaesthetics; intravenous opioids can be administered in combination with NSAIDs, which have a dose sparing effect for systemically administered opioids.

Pharmacological Options for Pain Management

Postoperative pain management should be stepwise and balanced as mentioned before. Laparoscopic surgery is a minimally invasive surgery, hence producing mild intensity pain. Postoperative pain can be controlled by simple noncomplicated techniques, which adds to the list of advantages to laparoscopic procedures.

Non-opioid analgesics: Paracetamol, NSAIDs, including COX-2 inhibitors are considered an effective choice for postoperative pain, especially in low-intensity pain procedures.

Weak opioid analgesics: Including tramadol alone or in combination with paracetamol.

Strong opioids: Are useful in moderate to severe postoperative pain control, including morphine, meperidine, and oxycodone.

Adjunctive analgesics: Ketamine, clonidine, gabapentine, pregabaline.[37]

Patient-Controlled Analgesia

Advances in computer technology have allowed the development of patient-controlled analgesia (PCA). By pushing a button, patients are able to self-administer precise doses of opioids intravenously (or intraspinally) on an as needed (PRN) basis. The physician programs the infusion pump to deliver a specific dose, the minimum interval between doses (lockout period), and the maximum amount of opioid that can be administered in a given period, and a basal infusion can be simultaneously delivered (Table 3.4).

Table 3.4 General guidelines for patient-controlled intravenous analgesia (PCIA) orders for the average adult (Adapted from Morgan et al.[37])

Opioid	Bolus dose	Lockout (min)	Infusion rate
Morphine	1–3 mg	10–20	0–1 mg/h
Meperidine (Demerol)	10–15 mg	5–15	0–20 mg/h
Fentanyl (Sublimaze)	15–25 μg	10–20	0–50 μg/h
Hydromorphone (Dilaudid)	0.1–0.3 mg	10–20	0–0.5 mg/h

Studies show that PCA is a cost-effective technique that produces superior analgesia with very high patient satisfaction with reduced total drug consumption. Patients additionally like the control that is given to them; they are able to adjust the analgesia according to their pain severity, which varies with activity and the time of day. PCA therefore requires the understanding and cooperation of the patient; this limits its use in very young or confused patients. The routine use of a basal ("background") infusion is controversial.

Central Neuraxial Blockade

Epidural administration of local anesthetic–opioid mixtures is an excellent technique for managing postoperative pain following abdominal, pelvic, open, and laparoscopic surgical procedures. Patients often have better preservation of pulmonary function and are able to ambulate early, with the added benefit of early physical therapy and lower risk for postoperative venous thrombosis. In lengthy extensive laparoscopic urologic surgery such as cystectomy, nephrectomy, and prostatectomy, the preoperative insertion of epidural catheter provides titratable analgesia with extendable duration and level. The tip of the catheter should be placed as close as possible to the surgical dermatomes: T6–T10 for major intra-abdominal surgery, and L2–L4 for lower limb surgery. Diluted local anesthetic solutions combined with opioids shows synergistic effect. Bupivacaine 0.0625–0.125% (or ropivacaine 0.1–0.2%) combined with fentanyl 2–5 μg/mL provides excellent postoperative analgesia with lower drug requirements and fewer side effects. Patient controlled epidural analgesia (PCEA) is a term describing the patient-controlled administration of analgesic medications in the epidural space, to cover periods of increased discomfort.

Dosage of PCEA: A mixture of Bupivacaine 0.0625–0.125% (or ropivacaine 0.1–0.2%) combined with fentanyl 2–5 μg/mL

- Background infusion of 4–6 mL/h
- Controlled infusion bolus dose: 2 mL (2–4 mL) lumbar or thoracic
- Minimum lockout interval 10 min (10–30 min)

Epidurally administered, preservative-free morphine allows lumbar injection to provide proper analgesia in both thoracic and upper abdominal procedures, which is attributed to the rostral spread phenomena of hydrophilic opioids. Epidural clonidine in a dose of 3–5 µg/kg is an effective analgesic, but it can be associated with hypotension and bradycardia.[37]

Ketamine

Ketamine is a noncompetitive, use-dependent antagonist of N-methyl-D-aspartate (NMDA) receptors; it reduces the postoperative pain in opioid tolerant patients, and postoperative nausea and vomiting. At a serum level of 0.1 µg/mL or higher, pain threshold is elevated.[38] Ketamine reduces opiate requirements by 30% postoperatively.[39] An intravenous dose of 0.1–0.2 mg/kg followed by a continuous infusion of 5–7 µg/kg/min is considered a sub-anesthetic dose effective in reducing morphine requirements in the first 24 h after surgery.[40] Central nervous system (CNS) excitatory effects included sensory illusions, sympathoneuronal release of norepinephrine, elevated blood pressure, tachycardia, elevated intracranial pressure (ICP), blurred vision, and altered hearing.[41]

References

1. Morgan GE Jr, Mikhail MS, Murray MJ. Laparoscopic surgery. In: Foltin J, Lebowitz H, Boyle PJ, eds. *Clinical Anesthesiology*. 4th ed. New York: McGraw-Hill; 2006:522-523.
2. Clayman RV, Kavoussi LR. Endosurgical techniques for the diagnosis and treatment of non-calculus disease of the ureter and kidney. In: Walsh P, Retik A, Stamey T, et al., eds. *Campbell's Urology*. 6th ed. Philadelphia, PA: W.B. Saunders; 1992:2231.
3. Cunningham AJ, Nolan C. Anesthesia for minimally invasive procedures. In: Barash PG, Cullen BF, Stoelting RK, eds. *Clinical Anesthesia*. 5th ed. Philadelphia, PA: Lippincott Williams & Wilkins; 2006:2204-2220.
4. Joris JL. Anesthesia for laparoscopy. In: Fleisher LA, Johns RA, Savarese JJ, Wiener-Kronish JP, Young WL, eds. *Miller's Anesthesia*. 6th ed. Philadelphia, PA: Elsevier; 2005:2285-2300.
5. Walder AD, Aitkenhead AR. Role of vasopressin in the haemodynamic response to laparoscopic cholecystectomy. *Br J Anaesth*. 1997;78:264-266.
6. Safran D, Sgambati S, Orlando R. Laparoscopy in high-risk cardiac patients. *Surg Gynecol Obstet*. 1993;176(6):548-554.
7. Holzman M, Sharp K, Richards W. Hypercarbia during carbon dioxide gas insufflation for therapeutic laparoscopy: a note of caution. *Surg Laparosc Endosc*. 1992;2(1):11-14.
8. Bardoczky GI, Engelman E, Levarlet M, Simon P. Ventilatory effects of pneumoperitoneum monitored with continuous spirometry. *Anaesthesia*. 1993;48(4):309-311.
9. Eldar S, Sabo E, Nash E, Abrahamson J, Matter I. Laparoscopic cholecystectomy for acute cholecystitis. *Prospective trial World J Surg*. 1997;21(5):540-545.
10. Ishizaki Y, Bandai Y, Shimomura K, Abe H, Ohtomo Y, Idezuki Y. Safe intraabdominal pressure of pneumoperitoneum during laparoscopic surgery. *Surgery*. 1993;114(3):549-554.
11. Cunningham AJ, Turner J, Rosenbaum S, Rafferty T. Transoesophageal assessment of haemodynamic function during laparoscopic cholecystectomy. *Br J Anaesth*. 1993;70(6):621-625.
12. Branche PE, Duperret SL, Sagnard PE, Boulez JL, Petit PL, Viale JP. Left ventricular loading modifications induced by pneumoperitoneum: a time course echocardiographic study. *Anesth Analg*. 1998;86(3):482-487.

13. Richardson JD, Trinkle JK. Hemodynamic and respiratory alterations with increased intra-abdominal pressure. *J Surg Res*. 1976;20(5):401-404.
14. Dorsay DA, Green FL, Baysinger CL. Hemodynamic changes during laparoscopic cholecystectomy monitored with transesophageal echocardiography. *Surg Endosc*. 1995;9(2): 128-133.
15. Wahba RW, Béïque F, Kleiman SJ. Cardiopulmonary function and laparoscopic cholecystectomy. *Can J Anaesth*. 1995;42(1):51-63.
16. Joris JL, Noirot DP, Legrand MJ, Jacquet NJ, Lamy ML. Hemodynamic changes during laparoscopic cholecystectomy. *Anesth Analg*. 1993;76(5):1067-1071.
17. Puri GD, Singh H. Ventilatory effects of laparoscopy under general anaesthesia. *Br J Anaesth*. 1992;68(2):211-213.
18. Kerbl K, Clayman RV, McDougall EM, Kavoussi LR. Laparoscopic nephrectomy: the Washington University experience. *Br J Urol*. 1994;73(3):231-236.
19. Ortega AE, Peters JH, Incarbone R, et al. A prospective randomized comparison of the metabolic and stress hormonal responses of laparoscopic and open cholecystectomy. *J Am Coll Surg*. 1996;183(3):249-256.
20. Wolf JS Jr, Carrier S, Stoller ML. Gas embolism: helium is more lethal than carbon dioxide. *J Laparoendosc Surg*. 1994;4(3):173-177.
21. Barash PG, Cullen B, Stoelting RK. Anesthesia for minimally invasive procedures. In: Barash PG, Cullen BF, Stoelting RK, eds. *Clinical Anesthesia*. 5th ed. Philadelphia, PA: Lippincott Williams & Wilkins; 2006:1066-1068.
22. Fleisher LA, Beckman JA, Brown KA, et al. ACC/AHA 2007 guidelines on perioperative cardiovascular evaluation and care for noncardiac surgery. *Circulation*. 2007;116(17): e418-e499.
23. Eikelboom JW, Hirsch J. Bleeding and management of bleeding. *Eur Heart J*. 2006;8: G38-G45.
24. Merritt JC, Bhatt DL. The efficacy and safety of perioperative antiplatelet therapy. *J Thromb Thrombolysis*. 2004;17(1):21-27.
25. Burger W, Chemnitius JM, Kneissl GD, Rücker G. Low-dose aspirin for secondary cardiovascular prevention: cardiovascular risks after its perioperative withdrawal versus bleeding risks with its continuation – review and meta-analysis. *J Intern Med*. 2005;257(5):399-414.
26. Poldermans D, Bax JJ, Boersma E, et al. Guidelines for pre-operative cardiac risk assessment and perioperative cardiac management in non-cardiac surgery: The Task Force for Preoperative Cardiac Risk Assessment and Perioperative Cardiac Management in Non-cardiac Surgery of the European Society of Cardiology (ESC) and endorsed by the European Society of Anaesthesiology (ESA). *Eur J Anaesthesiol*. 2010;27:92-137.
27. Taylor E, Feinstein R, White PF, Soper N. Anesthesia for laparoscopic cholecystectomy: is nitrous oxide contraindicated? *Anesthesiology*. 1992;76:541-543.
28. Graf BM, Vicenzi MN, Bosnjak ZJ, Stowe DF. The comparative effects of equimolar sevoflurane and isoflurane in isolated hearts. *Anesth Analg*. 1995;81(5):1026-1032.
29. Searle N, Martineau RJ, Conzen P, et al. Comparison of sevoflurane/fentanyl and isoflurane/fentanyl during elective coronary artery bypass surgery. *Can J Anaesth*. 1996;43(9):890-899.
30. Kien ND, Moore PG, Jaffe RS. Cardiovascular function during induced hypotension by fenoldopam or sodium nitroprusside in anesthetized dogs. *Anesth Analg*. 1992;74(1):72-78.
31. Morgan GE Jr, Mikhail MS, Murray MJ. Adrenergic agonists and antagonists. In: Foltin J, Lebowitz H, Boyle PJ, eds. *Clinical Anesthesiology*. 4th ed. New York: McGraw-Hill; 2006:212-223.
32. Kaplan J. Clinical considerations for the use of intravenous nicardipine in the treatment of postoperative hypertension. *Am Heart J*. 1990;119(2):443-446.
33. Morgan GE Jr, Mikhail MS, Murray MJ. Anesthesia for patients with respiratory disease. In: Foltin J, Lebowitz H, Boyle PJ, eds. *Clinical Anesthesiology*. 4th ed. New York: McGraw-Hill; 2006:511-524.

34. Tepel M, van der Giet M, Schwarzfeld C, Laufer U, Liermann D, Zidek W. Prevention of radiographic-contrast-agent-induced reductions in renal function by acetylcysteine. *N Engl J Med.* 2000;343(3):180-184.
35. Playford HR, Sladen RN. What is the best means of preventing perioperative renal dysfunction. In: Fleisher LA, ed. *Evidence-Based Practice of Anesthesiology.* Philadelphia, PA: Saunders; 2004:181-190.
36. Curet MJ. Special problems in laparoscopic surgery. Previous abdominal surgery, obesity, and pregnancy. *Surg Clin North Am.* 2000;80(4):1093-1110.
37. Morgan GE Jr, Mikhail MS, Murray MJ. Postoperative pain. In: Foltin J, Lebowitz H, Boyle PJ, eds. *Clinical Anesthesiology.* 4th ed. New York: McGraw-Hill; 2006:346-374.
38. Nimmo W, Clements J, Ketamine. In: Prys-Robert CH, ed. *Pharmacokinetics of Anesthesia.* Boston, MA: Blackwell; 1984:235.
39. Guignard B, Coste C, Costes H, et al. Supplementing desflurane-remifentanil anesthesia with small-dose ketamine reduces perioperative opioid analgesic requirements. *Anesth Analg.* 2002;95:103-108.
40. Bell RF, Dahl JB, Moore RA, Kalso EA. Perioperative ketamine for acute postoperative pain. *Cochrane Database Syst Rev* 2006;(1):CD004603. doi:10.1002/14651858.CD004603.pub2.
41. Grabow T. Special techniques in pain management. In: Wallace MS, Staats PS, eds. *Pain Medicine and Management: Just the Facts.* New York: McGraw-Hill; 2005:255-363.
42. Schellpfeffer RS, Crino DG. Anesthesia for minimally invasive surgery. In: Duke J, ed. *Anesthesia Secrets.* 3rd ed. Philadelphia, PA: Mosby Elsevier; 2006:494-499.

Difficulties in Urologic Laparoscopic Instrumentation

4

Ahmed M. Al-Kandari and Inderbir S. Gill

Laparoscopy has tremendously evolved the way that urologists treat different conditions. This is mainly due to innovations in instrumentation that have led procedures to be performed efficiently and safely. As with any technical instruments and disposable equipment, there are some problems that the laparoscopic urologist must be aware of in order to manage the unusual, and sometimes serious, consequences. This chapter will discuss problems that may be encountered and potential solutions.

Reusable Veress Needles and Trocars

In countries where cost is a significant issue in laparoscopic surgery, many institutions try to minimize costs by employing reusable Veress needles and trocars. These devices need to be evaluated for:

- Complete cleanliness, especially in the inner parts as any blood residuals can be a source of contamination.[1]
- Sharpness, as sharp needles and trocars are essential for the ease of the procedure.

Insufflators

Various authors have recommended several ways to take the best advantage of insufflations during laparoscopy and avoid difficulties that may adversely affect the patient and operation outcome.[2]

- As laparoscopy is dependent on the use of CO_2 insufflation, some institutions have a central gas supply and others use a bottle supply. It is of utmost importance to confirm that the system dealing with gas supply is functioning properly and does not run out of gas during a lengthy laparoscopic procedure.

A.M. Al-Kandari (✉)

Department of Surgery (Urology), Faculty of Medicine, Kuwait University, Jabriyah, Kuwait
e-mail: drakandari@hotmail.com

A.M. Al-Kandari and I.S. Gill (eds.), *Difficult Conditions in Laparoscopic Urologic Surgery*,   **33**
DOI: 10.1007/978-1-84882-105-7_4, © Springer-Verlag London Limited 2011

- Ensure that the pressure and other parameters of the machine are functioning properly as continuously monitored safe pressure during laparoscopy is important for patient safety.

Cameras, Monitors, and Ergonomics

Camera

Degree of camera angle: It is important that the surgeon selects the appropriate camera angle for the procedure being performed. Many authors recommend a 0° lens for pelvic surgeries and a 30° lens for abdominal surgeries.

Camera image quality: Since laparoscopic surgery relies on a camera to accomplish procedures, it is the authors' opinion that investing in cameras with the highest image quality is essential to help surgeons work at their best. Nowadays many high-definition cameras are made by multiple manufacturers and are quite helpful in accurate and excellent visualization. Built-in chips can be advantageous, especially in laparoendoscopic single site surgery (LESS), and avoid a cumbersome and bulky camera and lens (Fig. 4.1).

Camera size: The authors most commonly use 10-mm cameras, but smaller ones, such as 5-mm cameras, can also be used. If both are available, then this adds to the versatility of all useful instruments, especially in difficult cases.

Clear vision of the camera is a must throughout laparoscopic surgery. Here are potentially helpful tips to avoid poor visibility and/or fogging:

- Maintain a warm operating room temperature. This may not be beneficial to the surgeon, but it is good for the patient and procedure since it can minimize lens fogging.
- Always have a covered flask of very hot water ready for use.
- Keep your insufflations tube away from the camera port.
- If possible, use a laparoscopic gas conditioning device. This is beneficial to the patient in avoiding hypothermia and for laparoscopic visibility (Fig. 4.2).
- Instruct an assistant or nurse to have a piece of gauze and an artery forceps ready to clean the ports when needed.
- Use lens antifogging solutions when possible.
- During irrigation and suction, instruct your camera operator to avoid the irrigation. This prevents a dirty lens and thus saves operative time.

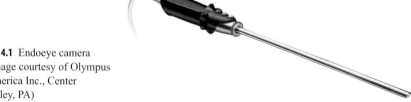

Fig. 4.1 Endoeye camera (Image courtesy of Olympus America Inc., Center Valley, PA)

Fig. 4.2 Insu*flow*® laparoscopic gas
conditioning device (Image courtesy of Lexion
Medical, St. Paul, MN. Reprinted with permission)

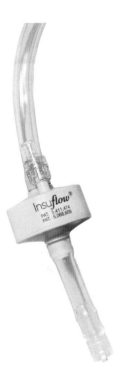

- If fog is due to cautery smoke, ask the assistant to vent quickly and gently to maintain pneumoperitoneum. The assistant can pull back in the port until the smoke has cleared.
- After a bleed has been controlled, clean the field with irrigation and suction or use a sponge. This minimizes the red color absorption that can affect the quality of vision.

Instrument and Assistant Ergonomics

- It is essential that the laparoscopic surgeon performs the procedure in the most comfortable and ergonomic way, which includes proper setup of the monitor for the surgeon, and, if possible, for the assistants. Also, placement of the other machines, such as the cautery, LigaSure® (Valleylab, Boulder, CO), or Ultracision Harmonic scalpel® (Ethicon Endo-Surgery, Inc., Cincinnati, OH), should be within comfortable reach. One of the main ergonomic problems associated with laparoscopy is the surgeon's non-neutral posture during laparoscopic procedures. There are five main issues that influence the posture of the surgeon: handheld instrument design, position of the monitor, the use of foot pedals to control diathermy, poorly adjusted operating table height, and static body posture.[3] All of these issues must be addressed in order to perform a laparoscopic procedure efficiently and comfortably. The surgeon must consider the long-term effects on his health in relation to difficult postures.

- Patient positioning should also be safe for the patient and enable the surgeon to easily use instruments without fighting with any part of the body. A good example is the arm positioning in an upper abdominal surgery such as laparoscopic pyeloplasty.
- An experienced camera operator is essential when performing complex procedures. If an experienced camera operator is unavailable, then the surgeon must guide the camera operator throughout the surgery to facilitate the procedure.[4]

Common Laparoscopic Instruments

Common laparoscopic instruments include bowel forceps, laparoscopic scissors, Maryland dissector, suction device, and needle holder. The surgeon and the operating room nurse must observe the following guidelines to avoid any intraoperative problems and difficulties:

- As previously mentioned, when reusable instruments are employed, ensure the instruments are properly cleaned prior to sterilization for patient safety.
- Ensure that scissors are sharp and that forceps are functional and hold well so as not to waste operative time.
- Make sure that the instruments' insulating sheaths are intact, especially on the scissors and hook, to prevent inadvertent electrical injury during electrocautery use, especially on the bowel.

Metal Clips

Metal clips are essential in most laparoscopic urologic procedures and are typically used to control vessels, usually of small or medium size. In many centers around the world, experts still use metal clips during laparoscopy nephrectomy for the renal artery. The following points should be kept in mind in order to avoid difficulties:

- Have an adequate supply of clips in both sizes (5 and 10 mm), especially for long and difficult cases.
- Avoid cross clipping as this may lead to weak clipping and clip slippage.
- Avoid clipping near where the endovascular gastrointestinal anastomosis (endo-GIA) stapler will be applied since clips will interfere with stapler closure. This may lead to an insufficient stapling effect and possible bleeding from the stapled vessels.
- Avoid clipping excess fatty tissue as this minimizes clipping efficiency.
- Avoid manipulating or holding the clips, as metal clips are prone to dislodgement. If clips fall off, attempt to remove them so that they do not interfere with other operative steps.
- Avoid blind clipping when bleeding is encountered. The surgeon should be able to visualize the bleed, then grasp it with the forceps and apply a clip.
- When faced with caval bleeding, avoid clipping across the cava as this can cause injury.

- Consider clipping from a different port if the port that is being used does not allow safe and easy access to the site to be clipped.
- If polymer or Hem-o-lok® clips (Teleflex Medical, Research Triangle Park, NC) are unavailable and metal clips are used, for example, to control the renal artery during laparoscopic radical nephrectomy, make sure that the artery is well skeletonized and clip at least three large (10 mm) clips on the aorta side and two on the kidney side.

Endovascular Gastrointestinal Anastomosis (Endo-GIA) Stapler

The endo-GIA stapler has been a great innovation in facilitating laparoscopic surgery. This device has made major organ retrieval possible, including the kidney and spleen, as well as bowel resection. The use of this device also carries additional risks that must be considered.

The endo-GIA stapler is useful in performing laparoscopic nephrectomy. However, malfunctions may occur and can be associated with significant blood loss and subsequent need for conversion to an open procedure. The majority of errors can be avoided with careful application and recognition. Many failures, especially when recognized before release of the device, can be managed without conversion to an open procedure.[5]

In one of the earliest reports, endo-GIA malfunction occurred in 10 cases (1.7%). In eight cases, the renal vein was involved and malfunctions affected the renal artery in two cases. The estimated blood loss ranged from 200 to 1,200 cc. Open conversions were necessary in two cases (20%). The etiology of the failure included primary instrument failure in three cases and preventable causes in seven cases. Open surgery was required in two patients and laparoscopic management was possible in eight.[5]

In a previously described report of approximately 460 laparoscopic cases, the authors encountered five problems (1%) with endovascular gastrointestinal anastomosis staplers. Fifty-five additional cases of Endo GIA failures occurred in 50 patients were documented in the Food and Drug Administration database. Of these 55 cases, 15 (27%) required open conversion to manage the problem, 8 patients (15%) received blood transfusions, and 2 patients (4%) died postoperatively.[6]

During laparoscopic live donor nephrectomy, various reports have illustrated that stapler malfunction can lead to bleeding vascular complication (0.6%). The first major vascular complication resulted from an endovascular stapler malfunction during transection of an accessory left renal artery[7]

Although the linear cutting stapler is easy to use, a 1.7% malfunction rate has been reported, and the consequences of this failure can be serious, including emergency conversion to an open procedure and even death.[5] Subsequently, caution and preparation is needed for emergent open conversion if endo-GIA stapler malfunction occurs to avoid patient morbidity or even mortality.

Different authors have recommended different techniques to ligate the renal vein without a stapler including holding it with the laparoscopic Babcock and bunching it for easy clipping with large Hem-o-lok® clips.[8] Others have used the same principle, but have ligated the vein first with suture and then applied the Hem-o-lok® clips.[9]

The following are important points to remember to avoid problems and difficulties with endo-GIA staplers:

- It is important for the surgeon, assistant, and operating nurse to be familiar with the technical details of the device, including the length of the stapler, width, opening mechanism, and angulation.
- If a new brand or type of endo-GIA stapler will be used, have an experienced user or a company representative assemble and guide the process during the operation to avoid problems. In the authors' experience, one real-life example of this problem occurred when an endo-GIA stapler positioned over the renal pedicle could not be removed until the surgeon and the nurse reviewed the device's instruction manual.
- Abnormal firing of the stapler and improper staple formation were the most common and morbid aspects of device malfunction.[6] Avoid using clips in the area where the endo-GIA stapler might be needed since clips will prevent stapler closure.

Polymer Clips (Hem-o-lok® Clips)

Polymer nonabsorbable clips have been used in laparoscopic surgery to control vessels of various sizes. They have become popular for renal vessel control in laparoscopic simple, radical, and donor nephrectomy. These clips are easy to apply and have locking feature that makes them secure for the renal pedicle (Fig. 4.3). A report published with data from the U.S. Food and Drug Adminstration (FDA) has mentioned some compli-

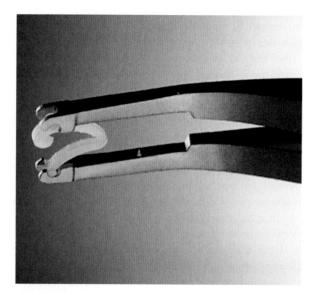

Fig. 4.3 Hem-o-lok® polymer clip (Teleflex Medical, Research Triangle Park, NC.) with applier (From Springer Science + Business Media: *Surgical Endoscopy*, Hem-o-lok plastic clips in securing the base of the appendix during laparoscopic appendectomy, Vol. 23, 2009, pp. 2851–2854, Delibegović S, Matović E, Fig. 1. With permission)

cations related to their use. No clear etiology for the events could be found, although in all situations, multiple clips had been applied with apparent initial vessel control intraoperatively. Cases of failure after laparoscopic nephrectomy require urgent exploration, although it is unclear whether device or user error is the underlying cause.[10]

On the other hand, other studies have documented the safety of Hem-o-lok® clips. Between October 2001 and June 2006, nine institutions with laparoscopically trained urologists performed 1,695 laparoscopic nephrectomies (radical nephrectomy, $N=899$; simple nephrectomy, $N=112$; nephroureterectomy, $N=198$; donor nephrectomy, $N=486$). Follow-up was a minimum of 6 months from the time of surgery. For each case, the authors used Hem-o-lok® clips to control the renal artery. The renal vein was controlled with Hem-o-lok® clips in 68 cases (radical nephrectomy, $N=54$; simple nephrectomy, $N=3$; nephroureterectomy, $N=5$; donor nephrectomy, $N=6$). The number of clips placed on the patient side of the renal artery was most often two, occasionally three. The number of clips placed on the patient side of the renal vein was most often two and rarely three. All cases used the large (L-purple) clip on the artery, and most cases of renal vein used the extra-large (XL-gold) clip on the vein. No clips failed. Based on this large retrospective review, properly applied Hem-o-lok® clips for vascular control during renal procedures may provide a safe option.[11] Others have reported the use of Hem-o-lok® clips only during laparoscopic renal surgery with excellent results in a more cost-effective manner.[12,13]

Suction Devices

A suction device is an important piece of equipment required in all laparoscopic procedures. The following points are important to avoid problems during using suction device in laparoscopic urologic procedures:

- Select an efficient suction device; the authors use a battery-activated suction device made by Stryker Endoscopy (San Jose, CA).
- If a reusable suction device is used, ensure that both the irrigation and suction are working properly.
- In some countries surgeons reuse a disposable suction device. Although the authors do not recommend this, the surgeon and the operating room nurse must ensure that the device is totally clean and is functioning well.
- When using the suction device, especially a reusable one, make sure that the tip is not sharp as sometimes the suction is used for blunt dissection. If the device is used for blunt dissection, this can cause trauma if not used carefully.
- When using the suction, some devices cause significant suction of the pneumoperitoneum, which leads to loss of visibility and may also cause the camera to get dirty, causing a loss of operative time.
- Assistants should be familiar with the suction device. Suction applied by the assistant from a side port can be helpful during a bleed to locate the source of the bleed, and also during urine accumulation in laparoscopic pyeloplasty.

Cautery Equipment

Hock

The hock is a commonly used piece of equipment during different laparoscopic procedures. The following are important aspects to remember in order to avoid problems:

- Remember that the hock is commonly connected to monopolar electricity which can have a spread injury effect. The surgeon should be careful to maintain distance to bowel to avoid thermal bowel injury.
- The hock has a good advantage of being fine with an angle that aids dissection in narrow areas. For example, in dissecting around the renal vessels, the hock is helpful in freeing the perivascular tissue. Remember that the hock can be traumatic—when pulling on tissues during dissection, avoid injuring bowel on the field.
- If a reusable hock is used, make sure that the insulating cover is intact to avoid proximal thermal injury.

Scissors

- Whenever possible, the authors recommend using new scissors for each case since they will be sharper and more efficient.
- If using reusable scissors or if disposable scissors are being reused, the surgeon and the operating room nurse should confirm the sharpness and integrity of the insulation cover.

Other Thermal Instruments

Ultrasonic Thermal Instruments

Ultrasonic thermal instruments are useful and help in hemostasis during dissection, expedite dissection with less thermal spread, and have cutting features. Recent studies have shown that ultrasonic devices have the potential to replace electrocautery without compromising safety in minimally invasive operations. With the combination of several functions into a single instrument, significant reduction in operative time and expense are possible and should increase acceptance of this new technology.[14] The following are important related points:

- It typically is recommended to use a new handle for each case as this guarantees efficiency.
- In cases where cost is an issue and it is decided to reuse a handle, test it before the procedure to confirm its efficacy.
- Ultrasonic thermal devices are effective in cutting Hem-o-lok® clips, especially when unnecessary clip removal is needed.

Electric Thermal Instruments

An effective electric thermal instrument used in laparoscopy is the LigaSure™, a bipolar radiofrequency generator. This new energy-based vessel-ligation device appears to be effective in advanced laparoscopic procedures.[15] It is used to control small sized vessels (less than 7 mm), and has 5 mm and 10 mm handles (Fig. 4.4). The LigaSure™ vessel-sealing system permanently seals veins, arteries, and tissue bundles in a consistent and reliable manner by fusing the collagen in vessel walls. By reducing sutures and the number of instrument exchanges in the operating theatre, LigaSure® decreases operating time and blood loss. The following are useful points to remember for maximum safety and efficiency:

- Avoid using reused handles; use a new handle per case.
- When coagulating a vessel with the 5 mm handle, try to coagulate a longer segment and cut in between.
- When using the Atlas LigaSure® device (Fig. 4.5), try to coagulate a longer segment and then cut.

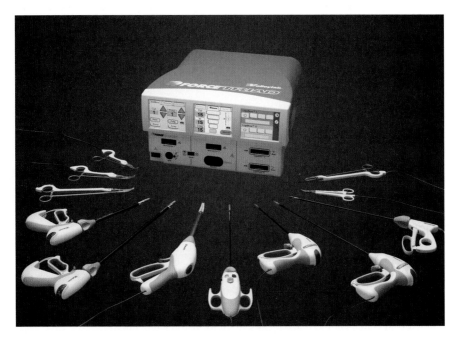

Fig. 4.4 LigaSure™ vessel-sealing system (Photo copyright ©2010 Covidien. All rights reserved. Reprinted with the permission of the Energy Based Devices Division of Covidien)

Fig. 4.5 Atlas LigaSure™
device (Photo copyright
©2010 Covidien. All rights
reserved. Reprinted with the
permission of the Energy
Based Devices Division of
Covidien)

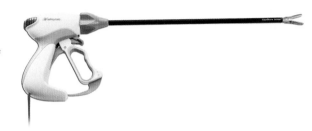

Retrieval Bags

Retrieval bags are important tools in the removal of various organs such as the kidneys, adrenals, prostate, and bladder, as well as stones from the urinary tract. Different companies produce different bag types; the following are important facts to remember for efficient usage:

For the Endo Catch™ Bag (Covidien, Dublin, Ireland)

- Use the appropriate size (10 or 15 mm), according to the size of the mass to be retrieved (Fig. 4.6).
- Remember that the trocar for the 15-mm bag comes in a separate pack, so make sure that the trocar is available before this bag is used.
- Use caution as the bag may separate from the ring. Some surgeons fix the bag edge to the ring with suture, but this may cause difficulty in folding and unfolding the bag into the metal handle.
- The help of an assistant is important for ease of organ entrapment within the bag.
- Once the mass is entrapped, avoid grasping the bag with instruments as the bag is not very strong and may be damaged. This can lead to loss of the organ and extra operative time loss.

Conclusion

Thorough understanding of all instruments and disposables used during laparoscopic urologic procedures are essential for safe and efficient surgery. For maximum efficiency, surgeons should do their best to utilize every possible technology that can make procedures safer and more efficient. Knowledge of the problems related to those instruments is important to avoid complications that may be caused by instrument failure.

Fig. 4.6 Endo Catch™ bag (Photo copyright © 2010 Covidien. All rights reserved. Used with the permission of Covidien)

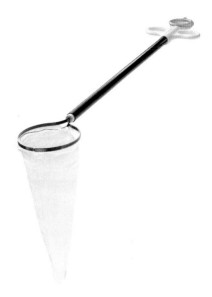

References

1. Fengler TW, Pahlke H, Kraas E. Sterile and economic instrumentation in laparoscopic surgery. Experiences with 6,000 surgical laparoscopies, 1990-1996. *Surg Endosc*. 1998;12(10): 1275-1279.
2. Jacobs VR, Morrison JE Jr, Kiechle M. Twenty-five simple ways to increase insufflation performance and patient safety in laparoscopy. *J Am Assoc Gynecol Laparosc*. 2004;11(3): 410-423.
3. Van Veelen, Jakimowicz K. Improved physical ergonomics of laparoscopic surgery. *Minim Invasive Ther Allied Technol*. 2004;13(3):161-166.
4. Chmarra MK, Kokman W, Jansen FW, Grimbergen CA, Dankelman J. The influence of experience and camera holding on laparoscopic instrument movements measured with the TrEndo tracking system. *Surg Endosc*. 2007;21(11):2069-2075.
5. Chan D, Bishoff JT, Ratner L, Kavoussi LR, Jarrett TW. Endovascular gastrointestinal stapler device malfunction during laparoscopic nephrectomy: early recognition and management. *J Urol*. 2000;164(2):319-321.
6. Deng DY, Meng MV, Nguyen HT, Bellman GC, Stoller ML. Laparoscopic linear cutting stapler failure. *Urology*. 2002;60(3):415-419.
7. Breda A, Veale J, Liao J, Schulam PG. Complications of laparoscopic living donor nephrectomy and their management: the UCLA experience. *Urology*. 2007;69(1):49-52.
8. Baumert H, Ballaro A, Arroyo C, Kaisary AV, Mulders PF, Knipscheer BC. The use of polymer (Hem-o-lok) clips for management of the renal hilum during laparoscopic nephrectomy. *Eur Urol*. 2006;49(5):816-819.
9. Janetschek G, Bagheri F, Abdelmaksoud A, Biyani CS, Leeb K, Jeschke S. Ligation of the renal vein during laparoscopic nephrectomy: an effective and reliable method to replace vascular staplers. *J Urol*. 2003;170(4, pt 1):1295-1297.

10. Meng MV. Reported failures of the polymer self-locking (Hem-o-lok) clip: review of data from the Food and Drug Administration. *J Endourol.* 2006;20(12):1054-1057.
11. Ponsky L, Cherullo E, Moinzadeh A, et al. The Hem-o-lok clip is safe for laparoscopic nephrectomy: a multi-institutional review. *Urology.* 2008 Apr;71(4):593-596.
12. Casale P, Pomara G, Simone M, Casarosa C, Fontana L, Francesca F. Hem-o-lok clips to control both the artery and the vein during laparoscopic nephrectomy: personal experience and review of the literature. *J Endourol.* 2007;21(8):915-918.
13. Izaki H, Fukumori T, Takahashi M, et al. Clinical research of renal vein control using Hem-o-lok clips in laparoscopic nephrectomy. *Int J Urol.* 2006;13(8):1147-1149.
14. Gill BS, MacFadyen BV Jr. Ultrasonic dissectors and minimally invasive surgery. *Semin Laparosc Surg.* 1999;6(4):229-234.
15. Leonard C, Guaglianone S, De Carli P, Pompeo V, Forastiere E, Gallucci M. Laparoscopic nephrectomy using Ligasure system: preliminary experience. *J Endourol.* 2005;19(8): 976-978.

Cost-Reductive Measures in Laparoscopy: Tips and Tricks for Developing Countries

5

Ahmed M. Mansour, Khurshid A. Guru, and Ahmed A. Shokeir

Introduction

> The enjoyment of the highest attainable standard of health is one of the fundamental rights of every human being without distinction of race, religion, political belief, or economic or social condition. (Constitution of the World Health Organization[1])

With major advances in the early 1980s due to the invention of the television-chip camera that allowed surgeons to operate with both hands, laparoscopic surgery has rapidly established itself and experienced unprecedented growth in well-developed countries. Urologists were ready for this revolution because of the endoscopic skills already acquired with transurethral surgery. Laparoscopic urologic surgery had an impact on minimizing morbidity and decreasing convalescence, which are essential to patient care. However, the spread of laparoscopy in third world countries has been hindered by the difficult management of hospital structures, insufficient medical and paramedical staff training, and, most importantly, limited financial resources.

The "cost-effectiveness" of laparoscopy versus open surgery has been investigated in many studies.[2,3] However, the evidence is inconclusive on whether or not laparoscopic surgery results in lower costs for the health-care system. Although laparoscopy does reduce hospital stay and periods of sick leave, laparoscopic operations cost more than open surgeries from the hospital's point of view. This is due to the initial investment in instruments and longer duration of operating and anesthesia times. Owing to these direct costs, some urologists in developing countries may encounter resistance from their hospitals regarding these start-up expenses. However, as laparoscopic skills are developed and assisting paramedical staff gain more experience, operating times are significantly reduced. In addition, with a steady increase in the number of cases performed, investment in reusable instrumentation may be an opportunity for cost-saving per case for the hospital.

A.M. Mansour (✉)

Department of Urology, Roswell Park Cancer Institute, Buffalo, NY, USA

A.M. Al-Kandari and I.S. Gill (eds.), *Difficult Conditions in Laparoscopic Urologic Surgery*, **45**
DOI: 10.1007/978-1-84882-105-7_5, © Springer-Verlag London Limited 2011

Out of sheer economic necessity, several cost-effective measures have emerged around the developing world aimed at reducing the costs of laparoscopic procedures. Expensive disposable instrument usage is kept to a minimum, and ordinary materials at hand are modified to serve new purposes. By working around the limits and restrictions of the tools available in the operating room, the gifted surgeon can take the least expensive tool and perform a certain task better than others using expensive disposable instruments. This chapter reviews reported tips and tricks that will reduce the costs of consumables, and may help urologists in developing world bring minimally invasive surgery into their everyday practices.

Reusable Laparoscopic Instrumentation

Laparoscopic instrumentation has evolved significantly in the last decade. Less traumatic access devices, improved high-definition, flexible-tip videolaparoscopes, a new generation of coagulation devices, and better tools for managing vessels are now available. However, minimal requirements for running a laparoscopic operating room in a developing country include a laparoscope and camera system, a monitor, an insufflation system, access instruments, trocars, and dissecting and needloscopic instruments.

It is now well known that reusable instruments are as safe as disposable ones.[4–6] Advocates of single-use instruments praise their high quality and criticize the time and expense necessary for cleaning and sterilization of the reusable instruments.[4] With single-use instruments, which are discarded after each operation, repairs are never necessary since there is no "wear and tear." With each successive operation one has optimal, unused material – scissors with sharp new blades, properly sealed trocars, and so forth. Moreover, the surgeon is certain that the latest model with the newest technologic refinements is at hand. However, these merits do not weigh the vast difference in the costs between reusable and single-use instruments.[5] Reusable instruments (Fig. 5.1) do require regular maintenance if their quality is to remain comparable to single-use instruments. This means more work, including necessary training, for hospital personnel who keep these instruments in top condition. Considering the significant cost savings and evidence of their comparable safety, reusable instruments for laparoscopy are strongly recommended.[6]

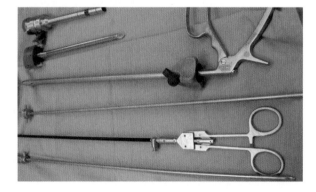

Fig. 5.1 Reusable laparoscopic instruments (from *left* to *right*): laparoscopic needle holder, MicroFrance® grasper (Medtronic, Minneapolis, MN), suction tip, Hem-o-lok® clip applier, metallic trocar, and cannula

Development of the Retroperitoneal Space: Homemade Balloon Technique

The retroperitoneoscopic approach was refined and popularized by Gaur et al. with the introduction of retroperitoneal dissection using the balloon technique.[7,8] Instead of disposable expensive commercial silicon balloons, a homemade balloon (Fig. 5.2) can be used in the development of the retroperitoneal space. The balloon can be fashioned from two fingers of a sterile number 7.5 or 8 surgical glove with one finger intussuscepted inside the other and tied over a 16–22 Fr catheter. Care must be taken to advance the catheter tip to the bottom of the finger balloon, which helps in early and prompt filling as well as in subsequent deflation of saline after the retroperitoneal space is created.[9] The balloon is introduced into the retroperitoneal space through a small incision below and behind the tip of the 12th rib. It is inserted just below the thoracolumbar fascia in the extraperitoneal space, and 300–500 cc of saline is injected into the balloon and left in situ for 5 min to achieve hemostasis. A 10-mm reusable metallic trocar is placed through the same incision site. Full thickness 1-0 silk sutures are then placed through all layers of the abdominal wall to keep the port in place and prevent dispersion of carbon dioxide between tissue planes. This step helps to avoid the use of a disposable sealing trocar.[9]

Cost-Reductive Measures for Vascular Control

In laparoscopic nephrectomy (simple, radical, or donor), renal vascular pedicle dissection, ligation, and transection are crucial steps. Various instruments have been devised to obviate the difficulty in controlling renal vessels with knots and thread. The most common laparoscopic devices used to secure the renal hilum include endovascular stapling devices, traditional titanium clips, and nonabsorbable polymer ligating (NPL) clips (Hem-o-lok®, Teleflex Medical, Research Triangle Park, NC). No large randomized prospective study

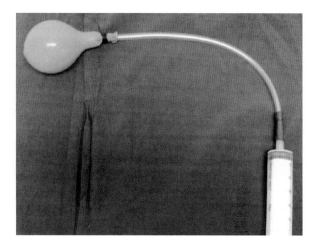

Fig. 5.2 Homemade balloon for development of the retroperitoneal space

has compared the techniques for renal hilar control to determine which device is the safest; hence, the use of a particular device is routinely chosen according to surgeon preference and previous exposure. In many centers, a vascular endo-GIA stapler is the preferred method for vascular control, especially for the renal hilum. However, using vascular staples increases the cost of a laparoscopic nephrectomy by approximately $800–$1,000.[10]

Hem-o-lok® clips are excellent, cost-effective devices for vascular control. They have become one of the most preferred methods owing to their low cost, good tissue handling, large size, and less chance of slippage because of distal locking.[11] A single disposable stapler device costs $400, while the cost of the Hem-o-lok® system is $32 for six clips, which undoubtedly can reduce the cost of the procedure.[12] Moreover, it is difficult to determine the correct closure on a blood vessel using the endo-GIA stapler until it is divided, while the Hem-o-lok® clip produces a click after it is secured correctly.

In 2006, Teleflex Medical, the manufacturer of the Hem-o-lok® clip, issued a warning stating that Hem-o-lok® clips are contraindicated in the control of the renal artery during laparoscopic donor nephrectomy after publication of a recall survey by Friedman and colleagues.[13] The survey included 893 members of the American Society of Transplant Surgeons and raised major concerns, prompting the manufacturer to release a contraindications statement. However, multiple publications have attested to the safety and feasibility of Hem-o-lok® clips for laparoscopic nephrectomies.[13–18] Based on a multi-institutional review, Ponsky et al. concluded that Hem-o-lok® clips, when applied correctly by laparoscopically trained urologists, are safe, effective, and reliable for use in all types of laparoscopic nephrectomies, despite the manufacturer's release of contraindications.[18] They recommended basic principles for Hem-o-lok® placement, including: complete circumferential dissection of the vessel, visualization of the curved tip of the clip around and beyond the vessel, confirmation of the tactile snap when the clip engages, maintenance of a visual stump below the most proximal clip, not squeezing clip handles too hard, careful removal of the applier after application as the tips are sharp and can cause a laceration of nearby vessels (i.e., renal vein), placement of a minimum of two clips on the patient side of the renal hilar vessel, and, finally, partial division to confirm hemostasis before complete transection (Fig. 5.3).[18]

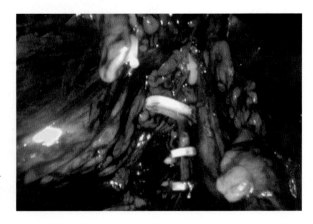

Fig. 5.3 Proper application of Hem-o-lok® clips for control of the renal artery

Large veins can be difficult to control using Hem-o-lok® clips, since the clip may not be long enough to completely occlude the vein. A trick reported by Janetschek et al.[19] suggests applying an extracorporeal ligature before application of the clip to reduce the caliber of the vein. A right angle dissector is passed posterior to the renal vein and a 2-zero 70 cm monofilament suture is fed to the dissector, which is withdrawn and pulled out. The other end of the suture is also grasped and drawn out through the same trocar, so that the suture is placed around the vein. One end of the suture is inserted extracorporeally into the convex side of a specially designed, round-eyed knot pusher (Latinovich, Tribuswinkel, Austria). It is then grasped by a mosquito and fixed under minimal tension by the assistant in the line of the trocar, ensuring that there is no kinking or twisting in whole length of the thread. The knot pusher is held with one hand (the nondominant hand in the authors' case) and the free end of the suture is held with the other hand to form a loop around the fixed part, as in open surgery. By maintaining minimal tension on each end of the thread, the loop is gently pushed down by the knot pusher to the level of the renal vein and then slightly tightened. This maneuver can be repeated 3–5 times to shrivel the vein. This can be followed by the application of Hem-o-lok® clips since the vein caliber has now been reduced.[19]

Specimen Retrieval: Technical Difficulties and Cost Reduction

Even with an experienced laparoscopist, specimen retrieval may encounter technical difficulties following extirpative laparoscopic surgery. This is specifically important in laparoscopic donor nephrectomy in which warm ischemia time is critical. The endo-catch bag provides an easy and rapid way to retrieve specimens. However, complications have been reported when using the endo-catch bag, including spleen and small bowel injuries.[20] Also, technical difficulties in retrieving the kidney using an endo-catch bag have resulted in prolonged warm ischemia time.[21]

Shalhav et al. have described a technique for manual retrieval of the kidney in laparoscopic live donor nephrectomy through a modified Pfannesteil incision. This technique shortens the warm ischemia time, avoids the technical difficulties associated with the endo-catch bag, and reduces the cost of the procedure.[22] Following complete kidney mobilization (leaving it only attached by the renal pedicle), the ureter is transected at the level of the iliac artery and the patient (in a 45° lateral decubitus position) is rotated lateral, so that the lower abdomen is in a more horizontal plane. A 7.5 cm Pfannestiel skin incision is made, followed by a 7.5-cm vertical incision in the linea alba. After the skin and fascia are incised, the rectus muscles are bluntly spread until the peritoneum (pushed by pneumoperitoneal pressure) is visualized bulging between the rectus muscles. The assistant's right hand is then wrapped, glove to elbow, with an adhesive drape to avoid fluid contamination through the sleeve and the laparoscope is then reinserted. Under direct vision, the assistant surgeon (using the fingers bluntly) inserts the hand through the peritoneum and into the abdominal cavity, avoiding the bladder and bowel. After the hand is in the abdominal cavity, pneumoperitoneum is reestablished and the patient is rotated medial to allow the bowel and spleen to reflect off of the kidney by gravity. The assistant's hand can be used for retraction of the medial bowel during control of the renal hilum, or can be used to hold up the kidney laterally if the bowels are well retracted by gravity alone. The best exposure is achieved by having the renal hilum between the second and third digit, while retracting the medial bowel with the thumb and the ureter lateral with the first digit. The renal vascular pedicle is then controlled, according to the surgeon's preference, and the kidney is then manually extracted.[22]

Similarly Ramalingam et al. delivered the kidney in a laparoscopic live donor nephrectomy through a 6–8 cm anterior subcostal flank incision without introducing the assistant's hand into the wound. Just before dividing the renal vessels, a 5-cm skin incision is made medial to the iliac fossa port. The incision is deepened to the level of the peritoneum, which is not breached. The renal pedicle is controlled and a fan retractor is used to push the kidney down towards the iliac fossa. The muscle was split and the peritoneum was opened. Two fingers (index and middle) were inserted through the incision to hold the perirenal fat lateral to the kidney, and the graft is gently retrieved.[23]

Hand-assisted laparoscopic live donor nephrectomy has been adopted in many transplantation centers with good results in regard to warm ischemia time. Pneumoperitoneum preserving devices, such as the GelPort® (Applied Medical, Rancho Santa Margarita, CA), LapDisc® (Hakko Medical, Tokyo, Japan), and Omniport® (ASC Limited, Wicklow, Ireland) have been successfully used.[24,25] However, problems related to high cost of these devices remain. Recently, Ramalingam et al.[23] described the use of hand-assisted laparoscopy without a pneumoperitoneum preserving device. Instead of the device, a double glove with a sponge between the inner and outer glove at the wrist acted as an obturating cuff. However, the safety and efficacy of this technique should be proved before its widespread adoption.

Training in Laparoscopy: Low-Cost Alternatives

Laparoscopic surgery requires the acquisition of additional skills beyond those needed for open surgery. The transfer of open surgical skills to the laparoscopic situation is not guaranteed.[26] Training alternatives have been developed, ranging from bench trainers to live animal models, to assist acquisition of laparoscopic skills in a safe environment. However, the use of animals is expensive and restricted in many countries. A variety of surgical simulators and trainers have been developed for laparoscopic training with different degrees of validity and reliability.[27] The high cost of these trainers, ranging between $500 and $2,500, has limited their availability to all urologists. The use of cheaper bench trainers, consisting of camera system and cardboard or plastic boxes, has been described as possible alternative.[28,29] These models, although less expensive than conventional commercially available video-laparoscopy pelvic trainers, still require significant investment. A cheap webcam was described as an alternative to the camera system in the pelvitrainer.[30] Chandrasekera et al.[31] described a low-cost alternative trainer consisting of a cardboard box with a section cut out of the top of the box to allow direct visualization, while the operator wears unilaterally blinded goggles to simulate two-dimensional vision. These cheap homemade trainers are good alternatives for developing countries and for trainees wishing to practice in their own homes or offices.

Robotic Surgery and the Developing World

Robotic technology is the latest innovation in minimally invasive surgery that has revolutionized the practice of urology in most of the developed world. In 1997, Intuitive Surgical, Inc. (Sunnyvale, CA) introduced a prototype robot named the "*da Vinci®*" which proved to be a breakthrough technology and has stood the test of time since its inception.[32] Robotic technology has provided urologists fundamental advantages, allowing those not laparoscopically trained the ability to offer their patients a minimally invasive alternative. For surgeons who are laparoscopically trained, robotic technology has provided a platform for operating at a technically superior level.

The robotic revolution has swept through the United States and Europe, and is now becoming popular in Asia and Latin America. Contemporary estimates of U.S. robot-assisted radical prostatectomy use range from 50% to 70%,[33-35] whereas a recent survey revealed a 25–75% decline in open and laparoscopic radical prostatectomy volume among urologists.[36] Robotic dissemination has been driven by patients and surgeons alike, both with a common goal of less invasive care with superior outcomes.

The high cost of purchasing and maintaining a robotic system is one of the biggest obstacles confronting developing countries in establishing robotic programs. There is one robot in the world with the required utilities and therefore the technology is at a premium price. The current cost of the *da Vinci®* system is $1.2 million with annual maintenance fees of $138,000.[37] Centers of excellence in developing countries should not ignore the robotic revolution. The authors believe that robotic surgery programs should be established, urologists should be trained, and cost-reductive measures should be innovated in order to overcome the high running costs. This will make investment in this technology effective and will positively affect patient care.

Conclusion

Laparoscopic surgery is rapidly growing in developing countries. Significant financial commitment is needed by hospitals and the laparoscopy teams to adopt laparoscopy in everyday practice. Several cost-effective measures and tricks for surgical access, vascular control, and organ retrieval has brought minimally invasive surgery to the forefront in many urologic extirpative procedures in the third world. The high cost of a robotic surgical system is still hindering its spread in developing countries.

References

1. World Health Organization. Constitution of the World Health Organization. Available at: http://www.who.int/governance/eb/who_constitution_en.pdf. Accessed May 10, 2010.
2. Hamidi V, Andersen MH, Oyen O, Mathisen L, Fosse E, Kristiansen IS. Cost effectiveness of open versus laparoscopic living-donor nephrectomy. *Transplantation*. 2009;87:831-838.
3. Winfield HN, Donovan JF Jr, Troxel SA, Rashid TM. Laparoscopic urologic surgery: the financial realities. *Surg Oncol Clin N Am*. 1995;4:307-314.
4. Reichert M. Laparoscopic instruments: patient care, cost issues. *AORN J*. 1993;57:635-662.
5. Schaer GN, Koechli OR, Haller U. Single-use versus reusable laparoscopic surgical instruments: a comparative cost analysis. *Am J Obstet Gynecol*. 1995;173:1812-1815.
6. Apelgren KN, Blank ML, Slomski CA, Hadjis NS. Reusable instruments are more cost-effective than disposable instruments for laparoscopic cholecystectomy. *Surg Endosc*. 1994;8: 32-34.
7. Gaur DD. Laparoscopic operative retroperitoneoscopy: use of a new device. *J Urol*. 1992;149:1137-1139.
8. Gaur DD, Agarwal DK, Purohit KC. Retroperitoneal laparoscopic nephrectomy: initial case report. *J Urol*. 1993;149:103-105.
9. Hemal AK. Re: laparoscopic nephrectomy via the retroperitoneal approach. *J Urol*. 1998;159:992-993.
10. Kumar A, Gupta NP, Hemal AK. A single institution experience of 141 cases of laparoscopic radical nephrectomy with cost-reductive measures. *J Endourol*. 2009;23:445-449.
11. Kapoor R, Singh KJ, Suri A, et al. Hem-o-lok clips for vascular control during laparoscopic ablative nephrectomy: a single-center experience. *J Endourol*. 2006;20:202-204.
12. Kumar A, Chaudhary H, Srivastava A, Raghavendran M. Laparoscopic live-donor nephrectomy: modifications for developing nations. *BJU Int*. 2004;93:1291-1295.
13. Friedman AL, Peters TG, Jones KW, Boulware LE, Ratner LE. Fatal and nonfatal hemorrhagic complications of living kidney donation. *Ann Surg*. 2006;243:126-130.
14. Yip SK, Tan YH, Cheng C, Sim HG, Lee YM, Chee C. Routine vascular control using the Hem-o-lok clip in laparoscopic nephrectomy: animal study and clinical application. *J Endourol*. 2004;18:77-81.
15. Eswar C, Badillo FL. Vascular control of the renal pedicle using the Hem-o-lok polymer ligating clip in 50 consecutive hand-assisted laparoscopic nephrectomies. *J Endourol*. 2004;18: 459-461.
16. Baumert H, Ballaro A, Arroyo C, Kaisary AV, Mulders PF, Knipscheer BC. The use of polymer (Hem-o-lok) clips for management of the renal hilum during laparoscopic nephrectomy. *Eur Urol*. 2006;49:816-819.
17. Baldwin DD, Desai PJ, Baron PW, et al. Control of the renal artery and vein with the nonabsorbable polymer ligating clip in hand-assisted laparoscopic donor nephrectomy. *Transplantation*. 2005;80:310-313.
18. Ponsky L, Cherullo E, Moinzadeh A, et al. The Hem-o-lok clip is safe for laparoscopic nephrectomy: a multi-institutional review. *Urology*. 2008;71:593-596.
19. Janetschek G, Bagheri F, Abdelmaksoud A, Biyani CS, Leeb K, Jeschke S. Ligation of the renal vein during laparoscopic nephrectomy: an effective and reliable method to replace vascular staplers. *J Urol*. 2003;170:1295-1297.
20. Capelouto CC, Kavoussi LR. Complications of laparoscopic surgery. *Urology*. 1993;42:2-12.
21. Kavoussi LR. Laparoscopic donor nephrectomy. *Kidney Int*. 2000;57:2175-2186.
22. Shalhav AL, Siqueira TM Jr, Gardner TA, Paterson RF, Stevens LH. Manual specimen retrieval without a pneumoperitoneum preserving device for laparoscopic live donor nephrectomy. *J Urol*. 2002;168:941-944.

23. Ramalingam M, Senthil K, Pai MG. Modified device-free HAL: an innovative cost-reductive approach [published online and ahead of print September 11, 2009]. *J Laparoendosc Adv Surg Tech A*. doi:10.1089/lap.2009.0203.
24. Wolf JS Jr, Tchetgen MB, Merion RM. Hand-assisted laparoscopic live donor nephrectomy. *Urology*. 1998;52:885-887.
25. McGinnis DE, Gomella LG, Strup SE. Comparison and clinical evaluation of hand-assist devices for hand-assisted laparoscopy. *Tech Urol*. 2001;7:57-61.
26. Figert PL, Park AE, Witzke DB, Schwartz RW. Transfer of training in acquiring laparoscopic skills. *J Am Coll Surg*. 2001;193:533-537.
27. Feldman LS, Sherman V, Fried GM. Using simulators to assess laparoscopic competence: ready for widespread use? *Surgery*. 2004;135:28-42.
28. Pokorny MR, McLaren SL. Inexpensive home-made laparoscopic trainer and camera. *Aust N Z J Surg*. 2004;74:691-693.
29. Chung SY, Landsittel D, Chon CH, Ng CS, Fuchs GJ. Laparoscopic skills training using a webcam trainer. *J Urol*. 2005;173:180-183.
30. Beatty JD. How to build an inexpensive laparoscopic webcam-based trainer. *BJU Int*. 2005;96:679-682.
31. Chandrasekera SK, Donohue JF, Orley D, et al. Basic laparoscopic surgical training: examination of a low-cost alternative. *Eur Urol*. 2006;50:1285-1291.
32. Menon M, Tewari A, Peabody JO, et al. Vattikuti Institute prostatectomy, a technique of robotic radical prostatectomy for management of localized carcinoma of the prostate: experience of over 1100 cases. *Urol Clin North Am*. 2004;31:701-717.
33. Klotz L. Robotic radical prostatectomy: fools rush in, or the early bird gets the worm? *Can Urol Assoc J*. 2007;1:87.
34. Moul JW. Will the global economic downturn affect prostate cancer care? Pelvic lymphadenectomy as an example. *Eur Urol*. 2009;55:1266-1268.
35. Lepor H. Status of radical prostatectomy in 2009: is there medical evidence to justify the robotic approach? *Rev Urol*. 2009;11:61-70.
36. Guru KA, Hussain A, Chandrasekhar R, et al. Current status of robot-assisted surgery in urology: a multi-national survey of 297 urologic surgeons. *Can J Urol*. 2009;16:4736-4741.
37. Morgan JA, Thornton BA, Peacock JC, et al. Does robotic technology make minimally invasive cardiac surgery too expensive? A hospital cost analysis of robotic and conventional techniques. *J Card Surg*. 2005;20:246-251.

Difficulties in Laparoscopic Simple Nephrectomy

6

Ahmed M. Harraz, Ahmed R. El-Nahas, and Ahmed A. Shokeir

The first transperitoneal laparoscopic nephrectomy was performed by Clayman et al. in 1990.[1] Since then, this surgery has been performed for various benign renal diseases. In 1992, Gaur et al. developed the balloon dissection technique for creation of the retroperitoneal space.[2] Since that time, retroperitoneoscopic nephrectomy has been demonstrated to be safe and effective for benign nonfunctioning kidneys.[3,4] Refinements such as entrapment bags and tissue morcellators have improved both the efficiency of specimen removal and the minimally invasive nature of the procedure. Laparoscopic nephrectomy offers less postoperative pain, shorter hospital stay and convalescence, and an optimal cosmetic result compared with traditional open surgery.[5,6]

Indications

Laparoscopic nephrectomy has become a routine procedure at specialized centers. It can be performed for all age groups, in obese patients and nearly all benign pathological conditions of the kidney.[7–10]

Removal of a nonfunctioning or poorly functioning kidney is indicated when it causes symptoms such as pain, urinary tract infection, or hypertension. It is also indicated in patients with chronic renal failure for removal of the left kidney before renal transplantation.[4,6,9,11–14] Laparoscopic nephrectomy was reported for the following benign pathologies:

- Hydronephrosis
- Chronic pyelonephritis
- Renovascular hypertension
- Reflux nephropathy
- Autosomal dominant polycystic kidney disease
- Renal dysplasia
- Post-traumatic atrophy of the kidney

A.A. Shokeir (✉)
Department of Urology, Urology and Nephrology Center, Mansoura, Egypt

A.M. Al-Kandari and I.S. Gill (eds.), *Difficult Conditions in Laparoscopic Urologic Surgery*,   **55**
DOI: 10.1007/978-1-84882-105-7_6, © Springer-Verlag London Limited 2011

Contraindications

Absolute contraindications to laparoscopic simple nephrectomy include active peritonitis, bowel obstruction, uncorrected coagulopathy, and severe cardiopulmonary insufficiency.[4,6,11,13] Relative contraindications include morbid obesity, severe inflammatory conditions affecting the kidney, such as xanthogranulomatous pyelonephritis (XGP), and renal tuberculosis.

Techniques of Laparoscopic Simple Nephrectomy

Transperitoneal Laparoscopic Nephrectomy

The patient is initially positioned supine for intravenous access, induction of general anesthesia, bladder catheterization, and nasogastric tube placement. The patient is then positioned in a modified lateral decubitus[6,15] or a standard lateral kidney position.[11,13] The table can be flexed as needed and padding is used to support all pressure areas (Fig. 6.1). The room setup is shown in Fig. 6.2. During the skin preparation and towel placement, the entire flank and abdomen are included in case conversion to an open procedure is required.

Access to the abdomen is obtained either with a Veress needle or with a Hasson canula. The needle is introduced at the lateral border of rectus muscle, at the level of the umbilicus.[11] Although the umbilicus is not the preferred site for needle placement during laparoscopic nephrectomy, it carries many advantages as the underlying peritoneum is fused to the overlying fascia, and it is the shortest distance between the skin and the peritoneum.[16] The intraperitoneal position of the tip of the needle can be ensured by the visual and tactile verification of release of the needle spring by the hanging drop test, and by injection of 2 mL of saline with failure of its retrieval upon suction. Patients with a history of multiple abdominal operations may have underlying adhesions and laparoscopic access is best

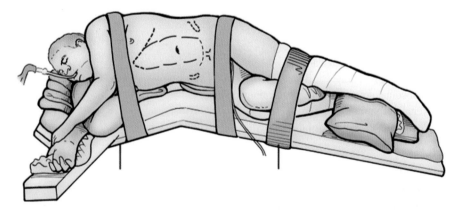

Fig. 6.1 Patient positioning for transperitoneal laparoscopic nephrectomy

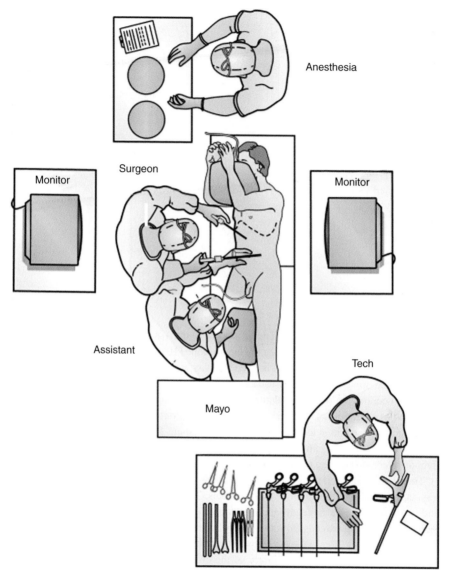

Fig. 6.2 Room setup for transperitoneal laparoscopic nephrectomy (From Bishoff and Kavoussi.[46] Copyright Elsevier 2007)

established by the open technique. The site of access is preferably via a small infra-umbilical or para-umbilical incision.[17]

Insufflation is started slowly, at a rate of 1 L/min until generalized resonance is achieved. The peritoneal cavity usually requires 3–6 L of CO_2 in adults and 1.5–3 L in children to be completely inflated. Then the flow is increased to maintain intraperitoneal pressure at 15 mmHg in adults and less than 12 in children using an automatic insufflator.[11]

Fig. 6.3 Port distribution for transperitoneal laparoscopic left nephrectomy

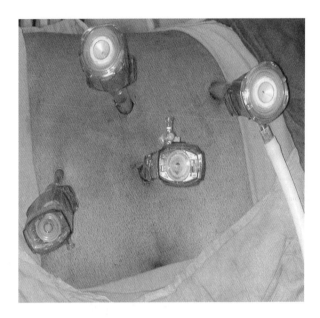

Four ports are used (Fig. 6.3). The first port (10 mm) is fixed at the site of the Veress needle. This port is used to introduce the laparoscope (10 mm, 0° lens). Under endoscopic guidance, the second port (12 mm) is fixed midway between the first port and the anterior superior iliac spine. This port is used to introduce dissecting electro-scissors, vascular stapler (to control the renal vasculature), and the endoscopic pouch (to entrap the kidney at the end of operation). The third port (10 mm) is inserted below the costal margin at the midclavicular line and is used to introduce the grasping forceps for tissue manipulation. The fourth port (5 or 10 mm) is inserted in the midaxillary line and is used for retraction of liver or spleen using a fan retractor.

Thorough inspection of the abdominal cavity is essential to exclude any inadvertent trauma, especially to the colon or blood vessels. The colon passes anterior to the kidney and the ureter. The peritoneum lateral to the colon (line of Toldt) is incised using diathermy scissors and extends from the level of the iliac vessels distally to above the colic flexures proximally (Fig. 6.4). A safety distance (about 1 cm) lateral to the colon should be respected to avoid diathermy injury of the colon. Using a combination of blunt and sharp dissection posterior to the colon, the colon is freed from the posterior abdominal wall and is reflected medially by the effect of gravity. The kidney becomes visible after reflection of the colon. The ureter passes anteromedial to the psoas muscle until it reaches the renal pelvis.

The upper ureter is easily identified and dissected with cephalad traction on the lower pole of the kidney. Using electrosurgical scissors, the periureteral fascia is dissected and the ureter is freed until it reaches the renal pelvis. Usually the ureter is divided at its lumbar level, about 5 cm below the level of the lower pole of the kidney. If its caliber is normal, it is divided between endoscopic clips. Otherwise, it can be ligated with endoscopic ligatures or clamped and incised with the endoscopic stapler.

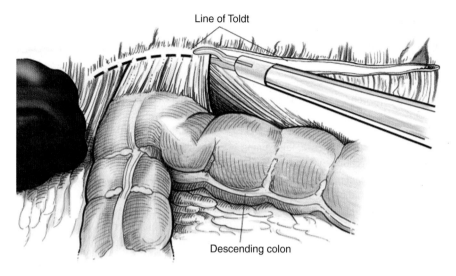

Fig. 6.4 Incision of the line of Toldt during left nephrectomy (From Bishoff and Kavoussi.[46] Copyright Elsevier 2007)

Proximal dissection of the ureter leads to the medial side of the renal pelvis where the renal artery and vein can be safely dissected. The renal vein is anteroinferior to the renal artery. In some cases, exposure of the vena cava in right-sided nephrectomy allows better visualization of the renal vein, whereas on the left side, the aorta is the landmark for the left renal artery. Exposure of the pedicle stump allows better and earlier control and avoids dealing with multiple branches and tributaries.

A toothed forceps (5 mm) is used to grasp the proximal end of the divided ureter. With caudal and lateral traction on the proximal end of the ureter, the anterior surface and medial border of the renal pelvis are dissected to expose the renal vessels. Using the endoscopic forceps, lateral traction along the medial aspect of the anterior surface of the kidney helps stretch the renal hilum to free it further, especially the upper, lower, and posterior sides. The renal vein appears first, followed by the renal artery posterosuperiorly.

Control of the Renal Pedicle

The renal artery is secured between endoscopic clips and cut, leaving two to three clips toward the stump side. In most cases the vein is too wide, so an endoscopic stapler is most useful. The stapler is used for simultaneous stapling and division of the vein. Another method to control the renal vein is to shrivel it using a ligature followed by clipping with a Hem-o-lok® (Teleflex Medical, Research Triangle Park, NC). This step combines advantages of suture ligation and clips with a locking mechanism and is important to shrivel a vein of any diameter to allow safe application of clips.[18] The main argument against the routine use of clips to ligate the pedicle is the relative ease with which clips may be dislodged. This drawback is overcome by using clips with a locking mechanism at the tip, such as the Hem-o-lok®, Laparo-clip (Tyco Healthcare, Mansfield, MA) and Absolok Plus (Ethicon Endo-Surgery, Cincinnati, OH). In addition, clip length is usually not adequate to occlude a large vein completely.[18]

Sometimes the vessels are surrounded by a dense fibrous reaction and an attempt to separate the artery from the vein seems difficult and hazardous. In this situation, division of the renal pedicle en mass using the endoscopic stapler may be accomplished. Although en bloc ligation of the renal pedicle has been potentially implicated in the postoperative development of arteriovenous fistula (AVF),[19] the possibility of its development is remote due to the presence of dense, intervening tissue between the vessels. This has been supported by other reports that have studied the possibility of AVF development after en bloc ligation of the renal hilum.[19–21]

In some cases, the gonadal vein is identified either crossing the right ureter anteriorly or lying medially alongside the upper left ureter. Both can be dissected and clamped with a 9-mm endoscopic clip and incised when necessary, but this must be done 2 cm away from the renal vein to avoid future problems with the applying the endoscopic stapler to the renal pedicle.

Gerota's fascia is identified by its orange yellow color and is incised to expose the renal surface. The plane between the fascia and the kidney is easily dissected with a combination of blunt and sharp dissection. One should avoid dissecting along the lateral border of the kidney initially, as early division of these attachments allows the kidney to drop medially and may hinder hilar dissection. To facilitate dissection of the upper pole, a fan-shaped retractor is passed to elevate the liver on the right side or the spleen on the left side.

After complete dissection of the kidney, a folded laparoscopic retrieval bag is introduced through the 12-mm port. The bag is folded around the 5-mm forceps in a clockwise direction. After introduction of the sac in the peritoneal cavity, it is unfolded in a counterclockwise direction. The mouth of the bag is kept open using two pairs of toothed forceps. Using a strong claw forceps, the kidney is thrown inside the sac. The mouth of the sac is closed by applying traction on the nylon thread, and it is pulled to the outside through the 12-mm port site. To extract the kidney, a combination of strong forceps and blunt-ended scissors is used to fragment the renal tissue. The kidney may be placed in an organ sack and retrieved intact through an extended skin incision.[6,13]

After the specimen retrieval is completed, a fingertip can be placed into the port through which the kidney was removed. Pneumoperitoneum is reestablished, and a final inspection of the intra-abdominal contents is performed. One must remember to decrease the intra-abdominal pressure to 7 mmHg to confirm hemostasis prior to exiting the abdomen. Fixation of an 18 F tube drain is done through the site of the most lateral port. The 5-mm ports are then removed under direct vision, and the remaining 10-mm port withdrawn with the laparoscope within it to observe the edges of the port during removal. All 12-mm ports should have fascial closure.

Advantages of the transperitoneal approach include more space to perform the surgery and easily identifiable anatomical landmarks. Therefore, the learning curve for the procedure is shorter and large kidneys are easier to manipulate in the large peritoneal space. However, there are some disadvantages, such as formation of intra-abdominal adhesions, contamination of the peritoneal cavity by urine, risk of injury to the intra-abdominal organs, and increased risk for bowel herniation compared to the retroperitoneal approach.[4,17]

Retroperitoneal Laparoscopic Nephrectomy

The same positioning steps in the transperitoneal approach are applicable for the retroperitoneal approach. The patient is placed in a lateral position (Fig. 6.5).

Creation of the Retroperitoneal Space

Gaur described the first technique for creation of the retroperitoneal space. The dissecting balloon is made with a number 8 red rubber catheter and a number 7 surgeon glove, where one end of the catheter is fed into the glove (which then becomes the balloon) while the other end is attached to the pneumatic pump of a blood pressure apparatus. A 2-cm skin incision is made just above the iliac crest in the midaxillary line. Blunt dissection is done down to the retroperitoneal space using artery forceps and occasionally, a finger. A curved artery forceps grasps the tip of the balloon and places it in the retroperitoneal space. The balloon is inflated using a pneumatic pump until a bulge appears in the abdomen. During this procedure, the balloon pressure is intermittently increased to 110 mmHg then decreased to 40–50 mmHg. The balloon is left inflated for 5 min to achieve hemostasis, then deflated and removed.[2]

Rassweiler et al. described another technique where a 15–18 mm skin incision is made in the lumbar (Petit's) triangle between the 12th rib and the iliac crest. A tunnel is created down to the retroperitoneal space using blunt dissection. Three methods were described to dissect the retroperitoneum: The first method uses a latex balloon formed from the middle finger of surgical glove on an 18 F catheter. The second method uses a balloon trocar system that consists of a latex balloon ligated to an 11-mm metal trocar sheath (Fig. 6.6). The third method uses the index finger exclusively to dissect the retroperitoneal space (Fig. 6.7).[4,22]

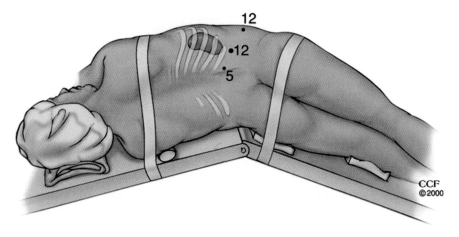

Fig. 6.5 Patient positioning for retroperitoneal laparoscopic nephrectomy (From Bishoff and Kavoussi.[46] Copyright Elsevier 2007)

Fig. 6.6 Creation of the
retroperitoneal space using
a balloon (From Hsu et al.[47]
Reprinted with permission
from Mary Ann Liebert,
Inc.)

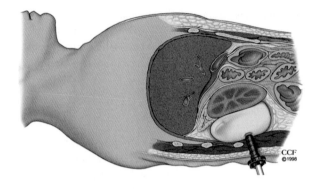

Fig. 6.7 Creation of the
retroperitoneal space using a
finger (From Hsu et al.[47]
Reprinted with permission
from Mary Ann Liebert,
Inc.)

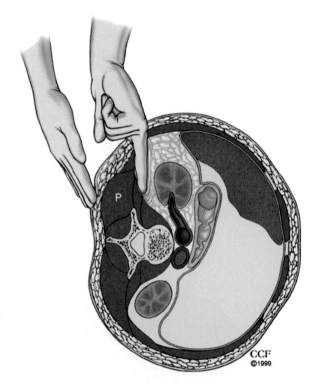

Gill et al. made a 1.5–2 cm incision immediately anterior to the tip of the 12th rib. The
posterior lumbodorsal fascia is incised between stay sutures, muscle layers are bluntly
separated and the anterior fascia is incised under vision. A fingertip is then inserted through
the incision, the lower pole of the kidney is palpated, and a retroperitoneal space is
created.[23]

El-Kappany et al. made a 2-cm subcostal incision one fingerbreadth below the tip of
the last rib. The incision is deepened by cutting or splitting the muscle until the white,

glistening lumbar fascia is identified. The fascia is sharply incised to reach the retro-peritoneum. Using the index finger for blunt dissection, a small retroperitoneal space is created to facilitate placement of the dissection balloon. A simple toy balloon of 1.5 L capacity is connected to an 18-F Nelaton catheter using double ligatures of number 0 silk sutures. The balloon is introduced into the retroperitoneum and inflated using sterile saline. It is kept inflated for 5–10 min to allow for more dissection and hemostasis of the retroperitoneum.[24]

El-Ghoneimi et al. published their experience in infants. They made an incision 1.5-cm long and at 1 cm from the tip of the twelfth rib. Gerota's fascia is approached by a muscle-splitting incision with blunt dissection, and then opened under direct vision. The first tro-car (5 or 10 mm) is introduced directly inside the opened Gerota's fascia. A working space is created by gas insufflation dissection and the first trocar is fixed with a purse-string suture applied around the deep fasciato to ensure an airtight seal.[25]

Port Distribution

A 10-mm blunt trocar is fixed at the site of the first incision. To prevent gas leakage, the muscles around the port must be closed using simple sutures, and two mattress sutures (number 1 silk) must be used to close the skin incision and fix the port in place. CO_2 insuf-flation is initiated through this port to maintain the pressure in the retroperitoneal space between 10 and 15 mmHg. The laparoscope is introduced through this port to facilitate fixation of another two ports under direct vision. The second port (12 mm) is fixed anterior to the first port at the same subcostal line. The third port (10 mm) is fixed one fingerbreadth above the anterior superior iliac spine. The third port is used for the laparoscope, and the first and second ports are used for dissection and manipulation (Fig. 6.8).

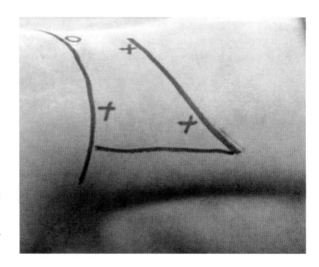

Fig. 6.8 Port distribution for retroperitoneal laparoscopic nephrectomy (From El-Kappany et al.[24] With kind permission of Springer Science + Business Media)

Operative Steps

The main landmark for orientation is the psoas muscle. This marks the posterior boundary of dissection, which is the first area to be tackled. A fibrous outer layer of Gerota's fascia is incised near the medial border of the psoas muscle to expose the perirenal fat. The incision is extended upward to expose the kidney, and downward to expose the ureter. The ureter appears as a white band anteromedial to the psoas muscle, with its surrounding vascular supply. The ureter is divided between endoscopic clips. If the ureter is followed up to the kidney (with dissection of the perirenal fat), the renal pelvis will be exposed. Here, the renal artery appears first and is posterosuperior to the renal vein. The gonadal vessel appears clearly on the left side of this vein. On both right and left sides, gonadal veins appear medial to the ureter when they reach the renal hilum. Then the procedure is completed as outlined in the transperitoneal technique.

The kidney is usually extracted without fragmentation from the initial subcostal incision in view of its small size. With average- or large-sized kidneys, entrapment and extraction are performed in a manner similar to the transperitoneal approach. Specimen extraction can be done by placing it in a laparoscopic retrieval bag or an organ entrapment bag, or intact removal of the specimen by enlarging the primary port or connecting two ports to make a large incision.

The retroperitoneal approach has many advantages. Since the peritoneal cavity is not entered, there is no risk of forming postoperative adhesions. There is also no risk of contamination of the peritoneal cavity with the contents of the urinary tract. There is a decreased risk of injury to the intraperitoneal organs and there is no need for retraction of the intra-abdominal viscera. As there is no need to mobilize the gut to expose the urinary tract, there is no postoperative ileus and hence a shorter convalescence.[26] Access to the site of lesion is direct as the kidney is a retroperitoneal structure. Less trocar punctures are needed as there are fewer requirements for retraction. The approach is safe even in patients with history of intraperitoneal surgery. There is less incidence of bowel herniation than with the transperitoneal approach.[3,4,17,27] Disadvantages include a smaller working space, and more difficult identification and exposure of some anatomical structures. More experience and a longer learning curve are needed for this approach as there are few landmarks in the retroperitoneum. This space is sometimes obliterated in patients with inflammatory pathologies such as pyelonephritis.[3,4,17]

Difficulties in Laparoscopic Nephrectomy

Laparoscopic Nephrectomy for Inflammatory Renal Conditions

Although the term "simple" is associated with nephrectomies that are performed for benign indications, this description continues to be one of the great misnomers in the field of urologic surgery. Inflammation, fibrosis, and scarring often affect the involved kidney, making the process of dissection much more difficult than that of the typical radical nephrectomy. When present, these factors make the laparoscopic approach to the simple nephrectomy a challenge for even the most experienced laparoscopic surgeons.

Perirenal and perihilar fibrosis is a common finding in infectious and inflammatory renal conditions such as pyonephrosis, tuberculosis, and XGP, making laparoscopic dissection challenging.[4,13] The theoretical advantages of the laparoscopic approach for inflammatory renal diseases have been questioned and were considered a relative contraindication to laparoscopy.[28]

The best laparoscopic approach for inflammatory renal conditions remains controversial. Whereas the retroperitoneal approach has been advocated for managing renal tuberculosis and other inflammatory renal conditions,[29,30] in many cases the transperitoneal approach provides superior exposure and more working space for difficult dissection. Thus, the transperitoneal approach has been advocated for XGP. A theoretical advantage of the retroperitoneal approach is the lack of intraperitoneal contamination with infectious material, as in pyonephrosis and tuberculous kidney. In previous series, two cases of spillage of tuberculous material were reported, although at follow up no disseminated or systemic disease was identified.[28,31] However, no difference was noted in the transperitoneal and retroperitoneal approaches for tuberculous kidneys.[30,31]

Technical Considerations in Laparoscopic Nephrectomy for Inflammatory Renal Diseases

1. Open access placement using the Hasson technique via the periumbilical or primary retroperitoneal approach has been recommended for tuberculous kidney. Alternatively, initial subcostal access may be achieved to establish pneumoperitoneum.[32]
2. Hydraulic distension using a balloon was found to be more effective than pneumatic distension during creation of the retroperitoneal space.
3. The hilum first approach is useful when dense perinephric adhesions are present as perihilar scarring makes dissection of the renal vessels difficult. A direct approach to the hilum without dissecting the kidney is crucial to minimize oozing.[33] The vessels are controlled outside the fascia just above the psoas muscle if it is not possible to identify the pedicle after incising the fascia. After controlling the pedicle, the kidney dissection continues inside the fascia. If adhesions make this impossible, the dissection is carried out outside the fascia as in radical nephrectomy.
4. En-bloc control of the renal hilum using the stapler can be performed. The hilum can be transected and secured with Endo-GIA staples without dissecting individual hilar structures.[32]
5. Subcapsular nephrectomy can be used with severe adhesions around the kidney. Adhesions between the renal capsule and parenchyma are not as serious as those between the kidney and perirenal tissues. This operational style avoids perirenal adhesions that may be present in the subcapsular space. The renal fibrous membrane is cut along the renal hilum, and the fat and fibrous tissues are separated to decrease the size of the renal pedicle. The renal pedicle is then thin enough to be controlled with an endoscopic linear cutter. This maneuver solves the problem of a broad renal pedicle that cannot be cut off in a laparoscopic operation.[34]
6. Dissection outside of Gerota's fascia has been reported to facilitate the procedure, especially in cases of chronic pyelonephritis with kidneys harboring stones. Intra-Gerotal dissection may be difficult. In such cases, dissection at the extra-Gerotal plane is better conducted to avoid the severe perirenal adhesions.

7. In patients with percutanous nephrostomy, after creation of the retroperitoneal space, division of the percutaneous nephrostomy tract in the retroperitoneum is helpful. This allows the kidney to be pushed forward and creates a larger retroperitoneal space.[33]

8. Recently, laparoscopic nephrectomy was reported in most cases of inflammatory renal conditions. A higher conversion rate and longer operative time should be expected. Early conversion may be required due to failure to progress, but blood loss, hospital stay, and analgesia requirements are lower compared to the open approach.[35]

Laparoscopic Nephrectomy in Patients with Previous Abdominal Surgery

Abdominal surgery promotes the formation of adhesions that may distort tissue planes, alter the position of anatomical landmarks and fix bowel to the anterior abdominal wall, making subsequent laparoscopic access and dissection more difficult. Therefore, it may be difficult to place the Veress needle due to abdominal wall adhesions. Abdominal scars may necessitate placing trocar sites at alternative suboptimal positions, potentially increasing the possibility of vascular injury while obtaining access, and hindering instrument manipulation during the procedure.[36]

Dissection of adhesions may increase the risk of bleeding and bowel injury. In addition, the distortion of normal anatomy may decrease visibility during the procedure. Technical considerations such as these have prompted many initial reports in the general surgical literature to cite previous abdominal surgery as an exclusion criterion to laparoscopy.[37]

Previous surgery at the same anatomical site is associated with longer operative time and increased hospital stay compared with patients with no history of surgery and surgery at a different location. Longer operative time was likely associated with the increased difficulty of laparoscopic surgery in an anatomical region previously subjected to operative dissection.[38]

Patients with previous history of abdominal surgery were more likely to receive blood transfusions. This trend was likely related to increased age and higher degree of medical co-morbidity. However, there were no significant differences in operative blood loss, the rate of operative conversion, or the rate or operative complication. Therefore, previous abdominal surgery does not appear to adversely affect the performance or safety of subsequent urological laparoscopy.[36]

In another report regarding transperitoneal laparoscopic simple nephrectomy in patients with history of previous abdominal surgery, there was no significant differences in operative time, estimated blood loss or overall complication rate. The only significant difference was a longer hospital stay in patients with previous abdominal surgery.[39]

Technical Considerations in Patients with Previous Abdominal Surgery

1. The retroperitoneal approach to laparoscopic nephrectomy is preferred over the transperitoneal approach as there is no difference in regard to operative times, blood loss or hospital stays between patients with a history of abdominal surgery and those with no history of abdominal surgery.[40]

2. The first port must be away from the scar of previous surgery.
3. Open insertion of the first port or using optical access trocars may prevent bowel injury.

Laparoscopic Nephrectomy for Giant Hydronephrosis

Giant hydronephrosis is defined as a kidney containing more than 1,000 mL fluid in the collecting system. Radiologically, these kidneys meet or cross the midline, occupy a hemi-abdomen or extend more than five vertebral lengths. The most common cause of giant hydronephrosis is ureteropelvic junction obstruction which is the etiology in about 80% of cases.[41]

Initial operator disorientation occurs because of the large hydronephrotic sac that occupies the retroperitoneum, obscuring the standard landmarks for surgery. Thus reorientation is needed once preliminary dissection is completed and the kidney is deflated.

Technical Considerations in Laparoscopic Nephrectomy for Giant Hydronephrosis

1. The transperitoneal approach is more appropriate than the retroperitoneum approach because of the larger cavity of the peritoneum.
2. Percutaneous aspiration of the fluid inside the hugely dilated pelvicalyceal system is advised to help develop adequate working space. Aspiration can be performed prior to pneumoperitoneum by passing a long percutaneous needle through the renal angle. Alternatively, using a Veress needle is an efficient way of achieving kidney decompression. In cases where the hydronephrotic kidney will not interfere with port placement, the kidney can be decompressed after initial dissection using laparoscopic suction because the tense hydronephrotic sac helps in the identification of the perirenal plane.
3. Adequate retraction of the collapsed renal sac is important to identify the renal pedicle. If further dissection cannot be achieved intracorporeally, bringing the sac out through an anterior port (extracorporeal retraction) aids in ease of retraction and hilar dissection. The port site needs to be enlarged to about 2–3 cm depending on the bulk of the kidney, since a large incision can lead to a gas leak. Once the kidney is fully mobilized and the vessels are clipped, it can be delivered through the same port by further enlarging the incision if needed. The laparoscopic retrieval bag is not needed in these cases as the collapsed kidney can be delivered after minimally enlarging the port site.[42]

Laparoscopic Nephrectomy in Obese Patients

Obese patients have higher rates of postoperative complications, including nosocomial infections, wound infections and wound dehiscence. However, Matin et al. did not find an association between body mass index (BMI) and surgical or postoperative complications.[43] Doublet et al. also documented that laparoscopic nephrectomy is safe and effective in obese patients.[44]

Technical Considerations in Laparoscopic Nephrectomy in Obese Patients

1. Extra care should be used in positioning obese patients.
2. Optimal ventilation is mandatory because pneumoperitoneum makes the already impaired respiratory movements in obese patients more difficult.
3. Adequate padding for pressure points is necessary.
4. Less bend is usually used in the operative table with obese patients.
5. Ports are inserted more laterally in patients with large abdominal girth.[45]

References

1. Clayman RV, Kavoussi LR, Soper NJ, et al. Laparoscopic nephrectomy: initial case report. *J Urol.* 1991;146:278-282.
2. Gaur DD. Laparoscopic operative retroperitoneoscopy: use of a new device. *J Urol.* 1992;148:1137-1139.
3. Pearle MS, Nakada SY. Laparoscopic nephrectomy: retroperitoneal approach. *Semin Laparosc Surg.* 1996;3:75-83.
4. Rassweiler J, Fornara P, Weber M, et al. Laparoscopic nephrectomy: the experience of the laparoscopy working group of the German Urological Association. *J Urol.* 1998;160:18-21.
5. Kerbl K, Clayman RV, McDougall EM, et al. Transperitoneal nephrectomy for benign disease of the kidney: a comparison of laparoscopic and open surgical techniques. *Urology.* 1994;43:607-613.
6. Doehn C, Fornara P, Fricke L, Jocham D. Comparison of laparoscopic and open nephroureterectomy for benign disease. *J Urol.* 1998;159:732-734.
7. Ehrlich RM, Gershman A, Fuchs G. Laparoscopic renal surgery in children. *J Urol.* 1994;151:735-739.
8. McDougall EM, Clayman RV. Laparoscopic nephrectomy for benign disease: comparison of the transperitoneal and retroperitoneal approaches. *J Endourol.* 1996;10:45-49.
9. Fornara P, Doehn C, Fricke L, Durek C, Thyssen G, Jocham D. Laparoscopic bilateral nephrectomy: results in 11 renal transplant patients. *J Urol.* 1997;157:445-449.
10. Fazeli-Matin S, Gill IS, Hsu TH, Sung GT, Novick AC. Laparoscopic renal and adrenal surgery in obese patients: comparison to open surgery. *J Urol.* 1999;162:665-669.
11. Eraky I, el-Kappany HA, Ghoniem MA. Laparoscopic nephrectomy: Mansoura experience with 106 cases. *Br J Urol.* 1995;75:271-275.
12. Doublet JD, Barreto HS, Degremont AC, Gattegno B, Thibault P. Retroperitoneal nephrectomy: comparison of laparoscopy with open surgery. *World J Surg.* 1996;20:713-716.
13. Keeley FX, Tolley DA. A review of our first 100 cases of laparoscopic nephrectomy: defining risk factors for complications. *Br J Urol.* 1998;82:615-618.
14. Shoma AM, Eraky I, El-Kappany HA. Pretransplant native nephrectomy in patients with end-stage renal failure: assessment of the role of laparoscopy. *Urology.* 2003;61:915-920.
15. Siqueira TM, Kuo RL, Gardner TA, et al. Major complications in 213 nephrectomy cases: the Indianapolis experience. *J Urol.* 2002;168:1361-1365.
16. Goel A, Hemal AK. Laparoscopic access. In: Hemal AK, ed. *Laparoscopic Urologic Surgery.* New Delhi, India: Churchill Livingstone; 2000:51-63.
17. Gill IS, Kavoussi LR, Clayman RV, et al. Complications of laparoscopic nephrectomy in 185 patients: a multi-institutional review. *J Urol.* 1995;154:479-483.

18. Janetschek G, Bagheri F, Abdelmaksoud A, Biyani CS, Leeb K, Jeschke S. Ligation of the renal vein during laparoscopic nephrectomy: an effective and reliable method to replace vascular staplers. *J Urol*. 2003;170:1295-1297.
19. Kouba E, Smith AM, Derksen JE, Gunn K, Wallen E, Pruthi RS. Efficacy and safety of en bloc ligation of renal hilum during laparoscopic nephrectomy. *Urology*. 2007;69:226-229.
20. Rapp DE, Orvieto MA, Gerber GS, Johnston WK III, Wolf JS Jr, Shalhav AL. En bloc stapling of renal hilum during laparoscopic nephrectomy and nephroureterectomy. *Urology*. 2004; 64:656-659.
21. White WM, Klein FA, Gash J, Waters WB. Prospective radiographic followup after en bloc ligation of the renal hilum. *J Urol*. 2007;178:1888-1891.
22. Rassweiler JJ, Henkel TO, Stoch C, et al. Retroperitoneal laparoscopic nephrectomy and other procedures in the upper retroperitoneum using a balloon dissection technique. *Eur Urol*. 1994;25:229-236.
23. Gill IS, Grune MT, Munch LC. Access technique for retroperitoneoscopy. *J Urol*. 1996;156:1120-1124.
24. El-Kappany H, Eraky I, Ghoneim MA. Laparoscopic nephrectomy. In: Novick AC, Marberger M, eds. *The Kidneys and Adrenals*. Philadelphia, PA: Current Medicine; 2000:151-163. Vaughan ED Jr, Perlmutter AJ, eds. *Atlas of Clinical Urology*; vol 3.
25. El-Ghoneimi A, Farhat W, Bolduc S, Bagli D, McLorie G, Khoury A. Retroperitoneal laparoscopic vs open partial nephroureterectomy in children. *BJU Int*. 2003;91:532-535.
26. Wolf JS, Carrier S, Stoller ML. Intraperitoneal versus extraperitoneal insufflation of carbon dioxide gas for laparoscopy. *J Endourol*. 1995;9:63-66.
27. Rassweiler JJ, Seemann O, Frede T, Henkel TO, Aiken P. Retroperitoneoscopy: experience with 200 cases. *J Urol*. 1998;160:1265-1269.
28. Bercowsky E, Shalhav AL, Portis A, Elbahnasy AM, McDougall EM, Clayman RV. Is the laparoscopic approach justified in patients with xanthogranulomatous pyelonephritis? *Urology*. 1999;54:437-442.
29. Gill IS. Retroperitoneal laparoscopic nephrectomy. *Urol Clin North Am*. 1998;25:343-360.
30. Hemal AK, Gupta NP, Kumar R. Comparison of retroperitoneoscopic nephrectomy with open surgery for tuberculous nonfunctioning kidneys. *J Urol*. 2000;164:32-35.
31. Kim HH, Lee KS, Park K, Ahn H. Laparoscopic nephrectomy for nonfunctioning tuberculous kidney. *J Endourol*. 2000;14:433-437.
32. Shekarriz B, Meng MV, Lu HF, Yamada H, Duh QY, Stoller ML. Laparoscopic nephrectomy for inflammatory renal conditions. *J Urol*. 2001;166:2091-2094.
33. Hemal AK, Gupta NP, Wadhwa SN, Goel A, Kumar R. Retroperitoneoscopic nephrectomy and nephroureterectomy for benign nonfunctioning kidneys: a single-center experience. *Urology*. 2001;57:644-649.
34. Zhang X, Zheng T, Ma X, et al. Comparison of retroperioneoscopic nephrectomy versus open approaches to nonfunctioning tuberculous kidneys: a report of 44 cases. *J Urol*. 2005;173: 1586-1589.
35. Manohar T, Desai M, Desai M. Laparoscopic nephrectomy for benign and inflammatory conditions. *J Endourol*. 2007;21:1323-1328.
36. Parsons JK, Jarrett TJ, Chow GK, Kavoussi LR. The effect of previous abdominal surgery on urologic laparoscopy. *J Urol*. 2002;168:2387-2390.
37. Lyass S, Perry Y, Venturero M, et al. Laparoscopic cholecystectomy: what does affect the outcome? A retrospective multifactorial regression analysis. *Surg Endosc*. 2000;14:661-665.
38. Savage SJ, Schweizer DK, Gill IS. Reoperative urologic laparoscopy: a critical analysis. Paper presented at: 17th World Congress of Endourology; September 2000; Sao Paulo, Brazil.
39. Seifman BD, Dunn RL, Wolf JS. Transperitoneal laparoscopy into the previously operated abdomen: effect on operative time, length of stay and complications. *J Urol*. 2003;169: 36-40.

40. Viterbo R, Greenberg RE, Al-Saleem T, Uzzo RG. Prior abdominal surgery and radiation do not complicate the retroperitoneoscopic approach to the kidney or adrenal gland. *J Urol.* 2005;174:446-450.

41. Friedland GW, Filly R, Gons M. Congenital anomalies of the urinary tract. In: Friedland GW, ed. *Uroradiology: An Integrated Approach.* New York: Churchill Livingstone; 1983: 1386-1391.

42. Hemal AK, Wadhwa SN, Kumar M, Gupta NP. Transperitoneal and retroperitoneal laparoscopic nephrectomy for giant hydronephrosis. *J Urol.* 1999;162:35-39.

43. Matin SF, Abreu S, Ramani A, et al. Evaluation of age and comorbidity as risk factors after laparoscopic urological surgery. *J Urol.* 2003;170:1115-1120.

44. Doublet JD, Belair G. Retroperitoneal laparoscopic nephrectomy is safe and effective in obese patients: a comparative study of 55 procedures. *Urology.* 2000;56:63-66.

45. Anast JW, Stoller ML, Meng MV, et al. Differences in complications and outcomes for obese patients undergoing laparoscopic radical, partial or simple nephrectomy. *J Urol.* 2004;172: 2287-2291.

46. Bishoff JT, Kavoussi MD. Laparoscopic surgery of the kidney. In: Wein AJ, Kavoussi LR, Novick AC, Partin AW, Peters CA, eds. Campbell-Walsh Urology, 9th ed. Philadelphia, PA: WB Saunders; 2007:1759-1809.

47. Hsu TH, Sung GT, Gill IS. Retroperitoneoscopic approach to nephrectomy. *J Endourol.* 1999;13:713-718.

Difficulties in Transperitoneal Laparoscopic Radical Nephrectomy

7

Rakesh V. Khanna and Robert J. Stein

Laparoscopic radical nephrectomy has gained widespread acceptance as the standard of care for localized renal cell carcinoma. Since its inception, the technique has continued to evolve and, therefore, it is not surprising that variations in technique exist.

Relative contraindications to laparoscopic radical nephrectomy include vena cava thrombus, bulky adenopathy, locally invasive tumors, and significant cardiopulmonary disease. Uncorrected coagulopathy is an absolute contraindication to laparoscopic nephrectomy.

Complications from laparoscopic transperitoneal nephrectomy (e.g., bowel injury, barotraumas) are discussed elsewhere in this book. The aim of the present chapter is to detail difficulties encountered intraoperatively and to provide practical methods on how they can be resolved. Each step of radical nephrectomy is described and potential difficulties dealt with.

Patient Positioning

The patient is positioned in a modified flank position with all pressure points padded. While the patient should be positioned over the break in the bed and the table flexed, excessive flexion is not required and may potentially increase the risk of rhabdomyolysis, especially in obese patients.

Access

A number of different approaches with regard to radical nephrectomy have been devised. In general this includes between three and five ports: one camera port, two working ports, one assistant port for retraction/elevation, and one port for liver retraction. Access

R.J. Stein (✉)
Center for Laparoscopic and Robotic Surgery, Glickman Urological and Kidney Institute, Cleveland Clinic, Cleveland, OH, USA
e-mail: steinr@ccf.org

A.M. Al-Kandari and I.S. Gill (eds.), *Difficult Conditions in Laparoscopic Urologic Surgery*, DOI: 10.1007/978-1-84882-105-7_7, © Springer-Verlag London Limited 2011

can be obtained either by using a Veress needle or an open Hassan technique. If using a Veress needle, prior to insufflation, a drop test, aspiration, and advancement test should be performed. Correct placement is confirmed under conditions of low flow of insufflant, low intraabdominal pressure (generally less than 8 mm Hg), and uniform abdominal distension.

If blood can be aspirated upon insertion of the Veress needle, raising concern of great vessel injury, the veress needle should be closed and left in place in order to identyfy the site of injury. A laparoscopic or open technique can be used to inspect the site of injury. Observation may be elected if there is a non-expanding henatomec. In general, if uncertainty exists with regard to Veress needle placement, an open Hassan technique should be performed.

In order to avoid injury to the epigastric artery, trocars should, in general, be placed either in the midline or lateral to the rectus muscle.

Bowel Mobilization

The line of Toldt is incised and the colon is mobilized medially to expose the kidney. On the right side, the duodenum is Kocherized and the liver is elevated and retracted cranially using a liver retractor or a grasper attached to the abdominal side wall. On the left side to provide optimal exposure, the pancreas and spleen must be mobilized medially. The lienorenal, phrenicocolic, and splenic attachments to the diaphragm should be divided so that the spleen is able to fall away medially with the aid of gravity.

When performing bowel mobilization, care should be taken to avoid injury to the duodenum or liver on the right side, and to the pancreas and spleen on the left side. Minor bleeding from the spleen or liver can be controlled by using argon beam coagulation or by applying compression with any of a number of hemostatic agaents. If an especially severe splenic laceration is noted, splenectomy can be considered with appropriate vaccinations administered prior to hospital discharge.

Difficulties with bowel mobilization consist initially of lysis of adhesions. Using a laparoscopic bowel grasper to provide gentle traction, adhesions are divided using cold scissors. Adhesions should be divided as close as possible to the peritoneal wall to avoid inadvertent bowel injury.

Attention is then turned to mobilization of the colon regardless of the side of nephrectomy. This is performed by identifying the lateral edge of the colon and dissecting this from the Gerota's overlying the kidney and ureter. A common mistake is to begin dissection lateral to the kidney. The lateral attachments of the kidney should be maintained until much later in the procedure in order to allow for optimal hilar exposure.

Identifying the correct plane between the mesentery of the bowel and Gerota's fascia can be difficult (Fig. 7.1). This is performed, however, by recognizing a difference in color and texture between the perirenal fat and the bowel mesentery. Additionally, the correct plane should be relatively avascular. Using a laparoscopic grasper, the bowel mesentery is grasped and pulled anteromedially in order to expose the plane of dissection. If significant

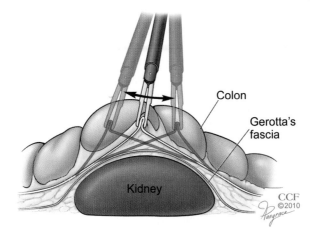

Fig. 7.1 Identifying the correct plane between the mesentery of the bowel and Gerota's fascia. This is performed by recognizing a difference in color and texture between the perirenal fat and the bowel mesentery. This is easier to appreciate by grasping the bowel mesentery using laparoscopic graspers and pulling the mesentery in an anteromedial direction (Reprinted with permission, Cleveland Clinic Center for Medical Art & Photography © 2010. All Rights Reserved)

bleeding is encountered, this is usually indicative that one is dissecting within an improper plane and one is within the bowel mesentery.

Identification of full-thickness bowel injury is critical. If this is noted, consideration can be given to primary repair in two layers with permanent sutures. It is the authors' standard practice to ask for an intraoperative general surgery consultation in this event. If there is only an injury in the serosal layer, oversewing with permanent suture should be performed.

Identification of the Ureter

The ureter is located anterior to the psoas muscle within the lower pole cone of Gerota's fat. The identification of the gonadal vein is a reliable landmark as the ureter will lie posterior and lateral to this vein. The ureter is isolated and traced superiorly to the renal hilum.

At times, especially when a lot of retroperitoneal fat is present, isolation of the ureter can be difficult. In such instances one should proceed by first identifying the psoas muscle and then the gonadal vein. The ureter will lie anterior to the psoas muscle and posterior to the gonadal vein. If uncertain, the ureter can be differentiated from the gonadal vein by recognizing that the ureter will often peristalse after manipulation.

On the right side, the insertion of the gonadal vein into the inferior vena cava can be a source of significant bleeding if avulsed. This can be avoided by dissecting the gonadal vein medially away from the ureter. Otherwise the gonadal vein can be clipped and divided.

If bleeding is encountered secondary to an avulsed gonadal vein, the area of bleeding should be grasped using a laparoscopic grasper or vascular clamp. This can then be controlled either by applying a clip or by suture ligation. Application of a Hem-o-lok® clip (Teleflex Medical, Research Triangle Park, NC) partially on the renal vein should not be attempted as the distal locking portion of the clip can severely injure the vessel. Instead, titanium clips can be attempted in this situation.

A critical point for left-sided nephrectomy is that the aortic pulse should be identified and all dissection carried out lateral to this. Dissection medial to the aorta increases the risk of inadvertent injury or transection of the superior mesenteric artery.

Hilar Dissection

A thorough review of preoperative imaging should be undertaken to provide an idea of: (1) relative position of artery and vein, (2) the number of arteries and veins, and (3) the possibility of renal vein thrombus. If a renal vein thrombus is suspected, intraoperative ultrasound must be available.

It must be stressed that the key to hilar dissection is to proceed in a meticulous fashion. In this respect, the authors prefer to use hook electrocautery, as opposed to scissors or the harmonic scalpel, as this provides for a more accurate dissection.

Hilar dissection requires that the kidney be retracted anterolaterally in order to place the hilum on gentle tension and that the bowel be fully mobilized medially in order to have optimal exposure.

Intraoperatively, the key to hilar dissection begins by first identifying the gonadal vein as on the left side it will lead to the left renal vein. The renal vein will usually be anterior to the renal artery. As one approaches the renal vein on the left side, often a posterior lumbar vein will be present. Care must be taken as significant bleeding can occur if this vein is disrupted. Often by clipping and dividing the lumbar vein, greater exposure will be achieved for identification and dissection of the renal artery. Furthermore, if the gonadal vein is to be ligated, this should not be done too close to the renal vein as clips may interfere with stapler firing and if hemorrhage occurs from the gonadal vein, a greater length of vein is available for control.

After the vein has been identified, focus is turned towards the renal artery. On the left side, before transecting an artery, it must be established that the artery is not the superior mesenteric artery. This can be established by ensuring that the artery travels to the kidney and that all dissection is being carried out lateral to the aorta.

Difficulties with this part of the procedure include (1) being unable to dissect the vein and artery separately, (2) dealing with a complex hilum (i.e., multiple arteries and veins), (3) the presence of a renal vein thrombus, (4) being unable to dissect the hilum secondary to hilar adenopathy, and (5) bleeding.

If access to the renal artery is difficult secondary to the presence of the renal vein, dissection may proceed by staying directly on the posterior aspect of the renal vein. Two tissue packets are created. The posterior packet will contain the artery and can be taken with the endovascular stapler followed by another firing on the anterior packet containing the renal vein (Fig. 7.2). When firing the stapler, one must stay lateral to the great vessels. In

Fig. 7.2 Difficult access to the renal artery. If unable to access the renal artery, dissection may proceed by staying directly on the posterior aspect of the renal vein. The tissue posterior to the renal vein will contain the renal artery and can be taken with the endovascular stapler (Reprinted with permission, Cleveland Clinic Center for Medical Art & Photography © 2010. All Rights Reserved)

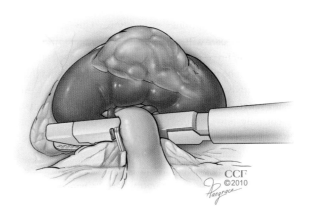

addition, before firing the endovascular stapler, one must ensure that the endovascular stapler is free of any clips and that the tissue packets are thin as these situations can cause misfiring. Otherwise, if partial arterial exposure can be achieved, a clip can be applied across the artery but not divided. Subsequently, the vein is stapled and divided to fully expose the renal artery. Additional clips to the artery can then be applied and the artery divided. Lastly, if the renal artery and vein packet cannot be separated, but can be thinned, consideration can be given to en bloc transection of the hilum using the endovascular stapler. An increased incidence of arteriovenous fistula formation has not been reported. However, if this is being performed and the stapler is being fired from a medial to lateral direction, the psoas muscle both superior and inferior to the renal vein should be visualized to ensure that the entire renal hilum has been taken.

If the artery and vein are taken separately, after division of the artery, a laparoscopic bowel grasper can be placed across the renal vein. If the renal vein remains collapsed, there is unlikely to be any additional arterial supply. However, if the renal vein fills, a search for accessory arteries should be performed.

In cases in which a renal vein thrombus is suspected, this can be confirmed by intraoperative ultrasound. Tumor thrombus will often retract after ligation of the renal artery. In right sided nephrectomies, one may isolate and clip the renal artery early in the procedure in the interaortocaval location. This not only may cause tumor thrombus retraction, and therefore provide a greater area in which the endovascular stapler may be fired, but will also aid in decreasing bleeding that may arise from large collateral vessels. After ligation of the renal artery, Doppler ultrasound of the renal vein is performed. The vascular stapler must be applied distal to the area of the thrombus. If unsure about stapler positioning, consideration should be given to performing an open procedure.

At times dissection of the hilum will be impossible (i.e., secondary to large adenopathy). In this circumstance, application of the stapler across the hilum and nodal tissue is not advised as a large tissue packet can result in stapler misfiring. In such a situation, if unable to perform a nodal dissection, strong consideration should be given to open conversion.

If bleeding is encountered, the first step is to remain composed. Grasping the lacerated vessel, pressure, packing with a surgical sponge, and application of a hemostatic matrix may be attempted. Furthermore, intra-abdominal pneumoperitoneum can be increased to

20 mmHg. A clip can be placed but only if safe placement is assured. As stated previously, placement of a Hem-o-lok® clip only partially across a vessel should not be done as the distal locking end will cause severe vascular injury. If unsure of safe placement of a Hem-o-lok® clip, a titanium clip can be attempted. If this results in control of bleeding, attention can be turned to another part of the case and this area can be reassessed at a later time. Otherwise, depending on one's level of expertise, intracorporeal suture ligation may be attempted. Application of a Hem-o-lok® clip to the distal suture end will aid in suturing by cinching down tissues and obviating the need for intracorporeal knot tying initially. Once a figure-of eight suture is placed, the Hem-o-lok® clip can be loosened and the clip cut from the suture and knots tied to secure the suture. In addition, another alternative includes insertion of an additional trocar. A laparoscopic Satinsky clamp may be placed through this trocar to obtain control. Definitive management can then be obtained, whether by clips, stapling, or suture ligature, under controlled conditions. On the right side, a laparoscopic vascular clamp must always be available in case emergency clamping of the vena cava is required. One must always keep in mind patient safety and if required one should not hesitate to convert to an open surgery. At least partial control of the hemorrhage with a laparoscopic instrument is optimal during open conversion in order to limit blood loss and also provide a landmark for rapid identification of site of hemorrhage once open exposure is established.

Upper Pole Mobilization

After hilar dissection, the remaining attachments of the kidney include the adrenal gland and the upper pole. The upper margin of dissection will depend on whether the adrenal gland is to be preserved.

Difficulties with this part of the procedure include dissecting within the correct plane between the adrenal gland and kidney (if the adrenal is to be preserved) or being unable to reach the upper part of the kidney secondary to a large tumor mass.

If the adrenal is to be removed en bloc with the kidney on the right side, the adrenal vein must be divided. Care must be taken as the adrenal vein on the right side drains directly into the inferior vena cava, is of short length, and can easily be avulsed. On the left side the medial edge of the adrenal gland should be identified and dissection should proceed superiorly and posteriorly.

Usually at this point in the procedure the kidney is freely mobile. Using a grasper, caudal traction can be placed on the kidney and the remaining attachments divided. If significant attachments remain, a stapler can be applied to fully mobilize the upper pole of the kidney. In situations with a large upper pole tumor, superior access can be difficult. Yet in nearly all cases a dissection plane exists between the mass and liver or spleen.

During upper pole dissection, care should be taken to avoid diaphragmatic injury. This should be suspected in the presence of increasing ventilatory difficulty or paradoxical diaphragmatic movements intraoperatively (the "bellows sign"). This can be closed using a figure-of-eight suture after a 14-F red rubber catheter is placed through one of the ports into the pleural space. The distal end of the catheter is placed under water. Pneumoperitoneum is reduced to 5 mmHg and the anesthesiologist is instructed to give the patient a large inspiration to expel the pleural air. After the air has been evacuated, the catheter is removed and the figure-of-eight suture tied down simultaneously.

Specimen Removal

After the upper pole has been mobilized, the ureter is divided and the specimen placed in an entrapment sac. It is the authors' practice not to morcellate the specimen when a radical nephrectomy is performed for tumor. The specimen may be removed though one of the port sites or a Gibson or Pfannensteil incision.

After specimen retrieval, hemostasis is verified with an intra-abdominal pneumoperitoneum of 5 mmHg. The trocars are removed under direct vision to ensure that no port site bleeding is present.

Conclusion

Though present for many years, laparoscopic transperitoneal nephrectomy remains a challenging technique. Patient safety and oncological control must not be compromised. However, it is hoped that after reading this chapter, the reader will have learned additional maneuvers to help perform this procedure.

Suggested Reading

Breda A, Finelli A, Janetschek G, Porpiglia F, Montorsi F. Complications of laparoscopic surgery for renal masses: prevention, management, and comparison with the open experience. *Eur Urol.* 2009;55(4):836-850.

De La Rosette JJMCH, Sternberg CN, Van Poppel HPA, eds. *Renal Cell Cancer: Diagnosis and Therapy.* London: Springer; 2008.

Kumar U, Gill IS, eds. *Tips and Tricks in Laparoscopic Urology.* London: Springer; 2007.

Rosenblatt A, Bollens R, Espinoza Cohen B. *Manual of Laparoscopic Urology.* Berlin-Heidelberg, Germany: Springer-Verlag; 2008.

Difficulties in Retroperitoneal Laparoscopic Radical Nephrectomy

8

Ricardo Brandina, Andre Berger, Robert J. Stein, and Inderbir S. Gill

Introduction

Laparoscopic radical nephrectomy is now routine practice for management of patients with localized renal cell carcinoma. Compared with open radical nephrectomy, the laparoscopic approach is associated with comparable operative time, decreased blood loss, superior recovery, improved cosmesis, and equivalent cancer control over a long-term follow-up.[1-3]

Even though the retroperitoneal approach has a smaller working space, it offers several unique advantages, including expeditious access to renal artery and vein allowing early ligation, extrafascial mobilization of the kidney, and en bloc removal of the adrenal gland, recapitulating the principles of open surgery.[4]

Technique

Preoperative Evaluation

The patient's cardiorespiratory status, coagulation profile, history of prior operations, and bone or spinal abnormalities needs to be assessed. The authors' preoperative bowel preparation comprises two bottles of magnesium citrate administered the evening before the surgery. The patient reports to the hospital on the morning of surgery. Broad-spectrum antibiotics are administered intravenously 2 h preoperatively and intermittent compression stockings are placed bilaterally.

I.S. Gill (✉)

Department of Urology, University of Southern California, Los Angeles, CA, USA

e-mail: igill@usc.edu; gillindy@gmail.com

A.M. Al-Kandari and I.S. Gill (eds.), *Difficult Conditions in Laparoscopic Urologic Surgery*, 79
DOI: 10.1007/978-1-84882-105-7_8, © Springer-Verlag London Limited 2011

Necessary Instrumentation

- One 10-mm 30° laparoscope
- One 10-mm trocar-mounted balloon dissection device (Origin Medsystems, Inc., Menlo Park, CA)
- One 10-mm Bluntip trocar (Origin Medsystems, Inc., Menlo Park, CA)
- Two 10–12-mm trocars
- One 5-mm electrosurgical monopolar scissors
- One 5-mm electrosurgical hook
- One 5-mm atraumatic grasping forceps (small bowel clamp)
- One 10-mm right-angle dissector
- One 10-mm three-pronged reusable metal retractor (fan-type)
- One 11-mm endoclip applier
- One 12-mm articulated ENDO GIA™ vascular stapler (Covidien, Mansfield, MA)
- One 5-mm irrigator/aspirator
- One 15-mm ENDO CATCH™ II bag (Covidien, Mansfield, MA)
- One Weck clip applicator with disposable clip cartridges (Teleflex Medical, Research Triangle Park, NC)

Patient Positioning

The patient is firmly secured to the operating table in a 90° full flank position after general anesthesia and Foley catheter placement. All bony prominences are meticulously padded and extremities carefully placed in neutral position to minimize postoperative neuromuscular sequelae. The kidney bridge is elevated moderately, and the operating table is flexed somewhat to increase the space between the lowermost rib and the iliac crest. To guard against development of neuromuscular spinal problems, the authors make every attempt to minimize the time period for which the patient is placed in the lateral decubitus flexed position.

Operation Room Setup

The surgeon and the camera operator (assistant) stand facing the patient's back. The surgeon stands toward the patient's feet, while the assistant stands toward the patient's head. The cart holding the primary video monitor, CO_2 insufflator, light source, and recorder is placed on the side of the table contralateral to the surgeon. The scrub nurse is positioned toward the foot end of the operative table.

Port Placement

During radical retroperitoneoscopic nephrectomy, three trocars are placed. The laparoscope is positioned in the primary port at the tip of the 12th rib. The surgeon works through the posterior and anterior secondary ports (Fig. 8.1).

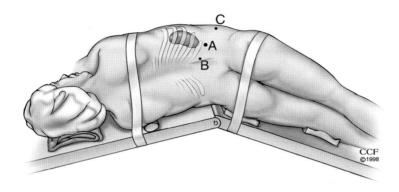

Fig. 8.1 Port placement during right retroperitoneoscopy radical nephrectomy. (A) Primary 10-mm port is placed at the tip of 12th rib. (B) 10-/12-mm port is placed at junction of lateral border of the erector spinae muscle with underside of 12th rib. (C) 10-/12-mm port is placed three fingerbreadths cephalad to iliac crest, between mid and anterior axillary lines (Reprinted with permission, Cleveland Clinic Center for Medical Art & Photography © 1998–2009. All Rights Reserved)

The open (Hasson cannula) technique is ideal for obtaining initial access. A horizontal 1.5-cm skin incision is made just below the tip of the 12th rib. Using S-shaped retractors, the flank muscle fibers are bluntly separated. Entry is gained into the retroperitoneal space by gently piercing the anterior thoracolombar fascia with the fingertip or hemostat. Limited finger dissection of the retroperitoneum is performed in a cephalad direction, remaining immediately anterior to the psoas muscle and fascia, and posterior to the Gerota's fascia to create a space for placement of the balloon dilator.[5] At this juncture the tip of the lower pole of the kidney can often be palpated by the finger. The authors insert a trocar-mounted balloon dissection device to rapidly and atraumatically create a working space in the retroperitoneum in a standardized manner (Fig. 8.2a).

The volume of air instilled into the balloon is typically 800–1,000 mL in adults (40 pumps of the sphygmomanometer bulb). The balloon dilatation outside Gerota's fascia (i.e., in the pararenal space between the psoas muscle posteriorly and Gerota's fascia anteriorly) effectively displaces the Gerota's fascia covered kidney anteromedially, allowing direct access to the posterior aspect of the renal hilum (Fig. 8.2b).

Laparoscopic examination from within the transparent balloon confirms adequate expansion of the retroperitoneum. Secondary cephalad or caudad balloon dilatation, as required by the clinical situation, further enlarges the retroperitoneal working space.

Following balloon dilatation and removal, a 10-mm Bluntip trocar is placed as the primary port. This trocar has an internal fixed fascial retention balloon and an external adjustable foam cuff, which combine to eliminate air leakage at the primary port site. The internal fascial retention balloon of the cannula is inflated with 30 cc of air, and the external adjustable foam cuff is cinched down to secure the primary port in an airtight manner.[6] Pneumoretroperitoneum is established to 15 mmHg, and a 10-mm, 30° laparoscope is inserted. The psoas muscle and Gerota's fascia are identified immediately. Two secondary ports are placed under 30° laparoscopic visualization. The immediately adjacent undersurface of the flank abdominal wall is visualized endoscopically.

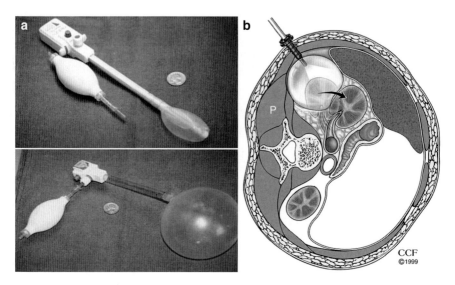

Fig. 8.2 (**a**) Trocar-mounted preperitoneal dilator balloon (uninflated and inflated) device. (**b**) Balloon dilator positioned between psoas fascia posteriorly and Gerota's fascia anteriorly. The distended balloon (800 cc) displaces Gerota's fascia/kidney antero-medially, allowing access to renal vessels (Reprinted with permission, Cleveland Clinic Center for Medical Art & Photography © 1998–2009. All Rights Reserved)

A 10-/12-mm port is placed three finger breadths cephalad to the iliac crest, between the mid and anterior axillary lines. A second 10-/12-mm port is placed at the lateral border of the erector spinae muscle just below the 12th rib.[7] A frustrating "clashing of swords" occurs if the trocars (and therefore the laparoscopic instruments) are located in close proximity. Thus, the port placed between mid and anterior axillary lines can be positioned even more anteriorly to the anterior axillary line; however, the lateral peritoneal reflection must be clearly visualized laparoscopically and avoided before the port is inserted. If necessary, the lateral peritoneal reflection can be bluntly mobilized further anteriormedially from the undersurface of the flank abdominal wall using the laparoscope's tip.

Renal Hilum Control

The kidney is retracted anterolaterally with a laparoscopic small bowel clamp or the fan retractor in the nondominant hand of the surgeon, placing the renal hilum on traction. Gerota's fascia is incised longitudinally in the general area of the renal hilum, parallel and 1- to 2-cm anterior to the psoas muscle. Care must be taken to avoid dissection close to the psoas muscle, which may lead the surgeon to reach the retrocaval or the retroaortic space. The longitudinal incision of the Gerota's fascia opens the retroperitoneal space, thereby adding to the effect of the carbon dioxide insufflation, and exposing the renal hilum. Blunt and sharp dissection in this avascular area of loose areolar fatty tissue is performed to identify renal arterial pulsations. Visualization of the vertically oriented, distinct arterial

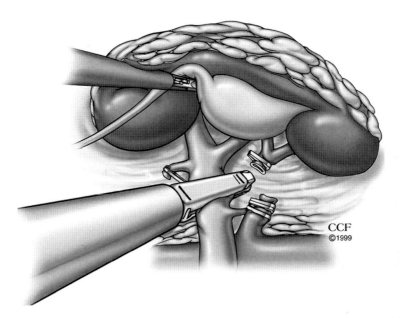

Fig. 8.3 Renal artery has been clip-ligated and divided. Renal vein is circumferentially mobilized and controlled with a gastrointestinal anastomosis stapler (Reprinted with permission, Cleveland Clinic Center for Medical Art & Photography © 1998–2009. All Rights Reserved)

pulsations indicates the location of the renal artery, which is circumferentially mobilized, clip-ligated (11-mm titanium clips; three on the "stay side" and two on the "go side") and divided. Subsequently, the renal vein is stapled and divided with an ENDO GIA™ stapler (Fig. 8.3).

Usually after division of the renal vein, some flimsy hilar attachments remain between the kidney and the great vessels. In order to avoid traction injury, which may lead to venous tear and bleeding, these remaining attachments should be precisely clipped and transected.

Circumferential Extrafascial Mobilization of the En Bloc Specimen

Suprahilar dissection is performed along the medial aspect of the upper pole of the kidney, and the adrenal vessels, including the main adrenal vein, are precisely controlled with clip-ligation. Dissection is next redirected towards the supralateral aspect of the specimen, including en bloc adrenal gland, which is readily mobilized from the underside of the diaphragm. In the avascular flimsy areolar tissue in this location, inferior phrenic vessels to the adrenal gland are often encountered and controlled. The anterior aspect of the specimen is mobilized from the underside of the peritoneum envelope. During this dissection, use of electrocautery must be avoided in order to avoid transmural thermal damage to the bowel located just beside the thin peritoneal membrane. The ureter, with or without the gonadal vein, is secured, and the specimen is completely freed by mobilization of the lower pole of the kidney. The entire dissection is performed outside Gerota's fascia, mirroring established oncologic principles of open surgery.

Specimen Entrapment

Organ entrapment is rapidly performed by using an ENDO CATCH™ bag. This bag is an impermeable plastic and nylon sac designed to prevent tumor spillage during intact specimen removal. This bag should never be employed during tissue morcellation.[8] The specimen is tented up by the nondominant hand. The bag is introduced through the anterior port, the spring-loaded mouth of the sac is opened in the retroperitoneun, and the specimen placed within. After specimen entrapment, the mouth of the bag is detached from the metallic ring and closed (under laparoscopic visualization) by tightening the drawstring (Fig. 8.4).

Specimen Extraction

In order to achieve a superior cosmetic result while providing an intact specimen for precise pathologic staging, the authors usually employ a low muscle-splitting Pfanensteil incision.[9] For the appropriate female patient, a vaginal extraction[10] of the specimen can be safely performed.

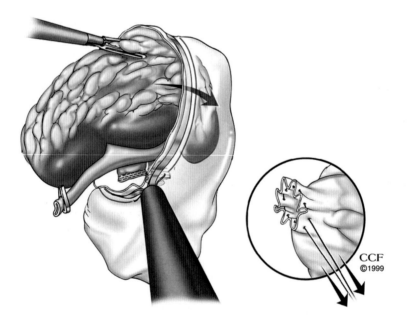

Fig. 8.4 After specimen entrapment, the mouth of the bag is detached from metallic ring and closed by pulling on the built-in drawstring (Reprinted with permission, Cleveland Clinic Center for Medical Art & Photography © 1998–2009. All Rights Reserved)

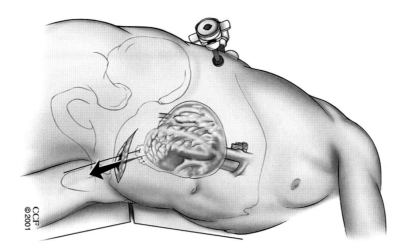

Fig. 8.5 A Pfanensteil skin incision (at or just below the level of the pubic hairline) is used to retrieve the intact specimen entrapped in a bag (Reprinted with permission, Cleveland Clinic Center for Medical Art & Photography © 1998–2009. All Rights Reserved)

A Pfannensteil skin incision (slightly lateralized towards the nephrectomy side) is made at or just below the level of the pubic hairline. Subsequently the anterior rectus fascia is incised obliquely, rectus muscle fibers are retracted medially, the posterior rectus fascia is incised, the peritoneal membrane is reflected cephalad using finger dissection, and extraperitoneal access is gained to the retroperitoneal space to extract the intact entrapped specimen (Fig. 8.5)

For a vaginal extraction, after the specimen is entrapped in an ENDO CATCH™ II bag, a generous longitudinal peritoneotomy is intentionally created along the undersurface of the anterior abdominal wall. The operating table is placed in a steep Trendelenburg position, and rotated such that the flank position is decreased to 60°. Bowel loops are retracted cephalad. A sponge-stick is externally inserted into the sterilely prepared vagina and tautly positioned in the posterior fornix. Laparoscopically, a transverse posterior 3-cm colpotomy is created at the apex of the tented-up posterior fornix, and the drawstring of the entrapped specimen is delivered into the vagina (Fig. 8.6).

After laparoscopic exit is completed, the patient is placed in a supine lithotomy position. The specimen is extracted intact per vaginum, and the posterior colpotomy incision repaired transvaginally. This approach is contraindicated in patients with even a mild degree of pelvic or intraperitoneal adhesions from any etiology.

Hemostasis

Hemostasis is confirmed under lowered retropneumoperitoneun (Fig. 8.7) and ports are removed under laparoscopic visualization. Fascial closure is performed for all 10-mm or larger port sites.

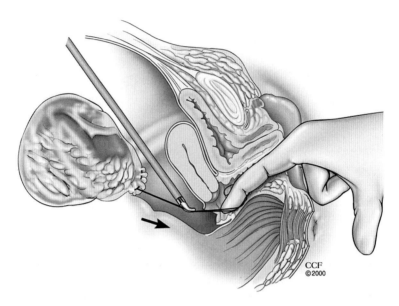

Fig. 8.6 The drawstring of the closed Endocatch II bag, previously grasped by the laparoscopic clamp, is delivered into the vagina (Reprinted with permission, Cleveland Clinic Center for Medical Art & Photography © 1998–2009. All Rights Reserved)

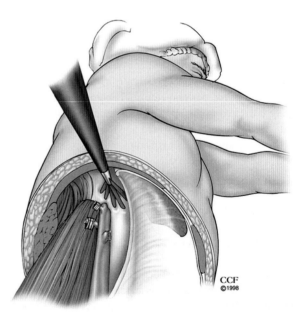

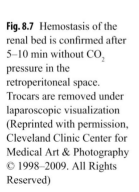

Fig. 8.7 Hemostasis of the renal bed is confirmed after 5–10 min without CO_2 pressure in the retroperitoneal space. Trocars are removed under laparoscopic visualization (Reprinted with permission, Cleveland Clinic Center for Medical Art & Photography © 1998–2009. All Rights Reserved)

Difficulties and Special Situations

Orientation in the Retroperitoneum

How to handle: The camera should be oriented such that the psoas muscle is always absolutely horizontal on the video monitor.[11] However, the retroperitoneal space is relatively small at this stage of the procedure. Anteromedial retraction of the kidney serves to increase the retroperitoneal space, exposing the psoas muscle that can be identified most easily caudal to the kidney.

Finding the Renal Hilum

How to handle: The surgeon should reinsert the laparoscope slowly and identify the psoas muscle. The psoas muscle should then be crossed from lateral-to-medial in a cephalad direction and a search conducted for arterial pulsation near its medial border. Pulsations of the fat-covered renal artery or aorta are usually identifiable. Gentle dissection with the tip of the suction device or hook is performed directly toward the pulsations. The renal artery is identified and traced directly to the renal hilum. One must always be mindful of aberrant major vessels, such as the superior mesenteric artery, which arises from the aorta more medially and superiorly than the left renal artery. Alternatively, the ureter can be identified and followed cephalad to the hilum. Dissection through the perirenal fat may identify the surface of the kidney, which can then be dissected toward its hilum.

Endovascular Gastrointestinal (GIA) Stapler Malfunction

The endovascular gastrointestinal (GIA) stapler is standard for control of the renal hilum. However, failure of the device can be associated with severe consequences, including emergency conversion to open procedure. Inadvertent placement of the device over a previously placed surgical clip is the most common cause of GIA stapler failure.[12]

How to handle: Extreme care must be taken when positioning and firing the GIA stapler in the presence of surgical clips in the area of the renal hilum.

Inadverted Peritoneotomy

A peritoneotomy does not necessarily mandate conversion to transperitoneal laparoscopy. Usually it does not cause significant problems, and the procedure can be completed retroperitoneoscopically.

How to handle: If it compromises operative exposure, a fourth port can be inserted to provide additional retraction of the billowing peritoneal membrane. Also, intra-abdominal viscera must be thoroughly inspected by inserting the laparoscope through the peritoneotomy to rule out iatrogenic injury.

Entrapment of Larger Specimens

How to handle: An intentional peritoniotomy may be created strictly for entrapment of large specimens. The large specimen is inserted within the peritoneal cavity where it is entrapped within the 15-mm ENDO CATCH™ II bag.

Persistent Renal Hilar Bleeding After Division of the Renal Artery and Vein

This usually indicates the presence of an overlooked accessory renal artery. The renal vein should appear flat and devoid of blood after flow is controlled from the main renal artery. A normally distended renal vein at this juncture indicates continued arterial inflow through an accessory renal artery. In this circumstance, division of the distended renal vein with an ENDO GIA™ stapler interrupts renal outflow, with a resultant increase in intrarenal venous back pressure. This causes persistent oozing during the remainder of the dissection. One should search for an accessory renal artery in this situation.

Retroperitoneoscopy in Obese Patients

Although the excessive retroperitoneal fat increases the degree of technical difficulty, adherence to a standardized stepwise anatomical approach[13] allows retroperitoneoscopy to be performed effectively in markedly obese or morbidly obese patients. In fact, the retroperitoneal flank approach allows gravitational pull to shift much of the weight of the pannus anteriorly, away from the ipsilateral flank. In the authors' series, 35% of the patients had body mass index (BMI) equal or greater than 30. However, the reader should be cautioned that these challenging procedures should be performed by surgeons facile with the laparoscopic technique (Table 8.1).

Conclusion

Retroperitoneoscopy does offer straightforward and rapid exposure and control of the renal hilum, and nonviolation of the peritoneum, thus minimizing the chances of intraperitoneal organ injury. For efficacious performance of retroperitoneoscopic surgery, proper development of the retroperitoneal space and constant orientation with various anatomical landmarks is critical which can be readily developed as the laparoscopic dissection proceeds.

Table 8.1 Technical difficulties in retroperitoneal laparoscopic nephrectomy

Port placement	Air leakage	• 10- mm Bluntip trocar with internal retention balloon
Renal hilum control	Problems with orientation in the retroperitoneum	• Anteromedial retraction of the kidney to increase space (expose the psoas) • Camera should be oriented such that the psoas muscle is always horizontal on the video monitor
	Difficulty in finding the renal hilum	• Search for arterial pulsation on psoas muscle lateral-medial in a cephalad direction • Gentle dissection with the tip of the suction • Follow ureter to the hilum • Dissection of the perirenal fat
	Persistent renal artery bleeding after division of the renal artery and vein	• Beware of normal distended vein after control of main renal artery (inflow through an accessory renal artery) • Search for accessory renal artery before controlling renal vein
	GIA stapler malfunction	• Extreme care must be taken when positioning and firing the GIA stapler in the presence of surgical clips in the area of renal hilum
Circumferential extrafascial mobilization	Inardverted peritoneotomy	• Fourth port to provide additional retraction • Use of laparoscope through peritoneotomy for inspection
Specimen entrapment	Large specimens	• Entrapment of specimen in the peritoneal cavity through a peritoneotomy

References

1. Gill IS, Meraney AM, Schweizer DK, et al. Laparoscopic radical nephrectomy in 100 patients: a single center experience from the United States. *Cancer.* 2001;92:1843-1855.
2. Colombo JR Jr, Haber GP, Aron M, et al. Oncological outcomes of laparoscopic radical nephrectomy for renal cancer. *Clinics (Sao Paulo).* 2007;62(3):251-256.
3. Hemal AK, Kumar A, Kumar R, Wadhwa P, Seth A, Gupta NP. Laparoscopic versus open radical nephrectomy for large renal tumors: a long-term prospective comparison. *J Urol.* 2007;177(3):862-866.

4. Gill IS, Rassweiler JJ. Retroperitoneoscopic renal surgery: our approach. *Urology*. 1999;54: 734-738.

5. Gaur DD. Laparoscopic operative retroperitoneoscopy: use of a new device. *J Urol*. 1992;148:1137-1139.

6. Gill IS. Retroperitoneal laparoscopic nephrectomy. *Urol Clin North Am*. 1998;25:343-360.

7. Gill IS, Schweizer D, Hobart MG, Sung GT, Klein EA, Novick AR. Retroperitoneal laparoscopic radical nephrectomy: the Cleveland Clinic experience. *J Urol*. 2000;163:1665-1670.

8. Urban DA, Kerbl K, McDougall EM, Stone AM, Fadden PT, Clayman RV. Organ entrapment and renal morcellation: permeability studies. *J Urol*. 1993;150:1792-1794.

9. Kaouk JH, Gill IS. Laparoscopic nephrectomy: morcellate or leave intact? Leave intact. *Rev Urol*. 2002;4(1):38-42.

10. Gill IS, Cherullo EE, Meraney AM, Borsuk F, Murphy DP, Falcone T. Vaginal extraction of the intact specimen following laparoscopic radical nephrectomy. *J Urol*. 2002;167:238-241.

11. Desai MM, Strzempkowski B, Matin SF, et al. Prospective randomized comparison of transperitoneal versus retroperitoneal laparoscopic radical nephrectomy. *J Urol*. 2005;173(1): 38-41.

12. Chan D, Bishoff L, Ratner L, Kavoussi LR, Jarrett TW. Endovascular gastrointestinal stapler device malfunction during laparoscopic nephrectomy: early recognition and management. *J Urol*. 2000;164:319-321.

13. Fazeli-Matin S, Gill IS, Hsu TH, Sung GT, Novick AC. Laparoscopic renal and adrenal surgery in obese patients: comparison to open surgery. *J Urol*. 1999;162:665-669.

Difficulties in Laparoscopic Live Donor Nephrectomy

9

Jihad H. Kaouk and Wesley M. White

Introduction

End stage renal disease (ESRD) is a leading cause of morbidity and death among Americans and represents a significant financial burden to the health care system of the United States.[1] Traditionally, renal replacement therapy has come in the form of hemodialysis or renal transplantation. Certainly, the latter is associated with not only significantly better longevity but also a tangibly improved quality of life.[2,3] Unfortunately, the pervasiveness of hypertensive and diabetic nephropathy in the Western culture has disproportionately exceeded the supply of available allografts.[4] Within the context of this mounting shortage, the rate of deceased donor renal transplants has remained relatively stagnant.[5] As a consequence, there exists a distinct and pressing need for increased accrual of living kidney donors.

Live donor nephrectomy was originally achieved through an open transperitoneal subcostal or extraperitoneal flank incision. While graft outcomes were excellent with this approach, these positive results came at the expense of considerable morbidity to the donor, including significant postoperative pain, prolonged convalescence, and poor cosmesis.[6,7] Indeed, the morbidity of live open donor nephrectomy was considered a major deterrent to kidney donation and an obstacle to its widespread application. In response to this public health concern, Gill and colleagues performed the first laparoscopic donor nephrectomy in an animal model in 1994.[8] One year later, Ratner et al. published their series on laparoscopic live donor nephrectomy in humans.[9] Evidence-based research over the ensuing decade ultimately confirmed laparoscopic live donor nephrectomy as a safe, feasible, and less morbid alternative to open procurement.[10,11] In 2007, the United Network for Organ Sharing (UNOS) reported 6,041 live donor kidney transplants with the vast majority of these allografts procured laparoscopically.[12]

Despite improvements in instrumentation, refinements in technique, and mounting experience, laparoscopic live donor nephrectomy remains one of the most challenging and admittedly stressful urologic procedures to perform. Although the common difficulties

W.M. White (✉)
Division of Urologic Surgery, The University of Tennessee Medical Center, Knoxville, TN, USA
e-mail: wwhite@utmck.edu

A.M. Al-Kandari and I.S. Gill (eds.), *Difficult Conditions in Laparoscopic Urologic Surgery*,
DOI: 10.1007/978-1-84882-105-7_9, © Springer-Verlag London Limited 2011

with laparoscopic donor nephrectomy are analogous to those of laparoscopic simple and radical nephrectomy, the nature of the operation engenders little margin for error and the implications of technical misadventures are profoundly magnified.[13] The operating surgeon is not only responsible for the safety of the donor who is altruistically undergoing a fundamentally elective procedure, but also for the quality and health of the allograft that will offer the recipient an improved and sustained life. Laparoscopic live donor nephrectomy demands attention to detail, technical proficiency and rigueur, and a thorough comprehension of the common difficulties experienced during the operation. This chapter will describe the authors' cumulative experience with laparoscopic live donor nephrectomy, offer insight into the nature and causes of difficulties experienced during the procedure, and tender practical suggestions on how to best avoid intra-operative complications.

Difficulties in Laparoscopic Live Donor Nephrectomy Lesson #1: Avoidance Through Preparation

Perhaps the most pragmatic way to overcome difficulties during laparoscopic live donor nephrectomy is with a systematic and meticulous preoperative evaluation, close collaboration with the transplant nurses and surgeons, and the assembly of a reliable and seasoned surgical team. Preparation and communication among the involved personnel is indeed critical for allograft procurement to be performed with favorable and reproducible outcomes.

Preoperative evaluation of the live donor candidate is multifaceted and, as previously stated, a close alliance between the nephrologists, transplant surgeons, and donor surgeons is crucial for outcomes to be optimized. All potential candidates must meet medical and psychological criteria as established by the American Society of Transplant Surgeons (ASTS).[14] In general, donor candidates will undergo screening at the behest of the transplant center that includes, but is not limited to, a baseline laboratory profile including serum creatinine, a 24-h urine assay for protein, creatinine, and volume, and a calculated estimate of the glomerular filtration rate (GFR) with subsequent confirmation based on a GFR isotope renal function test.[15] ABO histocompatibility testing and HLA cross-matching is performed to confirm the suitability and safety of the donation. The patient is screened for cytomegalovirus (CMV) and Epstein-Barr virus (EBV), as well as hepatitis C (HCV) and other blood-borne pathogens.[15]

After meeting baseline criteria for donation, the candidate is referred to the donor surgeon for consultation. The donor candidate's history should be focused and thorough. In general, the aforementioned medical and psychological testing selects for ostensibly healthy donor candidates with de facto favorable operative characteristics. This is in sharp contrast to the typical patient undergoing radical nephrectomy whose past medical history is often a virtual litany of latent operative risk factors. In addition to a review of the patient's medical history, a thorough review of prior intra-abdominal surgeries is vital as is close inspection of the abdominal wall for evidence of prior surgeries and overall body habitus. Typically, an elevated body mass index (BMI) is not a contraindication to laparoscopic live donor nephrectomy, but can impact the location and number of ports needed for adequate visualization.[16] A significant history of intra-abdominal surgeries is likewise not a contraindication for donation, but may alter or dictate the preferred approach for procurement (retroperitoneal vs transperitoneal).[17]

Radiographic evaluation of the kidneys and vasculature is perhaps the most important and germane component of the preoperative evaluation, especially to the junior laparoscopist. In the modern era, helical computed tomography of the kidneys with three dimensional reconstruction (3-D CT of the kidneys) offers unparalleled detail and definition of the renal vascular anatomy and demonstrates very well the presence of any anatomic or pathologic abnormalities.[18] In addition, volume rendering of the kidneys is performed that largely dictates the appropriate kidney for donation. The importance of personally reviewing and rereviewing the aforementioned imaging studies preoperatively cannot be overemphasized as, in the authors' opinion, the vast majority of intraoperative complications may be obviated with a thorough spatial command of the patient's vascular anatomy. The operating surgeon must be thoroughly versed on the number and relative location of the main renal vessels, the presence of any accessory or polar vessels, and the distance to the first branch of the main renal artery. In the authors' experience, it is helpful to inform the transplant surgeons preoperatively of early arterial branching (<1 cm), as their approach to bench preparation and implantation may be impacted by such a finding.

The decision to perform a left- or right-sided laparoscopic donor nephrectomy is governed in large part by the patient's anatomy as depicted on the aforementioned 3-D CT, as well as the collaborative opinion of the donor and recipient surgeons. Traditionally, the left kidney has been procured given its disproportionately longer renal vein.[14] However, ease of harvest and implantation should never be prioritized at the expense of the donor's future renal function. Among patients with renal volume discordance (more than 20% difference in renal volume), a nuclear renal scan should be performed to prove or disprove functional equivalence.[19] If the left kidney contributes more than 60% to the overall renal function, the right kidney should be considered for procurement. Additional relative indications for right-sided donor nephrectomy include, complex left renal vasculature, and/or an anomalous left collecting system.[14,20] If the right kidney is ultimately chosen for procurement, adequate vein length from the edge of the vena cava (> 2 cm) must be assured on 3-D CT (Fig. 9.1), and special concessions must be made intraoperatively and will be covered in detail later in this chapter.

Difficulties in Laparoscopic Live Donor Nephrectomy Lesson #2: Exposure

As stated, a methodical preoperative evaluation of the patient provides the donor surgeon with the information and strategic plan needed to effect a safe and successful procurement. Without reservation, the authors believe that optimized exposure during the operation ultimately allows this plan to be realized. While the preoperative evaluation should be consistent and systematic, obtaining adequate intraoperative exposure requires a more dynamic approach.

Following induction, a 16-F catheter is placed and the patient is positioned with the table break at the level of the iliac crest. The patient is converted to the full flank or modified flank position (45 °) with padding under the dependent hip and axilla as well as under

Fig. 9.1 Three-dimensional CT of the kidneys demonstrating the right renal vascular anatomy and approximate length of the right renal vein

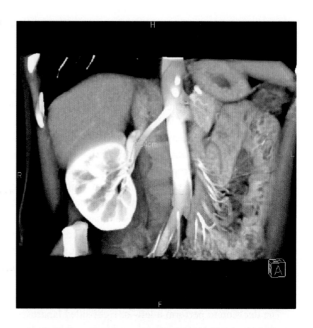

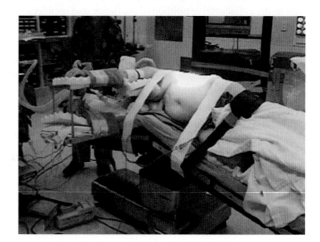

Fig. 9.2 Intraoperative photograph demonstrating patient positioning for laparoscopic left donor nephrectomy

and between the legs. The arms are placed on a double-arm board, padded, and taped. The authors prefer to flex the operating table slightly to accentuate the space between the costal margin and iliac crest but do not elevate the kidney rest. Once positioning is satisfactory, the patient is secured to the table with straps and 3-in. tape (Fig. 9.2). The abdomen is widely prepped from the xiphoid cephalad to the pubic symphysis caudad, laterally to the back and medially beyond the umbilicus. Drapes are secured to the patient with towel clips or a skin stapler to avoid contamination during extraction of the allograft. A sterile drape specifically designed for laparoscopy (prefabricated service pockets and Velcro® straps) is employed. When appropriately used, these drapes can provide order during the operative procedure and efficiency of instrument exchange.

In the authors' experience, adequate port position dictates adequacy of exposure and ultimately the outcome and efficiency of the case. Following the identification of relevant landmarks, a 12-mm incision is made vertically at or just above the level of the umbilicus and horizontally approximately halfway between the umbilicus and anterior superior iliac spine. Access to the peritoneum may be obtained with a Veress or Hasson technique. Once pneumoperitoneum is achieved at a pressure maximum of 15 mmHg, the first 12-mm trocar (right hand) is placed. The peritoneal cavity is widely inspected and the anterior abdominal wall evaluated for additional port placement. A second 12-mm port (left hand) is positioned at the subcostal margin at the lateral border of the rectus muscle. A third 12-mm port (camera port) is positioned at the level of the 12th rib again at the lateral border of the rectus muscle (Fig. 9.3). The authors' prefer to use a 10-mm laparoscope with a 30°-down lens.

With an atraumatic small bowel grasper in the left hand and athermal shears in the right hand, the descending colon is reflected off the left kidney along the white line of Toldt from the upper pole to beyond the lower pole. It is critically important to identify the appropriate plane of dissection between Gerota's fascia and the mesentery of the colon during this maneuver as dissection deeply into Gerota's fascia will generate unnecessary bleeding and/or trauma to the allograft and failure to dissect deeply enough will compromise exposure of the renal hilum. In addition, failure to reflect the mesentery medially may make subsequent identification of the gonadal vein "landmark" difficult. Additionally, it is not uncommon for the inferior mesenteric vein to be easily confused with the gonadal vein if the mesentery has not been adequately mobilized. If medial reflection of the colon remains difficult, it may be helpful to place an additional 12-mm port at the planned kidney extraction site through which a fan retractor or atraumatic grasper may be placed for additional exposure.

Once the colon has been adequately reflected, a plane between the upper/medial pole of the kidney and the spleen is easily identified. In most cases, the spleen may be completely

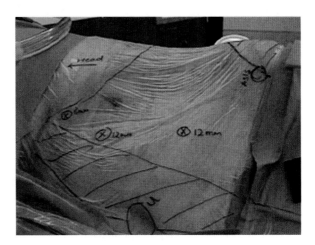

Fig. 9.3 Intraoperative photograph demonstrating relevant landmarks and port positioning during laparoscopic left donor nephrectomy

mobilized and reflected off the upper pole of the kidney by incising the splenocolic ligament. Typically, this plane of dissection should allow the tail of the pancreas, colon, and
the splenic vessels to be reflected en bloc away from the concave aspect of the kidney.
Again, if the mesentery was not adequately mobilized earlier, injury to these structures is
a possibility. In addition, one must be aware that the dependent portion (fundus) of the
stomach may sweep around the lateral aspect of the spleen and is therefore at risk for
injury when dissecting the splenophrenic attachments.

The ureter and gonadal vein are identified at the lower pole of the kidney in their normal
anatomic position atop the psoas muscle. It is important not to skeletonize the ureter as its
blood supply could become compromised with vigorous dissection. The authors find it
helpful to lift (but not directly manipulate) the gonadal vein/ureter package anteriorly with
the left hand while cleaning the psoas muscle up to and under the lower pole of the kidney
with a suction/irrigator in the right hand. Perivenous and periureteral tissue should be
swept anteriorly and laterally to ensure a healthy ureteral blood supply. The investments on
the anterior surface of the gonadal vein may be dissected thermally with the use of a fine-
tipped hook until the lumbar vein and main renal vein are identified. In order to gain adequate exposure during this critical step, the authors find it helpful to apply static anterior
traction on the aforementioned vein/ureter packet while cephalad torque is applied. This
maneuver allows the packet to be lifted, not only out of the operative field, but also places
tension on the tissue that requires dissection off the gonadal vein and approaching hilum.
Alternatively, a laterally positioned accessory 2- or 5-mm port may be placed to reflect the
packet anteriorly while the left hand is freed to apply tension to the tissue to be dissected.

As stated, dissection of the fine fibrous attachments on the anterior surface of the
gonadal vein typically affords visualization of the lateral edge of the aorta, the lumbar
vein, and the inferior surface of the renal vein. The authors prefer to leave the gonadal vein
intact at this point as judicious countertraction on the gonadal vein can make dissection of
the lumbar vein easier. Once the lumbar vein has been identified, the vessel is isolated and
skeletonized with a 10-mm right angle dissector. Care must be taken at this juncture as the
main renal artery is typically found in the angle between the lumbar vein, aorta, and main
renal vein. Once adequately isolated, the lumbar vein is doubly clipped with Hem-o-lok®
clips (Teleflex Medical, Research Triangle Park, NC) and transected. It is important to
place the proximal clip several millimeters away from the origin of the vein as clip dislodgement is a potentially disastrous complication. Further, placement of the clip too close
to the origin of the vessel may hinder secure deployment of the endovascular stapler during
division of the main renal vein. Once the lumbar vein has been controlled and transected,
the gonadal vein can typically be controlled with clips and transected. Once the gonadal
vein is divided, the renal artery and vein are generally well visualized.

Following dissection of the renal artery and vein (see Lesson #3), the posterior and
lateral attachments of the kidney may be taken down with blunt dissection and use of
monopolar shears or hook cautery. It is often helpful to dissect posteriorly and then attempt
to rotate the kidney further medially to access the remaining upper pole attachments.

When performing right-sided laparoscopic donor nephrectomy, several technical quali-
fications merit discussion. The liver typically obscures the operative field and the authors
have found that the placement of an additional 5-mm trocar near the xiphiod (through
which a locking laparoscopic Allis clamp may be placed) is helpful. It is important to

position this clamp under the "notch" in the liver to maximize exposure to the upper pole of the kidney. The ascending colon and liver attachments are freed and a Kocher maneuver performed. Following identification and isolation of the renal hilum, the renal artery is dissected lateral to the vena cava, controlled with Hem-o-lok® clips and transected. As renal vein length is of paramount importance when performing right-sided donor nephrectomy, several concessions must be made to ensure adequate vein length. Typically, the authors favor incorporating a portion of the lateral wall of the vena cava in the jaws of the endovascular stapler such that vein length is maximized (Figs. 9.4 and 9.5). Alternative maneuvers include retroperitoneal access, hand-assistance, and even control of the vena cava using a laparoscopic Satinsky clamp or through a small subcostal incision.[20,21] In the authors' experience, these latter maneuvers are difficult to master and may place the patient at a high level of risk.

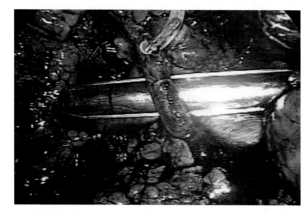

Fig. 9.4 Intraoperative photograph demonstrating incorporation of lateral edge of vena cava in the endovascular stapler to maximize vein length during right laparoscopic donor nephrectomy. The right renal artery is easily visible anterior to the vein

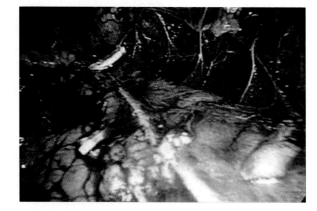

Fig. 9.5 Intraoperative photograph of vena cava immediately following stapler transaction of the right renal vein. The staple line is clearly visible and is flush with the lateral edge of the vena cava to maximize vein length during right-sided donor nephrectomy.

Difficulties in Laparoscopic Live Donor Nephrectomy Lesson #3: Vascular Control

There is no "best way" or "tricks" to simplify dissection of the renal artery and vein. The easiest way to avoid complications around the renal hilum is with adequate retraction and calculated and patient dissection. Fine-tipped hook cautery and blunt dissection of superficial fibro-adipose tissue should be employed to expose the limits of the main vessels. The authors find that alternating use of the suction/irrigator and 10-mm right angle dissector aid in dissection of the vessels. In order to effect safe and expeditious control of the renal hilum, the renal vessels must be freed of all ancillary investments such that a right angled dissector may be easily passed from each side of the vessel with adequate clearance from the aorta (artery) and inter-aortocaval region (vein) distally. Extensive or aggressive dissection to the level of the renal sinus is discouraged as this may induce arterial vasospasm. Early arterial branching as identified on preoperative imaging is also critical to recognize as aggressive distal dissection may insult these branches.

Once the recipient surgeon has confirmed readiness for acceptance of the allograft, 12.5 mg of mannitol is administered. The ureter is divided between Hem-o-lok® clips at or below the level of the iliac bifurcation. The gonadal package is taken down with an endovascular stapler or with Hem-o-lok® clips. At this point, the authors prefer to make an 7-cm Pfannenstiel incision, which is carried down to the peritoneum. It is important not to violate the peritoneum at this juncture as insufflation will be compromised.

Prior to division of the renal hilum, the authors perform a quick checklist that will obviate unnecessary complications and/or prolong the warm ischemia time. It is important to confirm that the CO_2 tank is filled such that insufflation is not lost during pedicle division. In addition, the authors prefer to have two endovascular staplers and a laparoscopic Satinsky clamp ready should stapler misfire be encountered. Once ready, the kidney may be lifted laterally to place the artery and vein on slight tension. The origin of the renal artery is identified, two Hem-o-lok® clips are placed proximally, warm ischemia time is called for, and the artery is divided with laparoscopic scissors (Fig. 9.6). It is vital to move efficiently but not haphazardly through this portion of the operation. The endovascular stapler is next

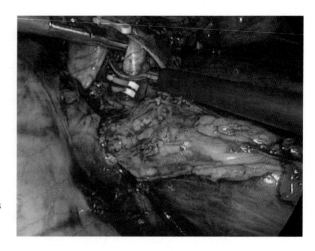

Fig. 9.6 Intraoperative photograph demonstrating control of the left renal artery with Hem-o-lok® clips just prior to arterial transaction

deployed across the renal vein as it crosses the aorta. The authors prefer to staple and divide the caudad two-thirds of the vein only. Two Hem-o-lok® clips are placed on the remaining one-third of the vein, the vein is divided, and the kidney allowed to "vent." Though speculative, the authors feel that such a maneuver decreases the risk of venous thrombosis by rapidly evacuating the kidney of venous blood. In addition to "venting" the kidney, partial transection of the vein keeps the endovascular stapler a safe distance from the superior mesenteric artery that is often found at the superior border of the renal vein and offers a margin of safety in the setting of stapler misfire by preventing venous retraction.

Certainly, control of the renal hilum and/or the management of intraoperative oozing and bleeding represent, in the authors' experience, the most common difficulties experienced during laparoscopic donor nephrectomy.[10,22,23] Although avoidance is easy to invoke, knowledge of how to address and manage untoward vascular events is vital. Generally, persistent venous oozing during dissection in and around the gonadal vessels and ureter is best controlled with direct pressure followed by careful observation. It is often helpful to initiate dissection in another area as this type of diffuse, insignificant bleeding will inevitably cease. Venous oozing around the renal hilum can be controlled in a similar fashion but is often best addressed when the renal vein is eventually controlled and divided. Small arterial bleeds should be directly compressed, the field evacuated of blood, and a hemostatic clip placed at the source. Injuries to the main renal vasculature are generally irreversible and typically require open conversion.[23] In such a circumstance, the operating surgeon must apply direct pressure to the area of transgression while the surgical team prepares open instruments and the anesthesia team resuscitates the patient.

Difficulties in Laparoscopic Live Donor Nephrectomy Lesson #4: Kidney Extraction

Once the renal hilum is transected, the peritoneum is incised and the kidney retrieved. A laparoscopic retrieval bag can be used, but the authors prefer to retrieve the kidney by hand under direct vision. The authors have found that the construct of many of the retrieval devices (specifically the rigid metal deployment ring) lend themselves to damage of the allograft. When the kidney is being removed, it is important to retract all ports to avoid inadvertent trauma to the allograft. Additionally, the upper pole of the kidney should be removed first to avoid avulsion of the ureter. Once the kidney is delivered, it should be handed directly to the recipient surgeon or his surrogate and placed immediately in an ice bath. Warm ischemia time may be stopped at this point. The fascia of the Pfannenstiel incision is closed and the abdomen re-insufflated and inspected for hemostasis.

Summary

Laparoscopic live donor nephrectomy is a challenging and technically demanding procedure, but is ultimately an extremely rewarding operation to perform. In the authors' experience, a meticulous preoperative evaluation, judicious and thoughtful intra-operative exposure, and "wisdom through experience" represent the most significant keys to success.

References

1. Hoyert DL, Kung HC, Smith BL. Deaths: Preliminary data for 2003. *Natl Health Stat Report.* 2005;53(15):1-48. http://www.cdc.gov/nchs/data/nvsr/nvsr53/nvsr53_15.pdf. Accessed on December 12, 2008.
2. Meier-Kriesche HU, Ojo AO, Port FK, Arndorfer JA, Cibrik DM, Kaplan B. Survival improvement among patients with end-stage renal disease: trends over time for transplant recipients and wait-listed patients. *J Am Soc Nephrol.* 2001;12:1293-1296.
3. Wolfe RA, Ashby VB, Milford EL, et al. Comparison of mortality in all patients on dialysis, patients on dialysis awaiting transplantation, and recipients of a first cadaveric transplant. *N Engl J Med.* 1999;341:1725-1730.
4. National Institutes of Health, National Institute of Diabetes and Digestive Kidney Diseases. U.S. Renal Data System 2004 annual data report: atlas of end-stage renal disease in the United States. http://www.usrds.org/atlas_2004.htm. Accessed December 30, 2008.
5. Sener A, Cooper M. Live donor nephrectomy for kidney transplantation. *Nat Clin Pract Urol.* 2008;5(4):203-210.
6. Barry JM. Open donor nephrectomy: current status. *BJU Int.* 2005;95(Suppl 2):56-58.
7. Streem SB, Novick AC, Steinmuller DR, Graneto D. Flank donor nephrectomy: efficacy in the donor and recipient. *J Urol.* 1989;141:1099-1101.
8. Gill IS, Carbone JM, Clayman RV, et al. Laparoscopic live donor nephrectomy. *J Endourol.* 1994;8:143-148.
9. Ratner LE, Ciseck LJ, Moore RG, Cigarroa FG, Kaufman HS, Kavoussi LR. Laparoscopic live donor nephrectomy. *Transplantation.* 1995;60:1047-1049.
10. Jacobs SC, Cho E, Foster C, Liao P, Bartlett ST. Laparoscopic live donor nephrectomy: the University of Maryland 6-year experience. *J Urol.* 2004;171:47-51.
11. Sundaram CP, Martin GL, Guise A, et al. Complications after a 5-year experience with laparoscopic donor nephrectomy: the Indiana University experience. *Surg Endosc.* 2007;21: 724-728.
12. United Network for Organ Sharing (UNOS)/Organ Procurement and Transplantation Network (OPTN). Donors recovered in the U.S. by donor type. http://www.optn.org/latestData. Accessed December 12, 2008.
13. Simon SD, Castle EP, Ferrigni RG, et al. Complications of laparoscopic nephrectomy: the Mayo Clinic experience. *J Urol.* 2004;171:1447-1450.
14. Bia MJ, Ramos EL, Danovich GM, et al. Evaluation of living renal donors: the current practice of U.S. transplant centers. *Transplantation.* 1995;60:322-326.
15. Kasiske BL, Cangro CB, Hariharan S, et al. The evaluation of renal transplantation candidates: clinical practice guidelines. *Am J Transplant.* 2001;S2:1-95.
16. Kuo PC, Plotkin JS, Stevens S, Cribbs A, Johnson LB. Outcomes of laparoscopic donor nephrectomy in obese patients. *Transplantation.* 2000;69:180-181.
17. Sundqvist P, Feuk U, Häggman M, Persson AEG, Stridsberg M, Wadström J. Hand-assisted retroperitoneoscopic live donor nephrectomy in comparison to open and laparoscopic procedures: a prospective study on donor morbidity and kidney function. *Transplantation.* 2004;78:147-153.
18. Pozniak MA, Lee FT Jr. Computed tomographic angiography in the preoperative evaluation of potential renal transplant donors. *Curr Opin Urol.* 1999;9:165-170.
19. Oh CK, Yoon SN, Lee BM, et al. Routine screening for the functional asymmetry of potential kidney donors. *Transplant Proc.* 2006;38:1971-1973.
20. Posselt AM, Mahanty H, Kang S, et al. Laparoscopic right donor nephrectomy: a large single center experience. *Transplantation.* 2004;78:1665-1669.

21. Turk IA, Giessing M, Deger S, et al. Laparoscopic live right donor nephrectomy: a new tech-nique with preservation of vascular length. *Transplant Proc.* 2003;35:838-840.
22. Toohei RL, Rao MM, Scott DF, et al. A systematic review of laparoscopic live-donor nephre-ctomy. *Transplantation.* 2004;78:404-414.
23. Manikandan R, Sundaram CP. Laparoscopic live-donor nephrectomy. *BJU Int.* 2006;97:1154-1160.

Staging procedures are particularly important with high-grade lesions and should include chest radiography, liver function tests, computerized tomography (CT) scan of the abdomen, and bone scan depending on the clinical stage of the lesion. If there is a risk of renal failure following removal of a renal unit, a nephrology evaluation should be undertaken preoperatively to aid with postoperative management and possible dialysis. A gentle mechanical bowel preparation with clear liquids and a mild laxative administered 1 day preoperatively will help prevent bowel distension. The patient should be typed and cross-matched, and is given prophylactic antibiotics.[24]

Surgical Techniques

As in open surgery, there are several technical modifications of the procedure with respect to nephrectomy as well as regarding the method of ureterectomy. Laparoscopic nephroureterectomy can be performed via transperitoneal or retroperitoneal access, in a pure laparoscopic, hand-assisted, or robot-assisted laparoscopic technique.

Patient Positioning

For the first step of securing the distal ureter, the patient is in a dorsal lithotomy position. For the second step of the nephroureterectomy itself, the patient is placed in a lateral decubitus position. All bony prominences must be padded. The downside axilla should be checked to ensure it is free of pressure. The upside leg should be elevated on one or two pillows until it is aligned smoothly with the upside flank. The patient is positioned on a radiolucent table top that has wedge-shaped, padded bolsters that secure the patient in position while offering excellent padding (Orthopedic Systems Inc., Union City, CA). The patient is strapped to the operating room table at three points: subaxillary, lower hip, and knee level. Egg crate padding is positioned beneath each strap where it crosses the body.

Patient Preparation

Before beginning laparoscopy, a nasogastric tube and a Foley catheter are always inserted. In men, gauze can be used to wrap the scrotum to prevent CO_2 from filling and distending the scrotum. Pneumatic stockings are placed on both legs. On call to the operating room, a single dose of a second-generation cephalosporin is given.

Preparation of the Bladder Cuff and Intramural Ureter

There are many alternatives for dealing with the distal ureter and ensuring a bladder cuff. Each has its own advantages and disadvantages.

Ureteral Stent Placement Without Ureteral Unroofing

External ureteral stent placement (e.g., 7.1-F pigtail catheter) is done to facilitate ureteral identification and dissection. The bladder cuff and distal ureter are taken through an open lower abdominal incision at the end of the procedure.

Ureteral Stent Placement with Ureteral Unroofing[25]

Using the flexible cystoscope and under fluoroscopic guidance, a 0.035-in. Bentson guide-wire is passed to the renal pelvis. The flexible cystoscope is withdrawn, and a 7-F ureteral dilating balloon (5-mm diameter, 10-cm length) catheter is inserted over the guidewire. The balloon is inflated to less than 1 atm of pressure with dilute contrast material mixed with indigo carmine to enhance visualization of the inflated balloon. A 24-F resectoscope equipped with an Orandi electrosurgical knife (Cirion-A, Santa Barbara, CA) is passed. Beginning at the presumed level of the luminal side of the ureterovesical junction, the ureteral tunnel and ureteral orifice are electrosurgically incised anteriorly over the balloon, exposing the underlying surface of the inflated balloon. The Orandi knife then is exchanged for a roller ball electrode and the edges of the incision are fulgurated to maintain hemosta-sis. The dilating balloon catheter is deflated and the roller electrode is used to fulgurate the posterior luminal portion of the now unroofed ureteral tunnel completely. The resecto-scope then is removed. Next, the dilating balloon catheter is removed, and a 7-F, 11.5-mm occlusion balloon catheter is inserted under fluoroscopic guidance over the Bentson guide-wire and is advanced into the renal pelvis. The balloon is inflated with 1 cc of dilute con-trast medium and is positioned at the ureteropelvic junction. The Bentson guidewire is replaced with a 0.035-in. Amplatz super-stiff guidewire. A sidearm adapter passed over the super-stiff guidewire, is affixed to the butt end of the occlusion balloon catheter, and is placed for drainage. A 16-F Foley urethral catheter is inserted alongside the 7-F occlusion balloon catheter. This procedure promotes ureteral identification and dissection in prepara-tion for eventual stapling of the bladder cuff, and limits any leakage of urine or spillage of TCC cells into the extraperitoneal space.[25]

Ureteral Orifice or Tunnel Resection into Fat: The Pluck Procedure

With the patient in a supine position, using a standard resectoscope, the ureteral orifice, tunnel, and intramural ureter are resected transurethrally until the perivesical fat is seen. This procedure is quick and facilitates the laparoscopic nephroureterectomy (LNU) proce-dure because no ureteral catheter is placed; instead of dissecting the distal ureter, the sur-geon can merely *pluck* the ureter cephalad from out of the pelvis during the laparoscopic nephrectomy. The only drawback to this approach is the concern over the leakage of malig-nant, cell-laden urine into the retroperitoneum until the ureter is occluded laparoscopi-cally.[26] Instances of seeding after a pluck procedure have been reported by several urologists.[27, 28]

Transvesical Laparoscopic Ureteral Dissection[16]

Under cystoscopic control, two 5-mm balloon tipped trocars are inserted suprapubically into the bladder. An endoloop tie is inserted through the ipsilateral suprapubic port and positioned around the targeted ureteral orifice. A ureteral catheter is cystoscopically passed through the endoloop into the ureteral orifice up to the renal pelvis (Fig. 10.1a). The targeted ureteral orifice is grasped with a grasper inserted through the contralateral suprapubic port and retracted anteriorly. This procedure tents up the ipsilateral hemitrigone, thus elevating the bladder base (Fig. 10.1b). A 24-Fr resectoscope fitted with a pointed coagulating electrode is inserted per urethra alongside the ureteral catheter to describe and detach circumferentially an adequate bladder cuff around the ureteral orifice in a full thickness manner using glycine irrigation. The anterior traction afforded by the suprapubic grasper is a critical adjunct in facilitating this circumferential detachment of the bladder cuff from the adjacent bladder, as well as delivering the freed intact extravesical ureter into the bladder. Extravesical fibrofatty attachments of the juxtavesical ureter are released with the coagulating electrode, thereby circumferentially mobilizing the most distal 3–4 cm of en bloc ureter (Fig. 10.1c). The intramural ureter is circumferentially occluded by cinching down the already placed endoloop tie, thus precluding local urine spillage.[16]

Nephroureterectomy

Three techniques for performing the nephrectomy have evolved over the past decade.

Transperitoneal Nephroureterectomy

Peritoneal access can be obtained by either the Veress needle (closed) technique or the Hasson cannula (open) technique, with the patient routinely in the lateral position. Typically, a four- to five-port approach is employed. For the laparoscope, a 12-mm primary trocar is inserted at the umbilicus or at the lateral border of the rectus muscle one to two fingerbreadths cephalad to the umbilicus (10 mm, 30°). Three secondary trocars are placed – a 5-mm port at the lateral border of the rectus near the costal margin, a 12-mm port at the lateral border of the rectus one to two fingerbreadths below the level of the umbilicus, and a 5-mm port for lateral retraction of the kidney inserted at the anterior axillary line near the costal margin (Fig. 10.2). For a right-sided nephrectomy, an additional 5-mm port is necessary at the costal margin for cephalad retraction of the liver.[29]

Using electrosurgical scissors and grasping forceps, the line of Toldt is incised from the hepatic or splenic flexure down into the pelvis across the iliac vessels. The incision is extended medial to the medial umbilical ligament. Dissection allows for complete mobilization of the bowel medially to expose the retroperitoneum. The dissection is then performed over the area of the iliac vessels to identify the ureter as it courses this region. Having secured the ureter in an umbilical tape for retraction, it is dissected down into the pelvis. The superior vesical artery is dissected as it crosses the ureter,

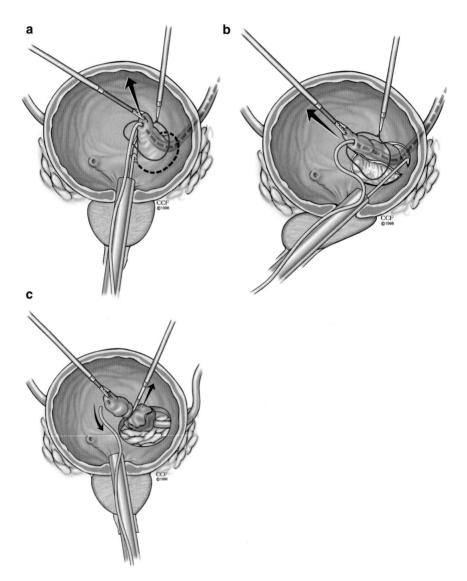

Fig. 10.1 (**a**) Figure illustrating the placement of two trocars (2 mm) in the bladder with ureteric catheter in the distal ureter and a loop encircling the orifice and Colin knife resectoscope, which creates the bladder cuff around the ureteric orifice. (**b**) Circumferential incision of the bladder mucosa and deep incision of the distal ureteric tissue are done with mobilization of the tissues further up to free the distal ureter. (**c**) Complete mobilization of the distal ureter with bladder cuff, followed by removal of the ureteric catheter and ligation of the distal ureter to avoid tumor spillage (Reprinted with permission, Cleveland Clinic Center for Medical Art & Photography © 1998–2010. All Rights Reserved)

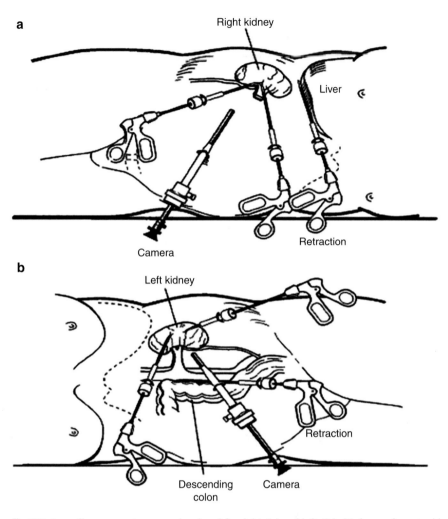

Fig. 10.2 A small accessory trocar can be placed for right- (**a**) and left- (**b**) sided procedures to aid with retraction of the liver, spleen, or bowel (This article was published in *Atlas of Laparoscopic Retroperitoneal Surgery*, Jarrett TW, Laparoscopic nephroureterectomy, pp. 105–120, Copyright Elsevier)

secured and transected. The medial umbilical ligament is also transected to complete the caudal dissection of the ureter down to the detrusor muscle. The ureter is completely freed until the detrusor muscle fibers at the ureterovesical junction are identified. At this point, by placing a grasping forceps through the lower anterior axillary line port, the ureter can be retracted superiorly and laterally, thereby tenting up the wall of the bladder to expose the ureterovesical junction. The open jaws of the endo-GIA stapler are placed across the cuff of bladder, then closed and fired to incise the tissue between staple rows.

Dissection cephalad along the ureter is then extended up to the renal hilar region. The renal artery and renal vein are circumferentially dissected and exposed. Vascular clips are used to secure the renal artery and a vascular endo-GIA stapler is used to secure the renal vein before transection. Dissection is performed outside of Gerota's fascia, freeing the kidney along the inferior, lateral, and posterior aspects. At the upper pole, dissection is completed through Gerota's fascia onto the upper pole of the kidney. In this manner the adrenal gland is left untouched and in situ.[30]

Sealed Laparoscopic Nephroureterectomy[17]

A new technique performed to avoid the disadvantages of transurethral bladder cuff excision and open/laparoscopic distal ureterectomy using the endo-GIA. First, a standard laparoscopic transperitoneal nephrectomy in a full flank position is performed. Three ports are used: one 10-mm trocar is placed by the Hasson technique supraumbilically, one 5-mm port is placed in the midclavicular line in the ipsilateral upper quadrant, and one 12-mm trocar is placed above the first one in the midline between the xyphoid and the first port. An optional fourth 5-mm trocar may be inserted above the former trocar on the right side and in the anterior axillary line on the left side. After mobilization of the colon, the ureter is identified and clipped without transsection to prevent inadvertent urine spillage. The renal artery and vein are dissected and divided, and the kidney is circumferentially mobilized, sparing the adrenal. The ureter is then dissected caudally into the pelvis. An additional two (5- and 10-mm) trocars are placed in the lower abdomen (Fig. 10.3a). After transection of the lateral umbilical ligament, dissection is continued caudally until the

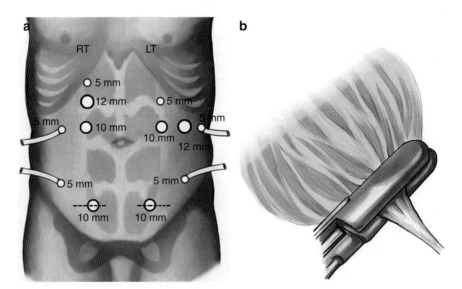

Fig. 10.3 (a) Schematics of trocar position. (b) The bladder cuff is incised by LigaSure Atlas™ (Valleylab, Boulder, CO). (Reprinted from Tsivian et al.[17], with permission from Elsevier)

detrusor muscle fibers at the ureterovesical junction are identified. The ureter is then retracted superior and laterally, tenting up the bladder wall at the ureterovesical junction. A 1-cm area of bladder adventitia around the ureterovesical junction is cleared, and a bladder cuff is incised with the use of a 10-mm LigaSure Atlas™ (Valleylab, Boulder, CO) (Fig. 10.3b). The bladder wall from one side and kidney together with the ureter and bladder cuff from the other side remain sealed after incision and detachment. Additional sutures on the bladder wall are not required.[17]

Technical Caveats

Dissecting instruments and grasping forceps should be placed at an approximately 45-degree angle to the scope. If placed too low, instrument handling will be impaired by the iliac bone and if too high, the instrument tips will be too close to the kidney.

Safe dissection of the renal hilum requires two conditions: (1) medial retraction of the colon and bowel by gravity or an additional retractor and (2) lateral retraction of the kidney by lifting it out of the renal fossa. Lateral retraction of the kidney with a grasper placed under the lower pole will place the vessels on tension. This is accomplished by gently placing the lateral grasper under the ureter and lower pole of the kidney until the grasper abuts against the abdominal sidewall. With the ureter and lower pole of the kidney elevated, layer-by-layer anterior dissection is performed with the irrigator aspirator until the renal vein is uncovered.

Transperitoneal: Hand-Assisted Nephroureterectomy

With hand-assisted NU, the kidney and proximal ureter are removed laparoscopically, and an incision is made for dissection of the distal ureter and bladder and intact specimen removal. This approach circumvents the difficulty in performing the most difficult portions of the procedure laparoscopically.[23] After pneumoperitoneum is achieved, the Pneumosleeve (Dexterity, Blue Bell, PA) device is assembled, which consists of a plastic wound protector that is inserted into the 7- to 8-cm incision and a clear plastic sleeve that is attached to the patient's skin by an adhesive ring similar to an ostomy disk. With this device, the surgeon's hand can be used for retraction and blunt dissection. This positioning works well for the right-handed surgeon working on a right kidney. For the right-handed surgeon working on a left kidney, however, a slightly higher periumbilical midline placement may be preferable. Relative to standard laparoscopic techniques, hand assistance seems to facilitate the operative speed and safety of laparoscopic nephrectomy (LN4) without significantly sacrificing the benefits of minimally invasive surgery.[31,32] It also makes intact removal of the specimen easy.

Retroperitoneal Nephroureterectomy

The retroperitoneal approach for nephroureterectomy for upper tract TCC recently was described by Gill and Salomon et al. Salomon et al. develops the retroperitoneal space with digital dissection, whereas Gill uses the trocar-mounted Origin balloon distension system (Origin Medsystems, Menlo Park, CA).[33,34] Patients were placed in the lateral decubitus position. 5 mm trocars (total 5 trocars) were used, including one 12 mm, two 10 mm, and three 5 mm. A 15-mm incision was made under the 12th rib on the posterior axillary line in front of the sacroiliac muscles. The retroperitoneum was entered by blunt dissection. The index finger was first used to push the peritoneum forward and then the index finger, protected by a latex finger cover, was placed in the retroperitoneum to guide the positioning of the other ports. A 10-mm trocar was placed at the apex of the 12th rib at the level of the anterior axillary line, a 5-mm trocar above the iliac crest at the level of the anterior axillary line, a 10-mm trocar above the iliac crest at the level of the median axillary line, and a 5-mm trocar above the iliac crest at the level of the posterior axillary line. The single 12-mm trocar was placed in the first incision made under the 12th rib on the posterior axillary line (Fig. 10.4). A pneumoretroperitoneum is created by applying 10–15 mmHg of CO_2 pressure. The initial maneuver is to clip ligate the upper ureter in continuity as a precaution to prevent urinary distention of the distal ureter. The renal artery and vein are individually controlled, and the renal specimen is circumferentially mobilized retroperitoneoscopically external to Gerota's fascia. If necessary, the adrenal gland is excised en bloc with the specimen. The ureter, along with en bloc gonadal vein and periureteral adipose tissue, are mobilized distally beyond the common iliac vessels. Gentle cephalad traction on the ureter with a laparoscopic 5-mm atraumatic small bowel clamp, combined with precise dissection with J-hook electrocautery, delivers the entire cystoscopically mobilized, intact distal ureter and bladder cuff into the upper retroperitoneum. Laparoscopic visualization of the prior intravesically placed endoloop tie around the intramural ureter provides assurance that the entire ureter has been retrieved without leaving any fragment of urothelium behind. The retroperitoneum is inspected for bleeding, a suction drain is inserted, and the pneumoretroperitoneum is exsufflated. The laparoscopic ports are removed and the puncture site is closed using 2-zero polyglycolic acid sutures.

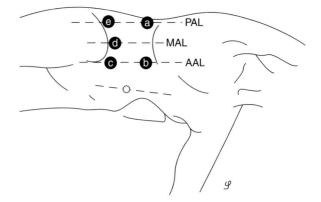

Fig. 10.4 Site of trocars. *a*, 12-mm trocar (suction-irrigation); *b*, 10-mm trocar (forceps); *c*, 5-mm trocar (forceps); *d*, 10-mm trocar (camera); *e*, 5-mm trocar (scissors). *PAL* posterior axillary line, *MAL* median axillary line, *AAL* anterior axillary line (Reprinted from Salomon et al.[34] With permission from Elsevier)

Specimen Entrapment and Delivery

The en bloc specimen is entrapped in an Endo Catch™ bag (Covidien, Dublin, Ireland) and extracted intact through an appropriate muscle splitting extension of the primary port site incision. The Endo Catch™ is a transparent sack that comes with a metal ring that readily opens the mouth of the sack when it is deployed (similar to a butterfly capture net), resulting in easy manipulation of the specimen into the sack. However, if a laparoscopic-assisted or open approach to the distal ureter has been used, then entrapment is not a necessary step because the specimen can be removed directly by the surgeon's hand.

Technical Caveats

During port placement, every effort should be made to separate out the ports as much as possible. Frustrating "clashing of swords" occurs if the trocars, and therefore the laparoscopic instruments, are located in close proximity. Thus, the anterior axillary line (AAL) port can be positioned even more anterior to the axillary line; however, the lateral peritoneal reflection must be clearly visualized laparoscopically and avoided before the AAL port is inserted. Similarly, care must be taken to avoid pleural injury during placement of the upper midaxillary line (UMAL) port. The 12-mm lower midaxillary line (LMAL) port must be located at a considerable distance (≥3 cm) cephalad to the iliac bone. The unyielding bone significantly compromises the torque capability of a trocar placed adjacent to it.

Detachment of the upper renal pole from the undersurface of the adrenal gland must be performed meticulously using a fore-oblique (30-degree) laparoscope and electrocautery for hemostasis. Persistent venous oozing from the adrenal bed can result in significant bleeding postoperatively.

Intraoperative Difficulties

Peritoneal Rent

A peritoneal rent may occur either initially during balloon inflation or subsequently during laparoscopic dissection. Usually a peritoneal rent does not cause significant problems, and the procedure can be completed retroperitoneoscopically. However, adequate medial retraction of the kidney by a fan retractor inserted through the UMAL port may be necessary to maintain operative exposure in the retroperitoneal space. Two points must be kept in mind: (1) intra-abdominal viscerae must be thoroughly inspected by inserting the laparoscope through the peritoneal rent to rule out iatrogenic injury, and (2) the peritoneal cavity must be drained of CO_2 prior to terminating the procedure.

Identification of the Renal Hilum

If the renal hilum cannot be located, the surgeon should reinsert the laparoscope slowly and identify the psoas muscle. The psoas muscle should then be crossed fromsss lateral-to-medial in a cephalad direction and a search conducted for arterial pulsations near its medial border. Pulsations of the fat-covered renal artery or aorta are usually identifiable. Gentle dissection with the tip of the suction device and electrosurgical scissors or hook is performed directly toward the pulsations. The aorta or renal artery are identified and traced to the renal hilum. Alternatively, the ureter can be identified and followed cephalad to the hilum. Dissection through the perirenal fat may identify the surface of the kidney, which can then be dissected toward its hilum.

Persistent Hilar Bleeding After Ligation of the Renal Pedicle

Persistent renal hilar bleeding generally indicates the presence of an overlooked, patent accessory renal artery. After flow is controlled from the main renal artery, the renal vein should appear flat and devoid of blood. A normally distended renal vein at this juncture indicates continued arterial inflow through an accessory renal artery. In this circumstance, division of the distended renal vein with an endo-GIA stapler interrupts venous outflow with a resultant increase in intrarenal venous back pressure. This causes persistent oozing during the remainder of the dissection. One should search for an accessory renal artery in this situation.

References

1. Oosterlinck W, Solsona E, van der Meijden APM, et al. EAU guidelines on diagnosis and treatment of upper urinary tract transitional cell carcinoma. *Eur Urol.* 2004;46:147-154.
2. Krogh J, Kvist E, Rye B. Transitional cell carcinoma of the upper urinary tract: prognostic variables and postoperative recurrences. *Br J Urol.* 1991;67:32-36.
3. Jemal A, Siegel R, Ward E, Murray T, Xu J, Thun MJ. Cancer statistics, 2007. *CA Cancer J Clin.* 2007;57:43-66.
4. Lehmann J, Suttmann H, Kovac I, et al. Transitional cell carcinoma of the ureter: prognostic factors influencing progression and survival. *Eur Urol.* 2007;51:1281-1288.
5. Sanderson KM, Cai J, Miranda G, Skinner DG, Stein JP. Upper tract urothelial recurrence following radical cystectomy for transitional cell carcinoma of the bladder: an analysis of 1, 069 patients with 10-year followup. *J Urol.* 2007;177:2088-2094.
6. Zigeuner RE, Hutterer G, Chromecki T, Rehak P, Langner C. Bladder tumour development after urothelial carcinoma of the upper urinary tract is related to primary tumour location. *BJU Int.* 2006;98:1181-1186.
7. Angulo JC, Hontoria J, Sanchez-Chapado M. One-incision nephroureterectomy endoscopically assisted transurethral stripping. *Urology.* 1998;52:203-207.
8. Rassweiler J, Henkel TO, Potempa DM, Coptcoat M, Alken P. The technique of transperitoneal laparoscopic nephrectomy, adrenalectomy, and nephroureterectomy. *Eur Urol.* 1993; 23:425-430.

9. McNeill A, Oakley N, Tolley DA, Gill IS. Laparoscopic nephroureterectomy for upper tract transitional cell carcinoma: a critical appraisal. *BJU Int*. 2004;94:259-263.

10. Tsujihata M, Nonomura N, Tsujimura A, Yoshimura K, Miyagawa Y, Okuyama A. Laparoscopic nephroureterectomy for upper tract transitional cell carcinoma: comparison of laparoscopic and open surgery. *Eur Urol*. 2006;49:332-336.

11. Landman J, Lev RY, Bhayani S, et al. Comparison of hand assisted and standard laparoscopic radical nephroureterectomy for the management of localized transitional cell carcinoma. *J Urol*. 2002;167:2387-2391.

12. Gill IS, Sung GT, Hobart MG, et al. Laparoscopic radical nephroureterectomy for upper tract transitional cell carcinoma: the Cleveland Clinic experience. *J Urol*. 2000;164:1513-1522.

13. Palou J, Caparros J, Orsola A, Xavier B, Vicente J. Transurethral resection of the intramural ureter as the first step of nephroureterectomy. *J Urol*. 1995;154:43-44.

14. Kurzer E, Leveillee RJ, Bird VG. Combining hand assisted laparoscopic nephroureterectomy with cystoscopic circumferential excision of the distal ureter without primary closure of the bladder cuff – is it safe? *J Urol*. 2006;175:63-67.

15. Vardi IY, Stern JA, Gonzalez CM, Kimm SY, Nadler RB. Novel technique for management of distal ureter and en block resection of bladder cuff during hand-assisted laparoscopic nephroureterectomy. *Urology*. 2006;67:89-92.

16. Gill IS, Sobel JJ, Miller SD, et al. A novel technique for the management of the en-bloc bladder cuff and distal ureter during laparoscopic nephroureterectomy. *J Urol*. 1999;161: 430-434.

17. Tsivian A, Benjamin S, Sidi AA. A sealed laparoscopic nephroureterectomy: a new technique. *Eur Urol*. 2007;52:1015-1019.

18. Rassweiler J, Frede T, Henkel TO, Stock C, Alken P. Nephrectomy: a comparative study between the transperitoneal and retroperitoneal laparoscopic versus the open approach. *Eur Urol*. 1998;13:489-496.

19. Cicco A, Salomon L, Hoznek H, et al. Carcinological risks and retroperitoneal laparoscopy. *Eur Urol*. 2000;38:606-612.

20. Rassweiler J, Tsivian A, Ravi Kumar AV, et al. Oncological safety of laparoscopic surgery for urological malignancies: experience with more than 1,000 operations. *J Urol*. 2003;169: 2072-2075.

21. Lee BR, Jabbour ME, Marshall FF, Smith AD, Jarrett TW. 13-year survival comparison of percutaneous and open nephroureterectomy approaches for management of transitional cell carcinoma of renal collecting system: equivalent outcomes. *J Endourol*. 1999;13:289-294.

22. Rassweiler JJ, Schulze M, Marrero R, Frede T, Palou Redorta J, Bassi P. Laparoscopic nephroureterectomy for upper urinary tract transitional cell carcinoma: is it better than open surgery? *Eur Urol*. 2004;46:690-697.

23. Jarrett TW. Laparoscopic nephroureterectomy. *Atlas Urol Clin North Am*. 2000;8:115.

24. Steinberg JR, Matin SF. Laparoscopic radical nephroureterectomy: dilemma of the distal ureter. *Curr Opin Urol*. 2004;14:61-65.

25. Shalhav AL, Elbahnasy AM, McDougall E, Clayman RV. Laparoscopic nephroureterectomy for upper tract transitional cell cancer: technical aspects. *J Endourol*. 1998;12:345-353.

26. Stephenson RN, Sharma NK. Tolley DA Laparoscopic nephroureterectomy: a comparison with open surgery. *J Endourol*. 1995;9(Suppl 1):99.

27. Arango O, Bielsa O, Carles J, Gelabert-Mas A. Massive tumor implantation in the endoscopic resected area in modified nephroureterectomy. *J Urol*. 1997;157:1839.

28. Hetherington JW, Ewing R, Philip NH. Modified nephroureterectomy: a risk of tumor implantation. *Br J Urol*. 1999;58:368-370.

29. Gill IS. Laparoscopic radical nephrectomy for cancer. *Urol Clin North Am*. 2000;27: 707-719.

30. McDougall EM, Clayman RV, Elashry O. Laparoscopic nephroureterectomy for upper tract transitional cell cancer: the Washington University experience. *J Urol.* 1995;154:975-979.
31. Nakada SY. Hand-assisted laparoscopic nephrectomy. *J Endourol.* 1999;13:9-14.
32. Wolf JS, Moon TD, Nakada SY. Hand assisted laparoscopic nephrectomy: comparison to standard laparoscopic nephrectomy. *J Urol.* 1998;160:22-27.
33. Gill IS. Retroperitoneal laparoscopic nephrectomy. *Urol Clin North Am.* 1998;25:343-360.
34. Salomon L, Hoznek A, Cicco A, Gasman D, Chopin DK, Abbou CC. Retroperitoneoscopic nephroureterectomy for renal pelvic tumors with a single iliac incision. *J Urol.* 1999;161: 541-544.

Difficulties in Laparoscopic Partial Nephrectomy

11

Ahmed M. Al-Kandari, Ricardo Brandina, Robert J. Stein, and Inderbir S. Gill

Introduction

Renal masses are more frequently diagnosed with the advent of routine abdominal imaging like ultrasound followed by computerized tomography (CT) scan, which has resulted in the need for more intervention. Among the different approaches, partial nephrectomy has proved the test of time. This has been duplicated by laparoscopic partial nephrectomy. Gill et al. have published the largest comparative study between laparoscopic partial versus open partial nephrectomy, in which they proved that laparoscopic partial nephrectomy (LPN) had a very comparable oncological benefit with superior functional outcome and minimal morbidity.[1] This highly advanced laparoscopic technique is being utilized in more centers around the world with very similar results to what has been published. In this chapter, the technique of laparoscopic partial nephrectomy that the authors utilize will be described and the important steps will be explained. This includes surgeon and patient preparation, intraoperative steps including laparoscopic approach, kidney dissection, intraoperative ultrasound, hilar control, partial nephrectomy, renal bed management, and finishing the procedure.[2] Difficult case scenarios that require special attention will also be discussed, such as renal impairment, solitary kidney, hilar mass, central mass, multiple renal arteries, renal masses with vascular pathology, and previously operated kidneys. LPN in obese patients, cystic masses, renal masses with ureteropelvic junction pathology, and horseshoe kidney will also be discussed. The authors' aim in this chapter is to provide practical guidelines and to review common and uncommon difficulties and explain ways to overcome them. This chapter will highlight important technical aspects of LPN that are done in the standard laparoscopic way; hand-assisted or robot-assisted techniques will not be discussed.

A.M. Al-Kandari (✉)

Department of Surgery (Urology), Faculty of Medicine, Kuwait University, Jabriyah, Kuwait

e-mail: drakandari@hotmail.com

A.M. Al-Kandari and I.S. Gill (eds.), *Difficult Conditions in Laparoscopic Urologic Surgery*,   **117**

DOI: 10.1007/978-1-84882-105-7_11, © Springer-Verlag London Limited 2011

Surgeon Preparation

It is of utmost importance that the laparoscopic surgeon, when considering a laparoscopic partial nephrectomy, should master certain skills and make various preparations:

1. Mastery of open partial nephrectomy skills
2. Mastery of intracorporeal suturing skills
3. Observe a video that illustrates the technique of laparoscopic partial nephrectomy
4. Prepare all the essential instruments to help complete the procedure (the instruments will be described later)
5. Include a good camera person and skilled laparoscopic nurse
6. Inform the anesthetist that the surgery will be time-consuming, especially at the beginning, and that a cooperative atmosphere is needed
7. Start with peripheral exophytic lesions
8. Prepare the sutures and other materials, such as hemostatic agents

Case Preparation

1. *Imaging review*: It is essential that thorough imaging review be done with prior operative planning to help anticipate difficulties and deal with them. Therefore, it is recommended that a CT scan of the abdomen with angiographic images be assessed for proper tumor size and location in respect to vascular and ureteral anatomy.
2. *Laboratory investigations*: Full blood tests, including complete blood count, coagulation profile, and blood for cross-match, should be performed. A renal function test should also be performed, as well as other full biochemical profiles, with routine urine tests.
3. *Consent form*: It is important to fully explain to the patient the possibility of an open conversion as well as the possibility of a total nephrectomy, as this is more likely in the beginning of the series.

Positioning

1. The authors commonly place a ureteric catheter after cystoscopy in order to access the integrity of the collecting system with retrograde methyelene blue.
2. The patient is placed in a modified flank position, with all pressure points supported, with antiembolic stockings and pneumatic compression devices for the lower limbs (Fig. 11.1).

Fig. 11.1 Patient position in modified flank position with pressure areas padded, antiembolic stockings and pneumatic compression on lower limbs applied

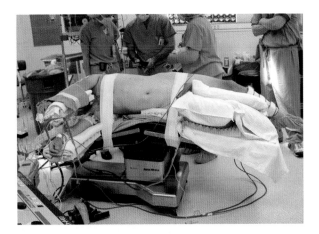

Standard Essential Equipment (Used by the Authors)

1. 30-degree lens laparoscope (Karl Storz, Tuttlingen, Germany)
2. Non-traumatic non-locking bowel forceps (Karl Storz, Tuttlingen, Germany)
3. Electrocautery scissors (Karl Storz, Tuttlingen, Germany)
4. Battery-activated suction/irrigation device (Stryker Endoscopy, San Jose, CA)
5. Needle holders (Ethicon, Inc., Somerville, NJ)
6. Laparoscopic Satinski clamp (Karl Storz, Tuttlingen, Germany)
7. 10-mm Endo Catch™ bag (Covidien, Dublin, Ireland)
8. Hemostatic agent (FloSeal™, Baxter International Inc., Deerfield, IL) with its applicator
9. Hem-o-lok® polymer clips (10 mm) with applier (Teleflex Medical, Research Triangle Park, NC)
10. Surgicel® (Ethicon, Inc., Somerville, NJ), which will be made into a bolster
11. 2.0 Vicryl™ on CT 1 needle 15-cm length (Ethicon, Inc., Somerville, NJ)

Standard Technique of Laparoscopic Partial Nephrectomy for Peripheral Lesion

1. The authors usually use a transperitoneal approach, with trocar placement as seen in Fig. 11.2. Then, after the colon is mobilized, the retroperitoneum can be accessed using electrocautery, such as the Harmonic Scalpel® (Ethicon Endo-Surgery, Cincinnati, OH) or the LigaSure™ device (Valleylab, Boulder, CO). The authors previously used a retroperitoneal approach, but have moved on to a transperitoneal approach as it allows a larger and better working space with minimal morbidity.
2. Renal mobilization is accomplished using blunt and sharp dissection, and the perinephric fat is removed from the kidney, except at the tumor site where it is left intact.

Fig. 11.2 Schematic picture showing the flank position and port sites for left LPN

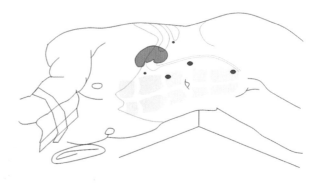

Fig. 11.3 Schematic drawings showing the hilar clamping with Satinski clamp, with different views illustrating the direction of the clamp in relation to the abdomen and vessels. (**a**) Outside view of the Satinski clamp showing the port used. (**b**) Outside and inside view of Satinski clamp. (**c**) View showing the suction device that can be used to carefully visualize the renal vessels during clamping. (**d**) Inside view of Satinski clamp showing complete and mass clamping of the renal vessels (Reprinted with permission, Cleveland Clinic Center for Medical Art & Photography © 1998–2009. All Rights Reserved)

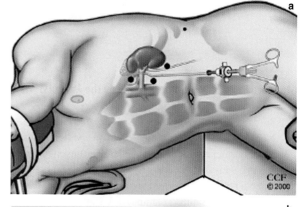

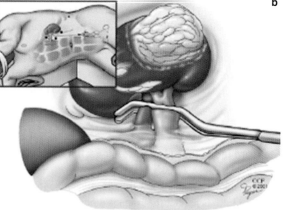

3. Hilar dissection is then carried out with aid of kidney traction. The authors do not isolate the renal artery or vein since a mass clamping is done at the time of the partial nephrectomy using the Satinski clamp (Fig. 11.3a–d).
4. Intraoperative laparoscopic ultrasound is routinely used to assess the tumor depth, aid in a precise excision, and also exclude any small intrarenal masses (Fig. 11.4a–c).

Fig. 11.3 (continued)

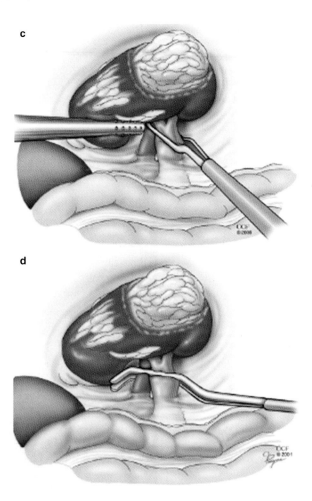

5. Strict stopwatch time calculation then begins to measure warm ischemia time, which should be as short as possible to minimize renal damage, which is done with a Satinski clamp. The authors commonly administer diuretics (furosemide, mannitol) to minimize the warm ischemia effect.

6. The site of resection is scored with a 5-mm margin around the tumor using the electrocautery scissors. Cutting of the mass is done as sharply as possible, taking care to avoid cutting into the mass.

7. The mass is then put aside or placed into a 10-mm Endo Catch™ bag and kept until the end of the procedure.

8. The bed of the resected area is sutured with 2.0 Vicryl™ on CT 1 needle to oversew bleeding vessels as a first layer.

9. The renal hilar ligation is removed to reperfuse the kidney while suturing the renal bed vessels; this minimizes warm ischemia time with acceptable visibility and bleeding.

Fig. 11.4 (**a**) Intraabdominal picture showing ultrasound probe. (**b**) Intraabdominal picture showing ultrasound probe (which helps decide the margins) of the tumor and hock used to score the margins. (**c**) Ultrasound of the tumor

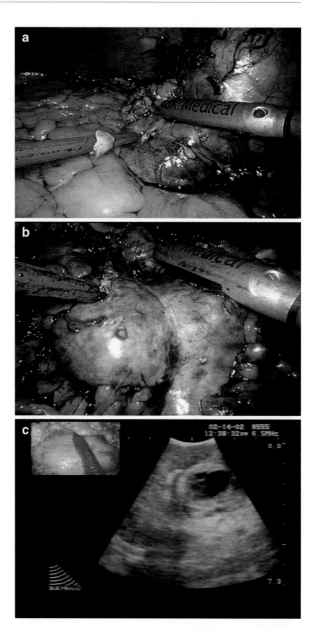

10. The integrity of the pelvicaliceal system is checked with methylene blue and the pelvicaliceal system is oversewn.
11. A pre-made Surgicel® bolster is inserted into the renal bed and is fixed with a suture with a Hem-o-lok® clip at one end. The suture is tightened with the Hem-o-lok® clip to save time.

12. A coagulating agent (FloSeal™) is applied at the renal bed.
13. The area is irrigated with normal saline and suction is applied. A drain is inserted near the area (Figs. 11.5–11.11).

Currently, the authors omit the Surgicel® bolster as others have described. Careful and efficient suturing of the collecting system and renal parenchyma combined with the application of FloSeal™ routinely produces excellent hemostatic results.

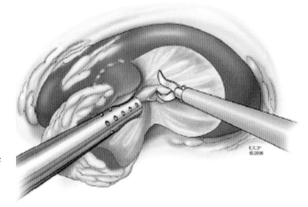

Fig. 11.5 Schematic drawing showing cold scissor cutting of the tumor (Reprinted with permission, Cleveland Clinic Center for Medical Art & Photography © 1998–2009. All Rights Reserved)

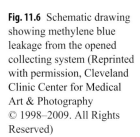

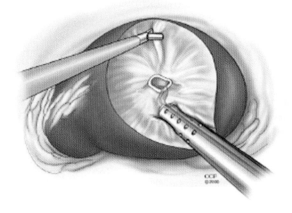

Fig. 11.6 Schematic drawing showing methylene blue leakage from the opened collecting system (Reprinted with permission, Cleveland Clinic Center for Medical Art & Photography © 1998–2009. All Rights Reserved)

Fig. 11.7 Schematic drawing showing first layer closure of the collecting system and bleeding vessels with CT-1 Vicryl™ running suture (Reprinted with permission, Cleveland Clinic Center for Medical Art & Photography © 1998–2009. All Rights Reserved)

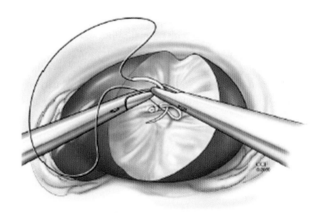

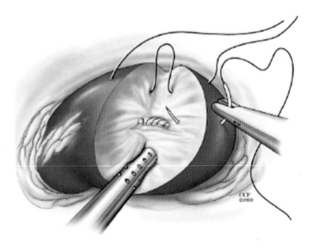

Fig. 11.8 Schematic drawing showing second layer closure with CT-1 Vicryl™ interrupted suture involving renal capsule and then use of Hem-o-lok® clips to hold sutures (Reprinted with permission, Cleveland Clinic Center for Medical Art & Photography © 1998–2009. All Rights Reserved)

Fig. 11.9 Schematic drawing showing the application of Surgicel® bolster under the second layer of suture line (Reprinted with permission, Cleveland Clinic Center for Medical Art & Photography © 1998–2009. All Rights Reserved)

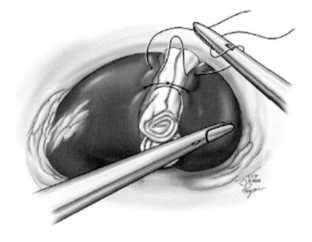

Fig. 11.10 Application of Surgicel® bolster

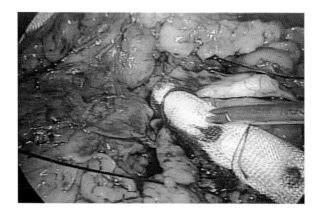

Fig. 11.11 Operative picture showing the application of FloSeal™ at the operated site

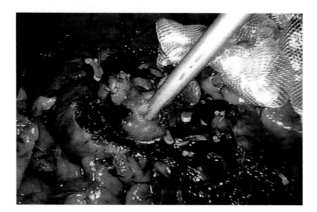

Common Difficulties in Laparoscopic Partial Nephrectomy

Bleeding

If the vascular pedicle is not clamped completely, then bleeding (both venous and arterial) can commonly occur. This can be quite bothersome and lead to difficulties in visualization. The assistant should be actively helpful in using suction to expose the field well and the surgeon should work promptly to oversew the bleeding point. Alternative ways of pedicle reclamping to include possible accessory vessels can be considered. The use of compressing gauze on a bleeding point by the assistant can also be helpful. If the surgeon still encounters a disturbing bleeder that inhibits visibility after implementing all of the above, then the option of open conversion should be considered since patient safety and achievement of oncologic control are the priorities in cancer treatment. On other occasions in which there is a normal contralateral kidney and a sizable tumor of around 6–7 cm, the option of total radical nephrectomy can be considered. Careful hemodynamic monitoring should be performed with blood transfusion when significant bleeding occurs, especially if hypotension is encountered. The decision of blood transfusion is commonly a joint decision between the anesthetist and surgeon.

Opening the Pelvicaliceal System During Deep Renal Resection

This is a common procedure during partial nephrectomy and should be anticipated during resection of deep tumors or polar lesions. The tissues' appearance should be noted along with any leakage of methelyne blue. Accurate closure is important to avoid urine leakage. This can be done with 2.0 Vicryl™ and also can be oversewn during renorrhaphy. Confirmation of absence of leakage is important to avoid complications. Difficulty can be encountered if the repair has to be done in the depth of resection where the needle cannot be rotated easily. In this case, consider bolster renorrhaphy, which will close the defect and solve the problem. Subsequently, it is important that the trajectory of the excised bed be wide to facilitate suturing.

Challenging Difficulties During Partial Nephrectomy

Renal Mass Near the Hilum

A hilar mass can be quite challenging during laparoscopic partial nephrectomy since proper hilar control is essential in order to perform the procedure and requires significant experience and can be tedious even in an open procedure. In a reported series of LPN, 6–19.1% of renal masses were hilar in location (Fig. 11.12).[2, 3] In this situation, one should try to dissect the renal vessels as medial as possible to allow application of the vascular clamp. In rare cases where the mass is adherent to a small part of the renal vein that requires excision, vascular repair may be necessary. Therefore, the authors suggest that

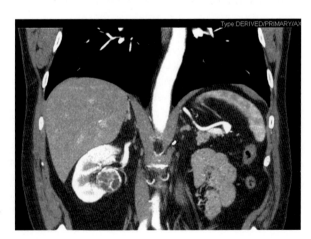

Fig. 11.12 CT scan image showing a renal mass at hilar location

these cases should be performed by surgeons with sufficient experience in laparoscopic partial nephrectomy. Total nephrectomy should be considered if the procedure cannot be safely completed, especially if there is a normal contralateral kidney. Extreme care in these cases is required to avoid cutting through tumor or leaving residual tumor; therefore, confirming negative margins is important in these cases.

Centrally Located Tumors

Centrally located renal masses comprise a reasonable percentage – nearly 40% of the masses that the authors manage with LPN (Fig. 11.13).[2] The authors typically utilize intraoperative ultrasound to localize the tumor and assess the depth of penetration. After hilar control (as previously described), the authors incise the renal parenchyma over the mass with cold shears and dissect around the mass with 5 mm of free margin. The procedure is then completed as routine. It is very important not to cut into the tumor in these cases, and that the margins be negative, which can be reviewed by frozen section pathological testing. Suture repair of the renal bed is done as previously described. Again, the use of bolster with parenchymal closure will usually be adequate for repair of the renal bed. The main major complication in this group was late-onset hematuria, which necessitated angiographic embolization. This facility should be available at centers where these advanced procedures are performed.[4] Again, experience is essential in these cases and the option of total nephrectomy must be considered if difficulty is anticipated.

Solitary Kidney and Compromised Renal Function Cases

A renal mass in a solitary kidney can be quite challenging (Fig. 11.14). Animal studies have described the relationship between the duration of warm ischemia and the magnitude of subsequent renal dysfunction. However, direct translation of these data to clinical practice is limited by significant anatomical and physiological differences among species. Current clinical data support a safe warm ischemia time limit of 30 min in patients with normal preoperative kidney function.[5] While laparoscopic partial nephrectomy is technically feasible

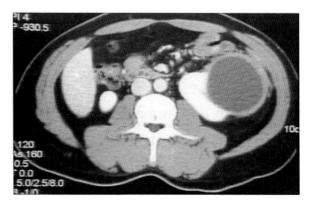

Fig. 11.13 CT scan showing a renal mass approaching the central part of the kidney

Fig. 11.14 Renal mass in a left solitary kidney

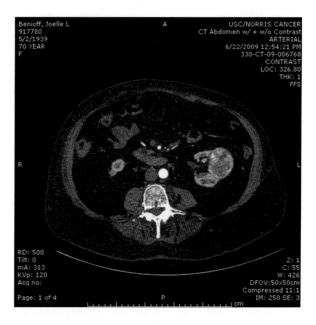

for a tumor in a solitary kidney, warm ischemia time was longer and complication rates higher compared with open partial nephrectomy in early series.[6] In addition, although average loss of renal function at 3 months is equivalent (after accounting for warm ischemia time), a greater proportion of patients required dialysis temporarily or permanently after laparoscopic partial nephrectomy in that series. Therefore, some authors suggest that, during early series of LPN, open partial nephrectomy may be the preferred nephron-sparing approach for patients at high risk for chronic kidney disease.[6] Of 485 patients undergoing LPN between September 1999 and August 2005 at the authors' institution, 48 (10%) had compromised baseline renal function (serum creatinine 1.5 mg/dL or greater, group I). Outcomes were compared with 437 patients undergoing LPN with normal baseline renal function (serum creatinine less than 1.5 mg/dL, group II). Both groups were compared regarding perioperative data, complications, and renal functional and oncologic outcomes. Group I patients were older (67.6 vs 58.6 years, $P < 0.001$) and had higher American Society of Anesthesiologists scores (2.8 vs 2.4, $P < 0.001$), higher Charlson Comorbidity Index (1.9 vs 0.7, $P < 0.001$), and larger tumors (3.3 vs 2.7 cm, $P = 0.01$). Intraoperative data, postoperative outcomes, overall complications, and pathologic data were similar between groups. At a mean follow-up of 21 months, the deterioration in serum creatinine and estimated glomerular filtration rate was similar between groups ($P = 0.99$ and 0.89, respectively). Dialysis was required in five patients (10%) in group I and three patients (0.6%) in group II ($P < 0.001$). Within group I, older patients (older than 70 years) with prolonged warm ischemia (greater than 30 min) had significantly worse renal functional outcomes. Comparing groups I and II, estimated 5-year overall survival was 78% versus 90% (log rank = 0.01) and cancer-specific survival was 100% versus 98% (log rank = 0.65). The authors concluded that older patients with compromised renal function and warm ischemia time greater than 30 min are at high risk for renal dysfunction after LPN.

Alternate nephron-sparing methods, including hypothermia or probe-ablation, should be considered in these patients.[7] Therefore, it is the authors' opinion that LPN in solitary kidney or with compromised renal function should be done by an experienced surgeon. To minimize the complications on renal function, cold ischemia through an open approach should be considered and patient counseling about possible temporary postoperative dialysis should be explained. If warm ischemia is considered, then the authors recommend early unclamping as described previously.

Presence of Vena Caval or Abdominal Aortic Pathology

Patients with vascular pathology involving the great vessels like abdominal aortic aneurysm, post aortic graft or vena caval pathology are prone to develop renal masses and require therapy. Those patients are typically elderly with comorbid medical conditions such as diabetes, hypertension, and mostly are on anticoagulants or antiplatelets. Subsequently they are high-riskanesthesia patients, requiring a careful approach and are considered challenging cases. The authors have reported on 17 cases of LPN in such a group of patients, with very acceptable and safe outcome.[8] The important aspects of managing such difficult patients is proper preoperative evaluation, including CT angiography to assess the renal vasculature and relation to the vascular pathology. Vascular surgeon consultation and possible intraoperative advice from that perspective is also important. Finally, the most important aspect is careful pre-, intra-, and postoperative anesthetic management with the need for invasive monitoring and intensive care unit (ICU) postoperative care for this group of high-risk patients. The careful surgical steps of LPN and accurate hemostasis is absolutely mandatory in this subgroup of patients who will mostly require antiplatelets or anticoagulants postoperatively.

Diaphragmatic Injury During Partial Nephrectomy

Inadvertent diaphragmatic injury can occur during laparoscopic renal or adrenal surgery, especially in difficult cases. The authors have reported a 0.7% risk in a large series of 1,850 cases of laparoscopic renal and adrenal surgery. Four cases of diaphragmatic injury occurred during LPN. These injuries were recognized immediately and managed with nonabsorbable running suture. The outcomes of these injuries were excellent in all cases. Although uncommon, managing these types of difficulties is an important aspect in performing laparoscopic partial nephrectomy safely.[9]

Laparoscopic Partial Nephrectomy in the Presence of Multiple Renal Arteries

The authors reported on LPN in kidneys with multiple arteries and compared those outcomes with LPN outcomes in patients with conventional renal arterial anatomy. In the authors' series, since September 1999, LPN was performed for tumors in 333 patients. From this prospectively maintained database, the authors identified 60 patients with multiple renal arteries and 273 patients with a single renal artery to the operated kidney. All patients underwent three-dimensional computed tomography preoperatively for accurate delineation of the tumor and renal vascular anatomy. The clinical and operative data were reviewed to assess critical outcomes. The baseline parameters, including tumor size ($P = 0.87$), were similar in the two groups. Intraoperatively, the method of vascular control, tumor parenchymal extension depth ($P = 0.40$), number requiring pelvicaliceal repair ($P = 0.62$), and specimen weight ($P = 0.49$) were similar between the two groups. Similarly, the warm ischemia time ($P = 0.60$), operative time ($P = 0.15$), blood loss ($P = 0.37$), and intraoperative ($P = 0.52$), postoperative ($P = 0.48$), and late complication ($P = 0.64$) rates were similar between the two groups. The authors' conclusion was that LPN can be efficaciously performed in the presence of multiple renal vessels. Preoperative evaluation with three-dimensional computed tomography is recommended to have preoperative knowledge of the renal vasculature and thereby minimize iatrogenic injury.[10] It is important that all the vessels to be included in the hilar clamp to minimize the intraoperative bleeding and subsequently the excision of the tumor and the renorrhaphy will be optimal.

Laparoscopic Partial Nephrectomy in Previously Operated Kidney

Previous renal surgery has been considered a relative contraindication to LPN because of perirenal surgical adhesions. The authors reported on their experience of LPN in previously operated kidneys in which 25 patients (3.7%) had undergone previous ipsilateral open or percutaneous renal procedures. Previous renal surgery included open surgery in 12 patients (nephro/pyelolithotomy in 8, pyeloplasty in 2, and partial nephrectomy in 2) and percutaneous surgery in 13 (percutaneous nephrolithotomy in 9 and renal biopsy in 4). The mean interval from previous surgery was 6.6 years (range 0.3–34). LPNs (16 transperitoneal and 9 retroperitoneal) were successful in all patients. The mean tumor size was 2.5 cm (range 1–5.6), the warm ischemia time was 35.8 min (range 22–57), and the estimated blood loss was 215 mL (range 25–600). The mean operative time was 3 h (range 1.5–4.5), and the hospital stay was 3.1 days (range 1–7.6). Histopathologic examination confirmed renal cell carcinoma in 19 patients (76%). No open conversions were needed, and no kidneys were lost. No intraoperative complications were reported, but three postoperative complications (12%) developed, including blood transfusion in one, nausea and epistaxis in one, and compartment syndrome requiring fasciotomy in one patient. The results of the authors' study have shown that, in select patients, LPN is feasible after previous ipsilateral renal surgery. However, the procedure can be technically challenging, and adequate previous experience with LPN is necessary.[11] As in any difficult situation, the patient must be informed of the possibility of total nephrectomy or open conversion, and priority must be given to the patient's safety and cancer control.

Laparoscopic Partial Nephrectomy in Obese Patients

Obesity is occasionally encountered during laparoscopic renal surgery and is considered technically challenging because of the anesthetic as well as the access issues related to laparoscopy. The authors reported their series from August 1999 to December 2004 in which 140 obese (group 1) and 238 nonobese (group 2) patients underwent laparoscopic partial nephrectomy at their institution. The demographics, operative data, and perioperative complications of these two groups were compared. Group 1 had a significantly greater incidence of hypertension and diabetes. In groups 1 and 2, respectively, the mean estimated blood loss was 310 mL (range 50–1,500) and 249 mL (range 50–2,500), the mean operating time was 3.4 h (range 2.5–6) and 3.4 h (range 1.5–6), and the mean warm ischemia time was 31 min (range 15–51) and 32 min (range 12–60). Intraoperative complications occurred in eight patients (5.7%) in group 1 and 20 (8%) in group 2 ($P = 0.19$), with a blood transfusion rate of 6% and 3%, respectively ($P = 0.42$). The postoperative complication rate was not significantly different between the two groups (13% vs 9%, $P = 0.77$). The mean hospital stay was 2.8 days (range 1–8) for group 1 and 3.5 days (range 1–32) for group 2. Retroperitoneal access was associated with a shorter operative time and hospital stay in both groups. The authors concluded that laparoscopic partial nephrectomy was performed safely in obese patients, with a perioperative complication rate similar to that of non-obese patients. The retroperitoneal approach was associated with a shorter operative time and hospital stay in the obese and non-obese patients.[12] In another series from the John Hopkins group on LPN, comparison of obese versus non-obese patients who underwent LPN revealed similar perioperative outcomes, with the exception of a greater blood loss in the obese patient cohort (391.7 ± 308.6 vs 280.9 ± 202.1 mL). Finally, in comparing perioperative data among non-obese patients who underwent open partial nephrectomy (OPN) versus LPN, those who underwent LPN were found to have improved operative times (248.9 ± 45.0 vs 181.1 ± 62.4 min), less blood loss (412.4 ± 274.6 vs 280.9 ± 202.1 mL), fewer intraoperative complications (21.4% vs 1.8%), and shorter length of hospital stay (6.3 ± 2.8 vs 3.2 ± 1.6 days). Laparoscopic partial nephrectomy has significantly better perioperative outcomes than open partial nephrectomy in both the obese and non-obese populations. As of late, the authors perform LPN via a transperitoneal approach in all patients, including obese patients, with excellent outcomes.[13]

Laparoscopic Partial Nephrectomy in Cystic Lesions

LPN in cystic lesions, which are typically complex renal cysts of Bosniak 3 or over, are best managed laparoscopically as this minimizes the morbidity of open surgery and achieves the diagnostic and therapeutic goals needed. But extreme care should be used when approaching the cyst so as not to puncture it and cause spillage, since malignancy is a serious risk of tumor spillage. The authors reported on their experience regarding cystic renal masses, which comprised 17.1% of their series and compared the outcomes to similar sized solid masses. No cyst spillage was encountered. Only one local recurrence was found during follow up, although the margins were negative. Surgical outcomes of LPN for suspicious cystic masses are similar to those of LPN for solid tumors. However, extreme caution and refined laparoscopic technique must be exercised to avoid cyst rupture and local spillage.[14] This includes the handling of the cyst during dissection and excision. Also, preparation of the retrieval bag is important to avoid accidental cyst rupture by the surgeon and assistant at the end of the procedure.

Laparoscopic Partial Nephrectomy in Horseshoe Kidney

Horseshoe kidney is an anatomically challenging kidney because of its vascular anatomy, specifically in relation to LPN. Subsequently, detailed preoperative imaging with CT angiography is essential to preoperatively identify the vascular pedicle close to the tumor area so that it may be clamped during tumor excision. Subsequently, the same technique is used to complete the procedure. Since the renal anatomy and position of the kidney is abnormal, extra care is required for deep tumors and repair of the collecting system is essential.[15]

Laparoscopic Partial Nephrectomy for Tumor in the Presence of Nephrolithiasis or Pelvi-Ureteric Junction Obstruction (PUJO)

Fifteen (3%) of 548 patients who underwent LPN (November 1999 to May 2005) had concomitant calculus/PUJO. The calculus/PUJO was treated in six, either before (one), during (three), or after (two) LPN, depending on the presence of obstruction. The remaining nine patients were monitored as they had a punctate and unobstructing stone burden. The mean (range) tumor size was 2.7 (1.4–4) cm, the operative duration was 3.8 (2–6) h, the warm ischemia time was 34.8 (22–53) min, and blood loss was 237 (50–600) mL. Two patients with concomitant PUJO had a single-session dismembered Anderson-Hynes pyeloplasty and LPN. Three patients with smaller stones (5–12 mm) had extracorporeal shock wave lithotripsy, percutaneous nephrolithotomy, or ureteroscopic removal before (one) or after (two) LPN. One patient with a larger 1.6-cm obstructing renal pelvic calculus had laparoscopic flexible pyeloscopy, but the stone was not visualized. At the end of all treatments, the 6-month tumor-free and stone-free rates were 15/15 and 11/13, respectively. The authors concluded that patients with a concomitant small renal mass and calculus/PUJO can be successfully managed in a simultaneous or staged manner using minimally invasive techniques. In managing such cases, it is very important to ensure patency of the ureter during LPN to avoid urine leakage complication.[16]

Laparosopic Partial Nephrectomy After Targeted Therapy

Targeted therapy is currently used in locally advanced renal cell carcinoma and metastatic disease. Subsequently surgical resection of renal tumors are indicated. The authors retrospectively identified patients with renal cell carcinoma treated with sunitinib, sorafenib, or bevacizumab plus interleukin-2 before tumor resection. Between June 2005 and August 2008, 19 patients were treated with targeted therapy and subsequently underwent resection. Surgical extirpation involved an open and a laparoscopic approach in 18 and 3 cases, respectively, for locally advanced (8), locally recurrent (6), and metastatic disease (3). Two patients with extensive bilateral renal cell carcinoma were also treated to downsize the tumors to enable partial nephrectomy. Perioperative complications were noted in 16% of patients. One patient had a significant intraoperative hemorrhage and disseminated intravascular coagulopathy from a concomitant liver resection. An anastomotic bowel leak and abscess were noted postoperatively in another patient who underwent en bloc resection of a retroperitoneal recurrence and adjacent colon. Two patients (11%) had minor wound complications, including a wound seroma and a ventral hernia. Pathological analysis of 20 specimens revealed clear cell, chromophobe, and unclassified renal cell carcinoma in 80%, 5%, and 10% of cases, respectively. One patient (5%) had a pathological complete response. Surgical resection of renal cell carcinoma after targeted therapy is feasible with low morbidity in most patients. However, significant complications can occur, raising concern for possible compromise of tissue and/or vascular integrity associated with surgery in this setting. Although the number of cases treated by LPN is small in this difficult subgroup of patients, it was technically feasible with more than average complications that need careful management.[17]

Decreasing Complications in Laparoscopic Partial Nephrectomy

Laparoscopic partial nephrectomy, in contrast, is a technically challenging procedure. Although the intermediate oncologic outcomes are comparable to those of the open experience, there are concerns related to warm ischemia time, and there is a risk of major complications such as urinary leakage and hemorrhage requiring transfusion.[2]

Centrally located renal tumors may be associated with more complications according to some series. Provided that there is adequate laparoscopic expertise, the outcome of laparoscopic partial nephrectomy for central tumors is comparable to that of peripheral tumors. The main major complication in this group was late-onset hematuria, which necessitated angiographic embolization. This facility should be available at centers where these advanced procedures are performed.[4]

Urine leakage after laparoscopic partial nephrectomy has been reported in some series to be 10.5%. Urine leak is a complication unique to partial nephrectomy that is more commonly noted when a larger endophytic mass involves the renal collecting system. Most leaks resolve with prolonged drainage or replacement of a ureteral stent.[18] The meticulous repair of the collecting system in a bloodless field and the renorrhaphy that the authors use has rarely lead to urine leakage in their series.

Hemorrhage during or after laparoscopic partial nephrectomy is reported to be less than in open series, and, with the renal hilar clamping as described in the authors' technique,[2] it is a very manageable issue. Hilar tumors in close proximity to the interlobar vessels can even be managed laparoscopically without difficulty but require experienced hands.[3]

Finally, renal impairment is a risk after laparoscopic partial nephrectomy. Multiple studies have considered the warm ischemia time of 30 min is satisfactory in not affecting renal function especially if there is a normal contralateral kidney. Lately, with improved technique, the authors reported halving the warm ischemia time by early unclamping while repairing the renal bed with excellent renal function preservation.[19] Others have reported on artery only occlusion with better renal function preservation, although only on a small series.[20]

In conclusion, the authors are pleased that, in their series, warm ischemia time of less than 30 min can be achieved in most cases of LPN, which subsequently will not harm the kidneys in most cases, but this technique requires significant surgical experience.

Overcoming Difficulties During Laparoscopic Partial Nephrectomy

The authors recommend the following steps to overcome difficulties during LPN:

1. Proper preoperative workup, including CT angiography, renal function tests, complete blood cell count (CBC), blood for cross-match.
2. Proper instruments, sutures, and hemostatic agents.
3. Intraoperative ultrasound assessment of tumor depth.
4. Careful hilar dissection and clamping in preparation for tumor excision.
5. Tumor excision with 5-mm margin, and then repair of the renal bed in efficient and expeditious way.
6. Careful postoperative evaluation of early outcome including renal function tests, CBC, and confirming absence or resolution of urine leakage and evaluation of surgical margin for oncologic control.

Conclusion

Laparoscopic partial nephrectomy has duplicated open surgery in a very competitive and comparable way. It does require significant laparoscopic surgical skills and careful pre-, intra-, and postoperative measures. Currently, more complex cases can be done laparoscopically with excellent results, but as previously stated, such cases require more experienced hands to achieve the best results.

References

1. Gill IS, Kavoussi LR, Lane BR, et al. Comparison of 1, 800 laparoscopic and open partial nephrectomies for single renal tumors. *J Urol*. 2007;178(1):41-46.
2. Haper GP, Gill IS. Laparoscopic partial nephrectomy: contemporary technique and outcomes. *Eur Urol*. 2006;49(4):660-665.
3. Lattouf JB, Beri A, D'Ambros OF, Grüll M, Leeb K, Janetschek G. Laparoscopic partial nephrectomy for hilar tumors: technique and results. *Eur Urol*. 2008;54(2):409-416.
4. Nadu A, Kleinmann N, Laufer M, Dotan Z, Winkler H, Ramon J. Laparoscopic partial nephrectomy for central tumors: analysis of perioperative outcomes and complications. *J Urol*. 2009;181(1):42-47.
5. Turna B, Frota R, Kamoi K, et al. Risk factor analysis of postoperative complications in laparoscopic partial nephrectomy. *J Urol*. 2008;179(4):1289-1294.
6. Gill IS, Colombo JR Jr, Moinzadeh A, et al. Laparoscopic partial nephrectomy in solitary kidney. *J Urol*. 2006;175(2):454-458.
7. Columbo JR Jr, Haber GP, Gill IS. Laparoscopic partial nephrectomy in patients with compromised renal function. *Urology*. 2008;71(6):1043-1048.
8. Lin YC, Haber GP, Turna B, et al. Laparoscopic renal oncological surgery in the presence of abdominal aortic and vena caval pathology: 8-year experience. *J Urol*. 2008;179(2):455-460.

9. Aron M, Colombo JR Jr, Turna B, Stein RJ, Haber GP, Gill IS. Diaphragmatic repair and/or reconstruction during upper abdominal urological laparoscopy. *J Urol*. 2007;178(6): 2444-2450.

10. Singh D, Finelli A, Rubinstein M, Desai MM, Kaouk J, Gill IS. Laparoscopic partial nephrectomy in the presence of multiple renal arteries. *Urology*. 2007;69(3):444-447.

11. Turna B, Aron M, Frota R, Desai MM, Kaouk J, Gill IS. Feasibility of laparoscopic partial nephrectomy after previous ipsilateral renal procedures. *Urology*. 2008;72(3):584-588.

12. Colombo JR Jr, Haber GP, Aron M, Xu M, Gill IS. Laparoscopic partial nephrectomy in obese patients. *Urology*. 2007;69(1):44-48.

13. Romero FR, Rais-Bahrami S, Muntener M, Brito FA, Jarret TW, Kavoussi LR. Laparoscopic partial nephrectomy in obese and non-obese patients: comparison with open surgery. *Urology*. 2008;71(5):806-809.

14. Spaliviero M, Herts BR, Magi-Galluzzi C, et al. Laparoscopic partial nephrectomy for cystic masses. *J Urol*. 2006;175(4):1577-1578.

15. Tsivian A, Shtricker A, Benjamin S, Sidi AA. Laparoscopic partial nephrectomy for tumour excision in a horseshoe kidney. *Eur Urol*. 2007;51(4):1132-1133.

16. Baccala A, Lee U, Hegarty N, Desai M, Kaouk J, Gill I. Laparoscopic partial nephrectomy for tumour in the presence of nephrolithiasis or pelvi-ureteric junction obstruction. *BJU Int*. 2009;103(5):660-662.

17. Thomas AA, Rini BL, Stephenson AJ, et al. Surgical resection of renal cell carcinoma after targeted therapy. *J Urol*. 2009;182(3):881-886.

18. Meeks JJ, Zhao LC, Navai N, Perry KT Jr, Nadler RB, Smith ND. Risk factors and management of urine leaks after partial nephrectomy. *J Urol*. 2008;180(6):2375-2378.

19. Nguyen MM, Gill IS. Halving ischemia time during laparoscopic partial nephrectomy. *J Urol*. 2008;179(2):627-632.

20. Gong EM, Zorn KC, Orvieto MA, Lucioni A, Msezane LP, Shalhav AL. Artery-only occlusion may provide superior renal preservation during laparoscopic partial nephrectomy. *Urology*. 2008;72(4):843-846.

Difficulties in Laparoscopic Adrenalectomy

12

Mahesh R. Desai and Arvind P. Ganpule

Introduction

Laparoscopic adrenalectomy is the method of choice in the majority of adrenal lesions. The open surgical approach for adrenal lesions requires a long skin incision, which at times may require muscle and rib cutting. The laparoscopic approach is quick and safe, the magnification offers excellent visibility, and blood loss is substantially decreased if the surgical technique is meticulous. Adrenalectomy is also one of the few laparoscopic procedures in which, due to the quick access to the area in question, has a shorter operative time.[1] Although there is general agreement on use of this approach for benign and small lesions, the issue of the laparoscopic approach in adrenocortical carcinomas remains unresolved.[2] This chapter discusses operative technique and troubleshooting measures. The steps, which require attention before and during adrenalectomy include:

1. Preoperative preparation of the patient
2. Preoperative imaging to ascertain the possible nature of the disease and the status of the contralateral gland
3. Port placements to ensure unhindered dissection
4. Tips and tricks to identify the adrenal vein and prevent hemorrhage during the procedure

Surgical Anatomy

The right gland is more superiorly located in the retroperitoneum. It is almost directly cranial to the upper pole of the right kidney. Surrounding structures include the liver anterolaterally, the duodenum anteromedially, and the inferior vena cava medially. It is also important to note that there is often a retrocaval extension of the gland on the right side. These facts are important for optimal port placement and dissection in relation to the vena

M.R. Desai (✉)
Department of Urology, Muljibhai Patel Urological Hospital, Nadlad, Gujarat, India
e-mail: mrdesai@mpuh.org

A.M. Al-Kandari and I.S. Gill (eds.), *Difficult Conditions in Laparoscopic Urologic Surgery*, 137
DOI: 10.1007/978-1-84882-105-7_12, © Springer-Verlag London Limited 2011

cava. The left gland is crescentic and medial to the upper pole of the left kidney. The upper and anterior aspects are related to the stomach, tail of the pancreas, and splenic vessels.[3] During dissection of the splenic flexure, the above structures need to be protected.

The arterial supply to the adrenal gland originates from three sources. Superiorly, from the inferior phrenic artery, few branches directly originate from the aorta. At times, branches from the aorta also supply the adrenal. Most of the time, no definite artery can be identified. Frequently, both the adrenals are drained by a single adrenal vein. The adrenal vein is the key structure to be identified during adrenalectomy. On the left side it enters the cranial aspect of the left renal vein. On the right side, the adrenal vein enters the vena cava directly on its posterolateral aspect.[3] The significance of this lies in securing the adrenal vein during adrenalectomy. The short stump of the adrenal vein and its origin from the cava require care when applying lateral traction. In regards to the left adrenal vein, it arises from the inferomedial aspect of the gland to enter the renal vein. This vessel has a close relation to the upper polar renal artery, upper polar branch of the main renal artery, and the inferior phrenic artery. One should be cautious of these structures while securing the adrenal vein.

The Surgical Procedure

The authors prefer the transperitoneal approach. All the laparoscopic adrenalectomies at the authors' center are carried out via the lateral transperitoneal approach.

Transperitoneal Approach

Left Side

Once the pneumoperitoneum is created, the ports are placed (Fig. 12.1), the white line of Toldt is incised and the colon reflected. The key step for adequate exposure is dissection of the splenorenal ligament right down to the splenic hilum (Fig. 12.2). The colon should be reflected optimally to expose the renal vein. The adrenal vein is identified from its origin from the renal vein. The authors prefer to secure the renal vein with the help of either Allport® (Ethicon Endo-Surgery, Inc., Cincinnati, Oh) or Ligaclips (Ethicon Endo-Surgery, Inc., Cincinnati, OH). In the authors' initial cases, the Hem-o-lok clip™ (Teleflex Medical, Research Triangle Park, NC) was used for ligation. The next step to be followed is dissection posterior to the clips along the psoas muscle (Fig. 12.3). Once this is done, the dissection should be outside the adrenal fascia; this helps in preventing fractures of the adrenal. The next step is dissection along the superior border of the aorta. As the adrenal does not have any definite blood supply, any suspicious blood vessels should be secured. The medial wall of the adrenal is dissected last. In all cases of adrenal lesions suspected to be pheochromocytomas, the adrenal vein should be secured first; in all other cases it is prudent to dissect and secure the adrenal vein last because of the concern that early ligation of the adrenal vein might cause congestion of the gland and subsequent oozing.

Port position and liver retraction

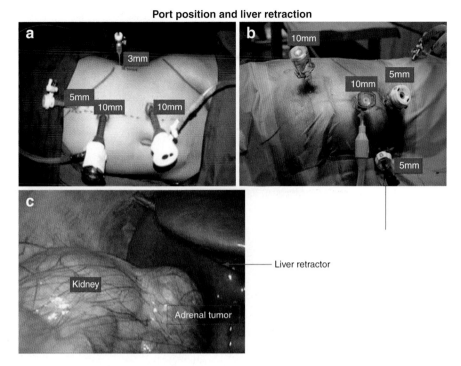

Fig. 12.1 (**a**) Left-side transperitoneal adrenalectomy with four ports (one 10 mm for camera, one 10 mm for working instruments, one 5 mm for retraction, and occasionally one 3 mm for lateral retraction). (**b**) Right transperitoneal adrenalectomy with 4-port approach. The ports mirror the left side; an additional 5-mm port helps in liver retraction. (**c**) 5 mm Allis locking forceps helps in retraction of the liver on the right side; note that the adrenal mass is easily visible through the peritoneum

Right Side

The port placement mirrors that on the left side, except an extra port is required for retraction of the liver (Fig. 12.1). The lie of the colon differs on the right side as compared to the left, the landmarks to be identified in these cases are the inferior vena cava and the renal vein (Fig. 12.3). Once the kocherization of the duodenum is done, the inferior vena cava is traced, this is followed by identifying the renal vein. The adrenal gland is dissected on the superior border of the vena cava. The dissection on the under surface of the liver needs to be aggressive for proper identification and securing of the adrenal vein. The adrenal vein can be secured with Hem-o-lok™ clips (Fig. 12.4).

All adrenalectomy specimens should be bagged before retrieval, typically they are retrieved by extending one of the ports.

Although a variety of approaches have been described, all of them have their own advantages and disadvantages. In a nonrandomized, background-matched analysis, the authors of a study concluded that if a tumor was more than 5 cm and the surgeon not

Fig. 12.2 (**a**, **b**) On the left
side, aggressive dissection
of the splenic flexure with
division of splenocolic
ligament makes the spleen
fall off and provides
exposure of the adrenal bed.
(**c**) On the left side, the
renal vein acts as a guide to
identify the adrenal vein.
(**d**) Dissection of adrenal
the vein

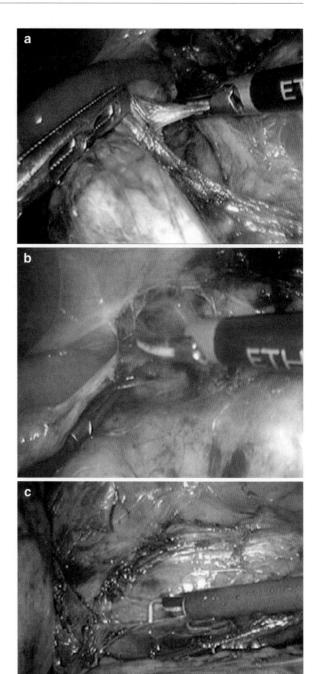

Fig. 12.2 (continued)

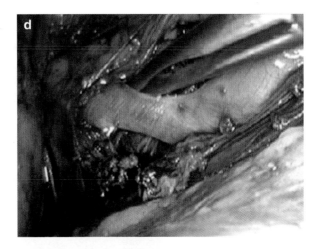

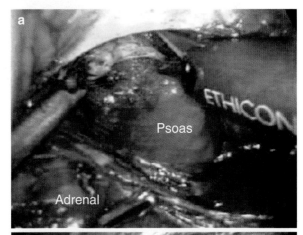

Fig. 12.3 (**a**, **b**) Once the adrenal vein is secured, the next step should be to identify the psoas; this helps in the dissection between the kidney and adrenal without injuring either. (**c**, **d**) The vena cava and renal vein are the landmarks for dissection on the right side

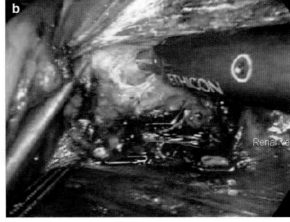

Fig. 12.3 (continued)

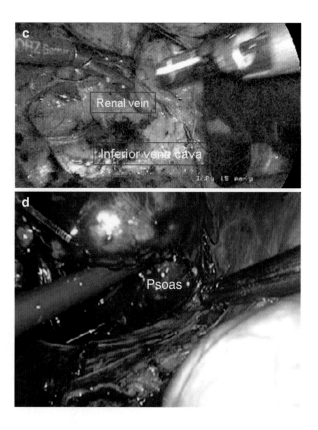

Securing the adrenal vein with Hem-o-lok™

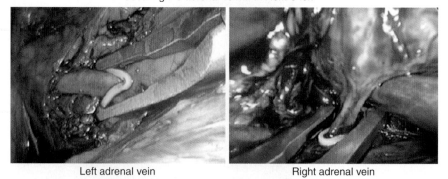

Left adrenal vein   Right adrenal vein

Fig. 12.4 The adrenal vein should be circumferentially dissected prior to clipping. This helps in proper application of clips

experienced, then the lateral transperitoneal approach was preferred. The lateral retroperitoneal approach was also preferred in cases with upper abdominal surgeries.[4, 5]

In the *anterior transperitoneal approach*, the patient is in semi-lateral position. On the right side the hepatocolic ligament is incised, while on the left side the phrenicocolic ligament is incised.

In the *lateral transperitoneal approach*, the patient is in full lateral position. In this approach, the dissection is carried out till the diaphragm close to the curvature of the stomach. The spleen falls off the operating field, which helps to improve the exposure. On the right side, mobilization of the triangular ligament is carried out. The dissection is continued up to the diaphragm. This helps in allowing good exposure as the liver is shifted away from the operating field.

Retroperitoneal Approach

The patient is placed in a lateral decubitus position. A 15-mm incision is made under the 12th rib. The space is created with the help of a balloon dilator after finger dissection. The camera port is inserted and the rest of the ports are inserted under vision; a five-trocar approach has been described (one is 12 mm, two are 10 mm, and two are 5 mm). The kidney remains in contact with its peritoneal attachment. The psoas muscle acts as a landmark. The renal vein on the left side and the vena cava on the right side are identified to ascertain the position of the adrenal vein. The suction drain is kept at the conclusion of the procedure. The specimen is always bagged.[6]

Key Steps to Avoid Problems in Laparoscopic Adrenalectomy

Preoperative Preparation of the Patient

Optimal preoperative preparation in patients undergoing surgery for pheochromocytoma is key to success and safety. The pillars of success are:

1. Correction of biochemical abnormalities
2. Volume repletion
3. Bowel preparation for transperitoneal approach

Patients to be operated for pheochromocytoma need special care. Alpha-adrenergic blockade should be started 2 weeks before surgery, preferably phenoxybenzamine, starting gradually with a dose of 10–20 mg twice per day. Some individuals may require beta blockade. Intraoperatively, high blood pressure can be treated with nitroprusside or a short-acting β(beta) blocker like esmolol. Volume repletion is important to prevent the postoperative hypotension secondary to loss of tonic vasoconstriction.

Patients with Cushing's syndrome require correction of electrolyte abnormalities and diabetes before surgery. It is prudent to estimate cortisol levels in these patients. These patients are prone to infection and they should be administered preoperative antibiotics. Occasionally they may need steroids, intraoperatively or postoperatively.[3]

Imaging Studies

It is generally accepted that the plain film of the abdomen has little value in identifying and evaluating adrenal tumors, although calcification within an adrenal mass is commonly thought to signal malignancy. Ultrasound, although effective, may be of limited benefit in obese patients and patients having overlying bowel gas. Computed tomography (CT) generally is considered the method of choice in the radiodiagnostic evaluation of adrenal disease. The location, size, and shape of adrenal masses and nodules as small as 1 cm generally are demonstrated using conventional CT techniques. However, using thin-section CT scanning, nodules as small as 3–5 mm can be identified. Magnetic resonance imaging (MRI) improves adrenal imaging and provides prognostic help by appearance of the lesion on T1 and T2 imaging modes.[7]

Exposure of the Adrenal Gland

Difficulties may arise due to inadequate exposure of the adrenal gland, leading to troublesome hemorrhage from the adrenal vein and the adrenal gland. These Most of the time the solution is proper port placement, adequate mobilization of the colon, and exposure of the splenorenal recess (Figs. 12.1–12.3).

Port Placement and Patient Positioning

The patient in a lateral position in a transperitoneal approach offers adequate exposure as the viscera tends to fall with gravity. The port position at the authors' center is as shown in Fig. 12.1. It resembles that of a transperitoneal nephrectomy, and typically the ports are placed more cranially as compared to the position in a nephrectomy. In addition, the colon should be reflected adequately so that the renal vein is adequately exposed. The adrenal bed is better exposed when the splenorenal ligament is taken down along the greater curvature of the stomach.

Placing an additional port, which may be either a 3- or 5-mm port, improves the exposure. A retractor inserted through this port helps in retracting the kidney and delineating the mass in a better way, but one needs to be careful of injuring the spleen/liver through such laterally placed ports on the left side.[8]

The port for retracting the liver should be inserted in the midline as high as possible near the xiphisternum and passed along the undersurface of the liver towards the lateral sidewall. Care must be taken to avoid injuring the gall bladder. Various instruments can be used to retract the liver; they include the fan retractors and locking Allis 5-mm clamps. The authors use the locking Allis clamp for the purpose. The Allis clamp is closed and locked, thereby creating a self-retaining retractor that does not require an assistant to hold it (Fig. 12.1).

Mobilizing the spleen is a safe and feasible way of gaining adequate exposure on the left. While mobilizing the spleen, care must be taken not to tear the splenic capsule or to injure the diaphragm. If, however, in spite of extensive mobilization one finds a floppy spleen, a suprapubic trocar can be inserted and a sponge holder with gauze can be used for retracting the spleen and the pancreas.

Dissection of the Adrenal Vein

The adrenal vein is identified on the left side by identifying the renal vein. At times the renal vein can be identified by tracing the origin of the gonadal vein (Fig. 12.2). The gonadal vein almost always enters the renal vein opposite the entry point of the left adrenal vein. Therefore, upon reaching the left renal vein along the gonadal vein, dissection is performed medially along the anterior surface of the renal vein to identify the left adrenal vein. The key point in the dissection of the adrenal vein is that it should be dissected for a considerable length. The adrenal vein should always be dissected till the limit of the adrenal gland is seen (Fig. 12.2).

The adrenal gland should be dissected outside the periadventitial plane, if this plane is not followed, one runs the risk of causing parenchymal fractures and persistent oozing from the adrenal surface. On the left side, a combination of blunt and sharp dissection helps to free the gland from the aorta and the upper pole of the kidney (Fig. 12.3). Particular care should be taken while coagulating small adrenal vessels as they may cause tears in the adrenal parenchyma.

On the right side, the adrenal gland is more easily identified through the peritoneum (Fig. 12.1). The lower aspect is separated from the renal vein (with care taken to preserve the upper polar renal artery), the medial aspect is cleared from the inferior vena cava.

Adrenalectomy in Difficult Situations

Obese Patients

Markedly obese patients have increased chance of surgical complications; this fact assumes importance in patients with Cushing's syndrome with truncal obesity.

In their study, Fazeli-Matin et al. concluded that, compared to open surgery, the laparoscopic approach offers decreased blood loss, quicker return of bowel function, less analgesia, and shorter convalescence. They observed that abdominal wall obesity is located in the pannus, which in flank position shifts from the operative side, thus flank position offers the opportunity to use routine ports. They felt that a retroperitoneoscopy approach offers a shorter and more direct route to the kidney compared to the transperitoneal approach. The points in operating on these patients include the following: experience of the surgeon; adequate padding of all pressure points; to maintain pneumoperitoneum, use of two carbon dioxide insufflators; and insufflation done with balloon dilators and kept anterior to the psoas fascia.[9]

Large Tumors and Malignancy

The opinions differ as far as adrenocortical carcinoma (ACC) is concerned. It is a deadly disease and complete resection is of utmost importance. Miller et al., in their retrospective study, concluded that laparoscopic approach should not be done in adrenocortical carcinomas.[10] The absolute contraindication for laparoscopic adrenalectomy is adrenocortical carcinomas with periadrenal invasion or venous thrombus. The relative contraindications include uncorrected coagulopathy, abdominal sepsis, intestinal obstruction, and unacceptable cardiopulmonary risk.[11] Although size alone is not a contraindication, there is considerable debate as to the size threshold for offering laparoscopic adrenalectomy as it is well known that the incidence of carcinoma increases with increasing size.[12] The estimation of risk of ACC for lesions more than 6 cm is 25% and for tumors between 4 and 6 cm is 6% and 2% for tumors <4 cm in size, as stated in the National Institutes of Health (NIH) consensus statement.[13] The authors' data revealed an incidence of 5.2% of ACC in tumors larger than 5 cm.[14] Other potential problems associated with offering laparoscopic adrenalectomy for large adrenal masses are anatomical considerations, handling of tumor, technical difficulty in dissecting large adrenal tumor, increased likelihood of complications and peritoneal dissemination of carcinoma. There is no well-defined arterial supply to the adrenal gland.[11] There will be more technical difficulty in dissection of the large adrenal mass, leading to higher chances of intraoperative hemorrhage. Direct handling of a larger tumor is more likely to lead to fracture during handling, resulting in troublesome bleeding and inadequate removal and peritoneal dissemination.[11]

The prerequisites include proper preoperative diagnosis as suggested by Suzuki; findings of heterogeneous mass lesions and irregular mass lesions on CT may suggest a malignancy. The lesion should be completely removed; incompletely removed lesions have a uniformly poor prognosis.[15]

Pediatric Patients

These patients should have a proper anesthesia checkup. It is advisable to have pediatric instruments (5-mm harmonic scalpel, pediatric suction and dissecting instruments). The working pneumoperitoneum pressures should be 8–10. The adrenal tumors are usually easily visible in the transperitoneal approach. In all these cases, a biochemical workup is prudent. The adrenal vein is secured with the help of an Allport® or Ligaclips.

Reports are available that describe this approach for neuroblastomas. Laparoscopic adrenalectomy for neuroblastomas is safe and feasible in children with good results; the prerequisite being adequate experience with advanced laparoscopy. In a study by de Lagausie, adrenalectomy was performed in nine patients. The mean operative time was 85 min with no deaths. There was no instance of recurrence or metastasis. The authors noted that a transperitoneal approach is recommended because of the necessity of exploring the entire abdomen to detect and inspect enlarged lymph nodes. This approach also facilitates exploration of the aortocaval space and the hepatosplenic region. The results are good for stage I tumors.[16]

Laparoscopic Adrenalectomy for Adrenal Metastasis

Most malignancies that metastasize to the adrenal are to the medullary portion (center) of the gland, rather than to the adrenal cortex. Adrenal metastases rarely penetrate through the capsule of the gland, making laparoscopic surgical resection much less likely to result in tumor fracture, which could potentially predispose a patient to increased rates of local recurrence or intraperitoneal dissemination To date, eight series totaling 98 patients have reported the use of laparoscopic adrenalectomy for metastasis with no port-site recurrences and only one patient (1%) developing peritoneal dissemination of disease.[17]

Postoperative Management

Electrolyte values are checked the night of surgery and each morning; this is especially important for patients with Conn's or Cushing's syndrome. The urinary catheter can usually be removed on the first postoperative day when the patient is ambulatory. If a nasogastric tube was placed for open surgery, it can be removed with return of bowel sounds. Diet resumption is usually started on the first postoperative day for laparoscopic surgery and when bowel sounds resume for open surgery.

Blood pressure is carefully evaluated for hypertension or hypotension. Unexplained hypotension, confusion, lethargy, nausea, vomiting, or fever could represent addisonian crisis (adrenal insufficiency). Adrenal insufficiency is most commonly seen after surgery for Cushing's syndrome as a result of contra lateral cortisol suppression.

Conclusion

The key steps in adrenalectomy include adequate adrenal exposure; working along landmarks such as the renal vein, vena cava and psoas; early adrenal vein identification and clipping; and bagging of all specimens. Difficult situations such as pediatric cases, adrenocortical carcinomas, etc., should be done with discretion, depending on the experience of the surgeon. The surgeon should choose the approach (retroperitoneal or transperitoneal) with discretion. The surgeon should also not hesitate to convert to open surgery when needed.

References

1. Janetschek G, Altarac S, Finkenstedt G, Gasser R, Bartsch G. Technique and results of laparoscopic adrenalectomy. *Eur Urol*. 1996;30:475-479.
2. Porpigilia F, Destefanis P, Fiori C, et al. Does adrenal mass size really affect safety and effectiveness of laparoscopic adrenalectomy? *Urology*. 2002;60:801-805.

3. Chow GK, Blute ML. Surgery of the adrenal gland. In: Wein, Kavoussi, Novick, Partin, Peters, eds. *Campbell-Walsh Urology*. 9th ed. Philadelphia, PA: Saunders; 2007:1869.
4. Terachi T, Matsuda T, Terai A, et al. Transperitoneal laparoscopic adrenalectomy: experience with 100 patients. *J Endourol*. 1997;11:361-365.
5. Suzuki K, Kayeyama S, Hirano Y, Ushiyama T, Rajamahanty S, Fujita K. Comparison of 3 surgical approaches to laparoscopic adrenalectomy: a nonrandomized background matched analysis. *J Urol*. 2001;166:437-443.
6. Gasman D, Droopy S, Koutani A, et al. Laparoscopic adrenalectomy: the retroperitoneal approach. *J Urol*. 1998;159:1816-1820.
7. Wajchenberg BL, Albergaria Pereira MA, Medonca BB, et al. Adrenocortical carcinoma: clinical and laboratory observations. *Cancer*. 2000;88(4):711-736.
8. Udaya K, Gill IS, eds. *Tips and Tricks in Laparoscopic Urology*. London: Springer-Verlag; 2007:147-156.
9. Fazeli-Matin S, Gill IS, Hsu TH, Sung GT, Novick AC. Laparoscopic renal and adrenal surgery in obese patients: comparison to open surgery. *J Urol*. 1999;162:665-669.
10. Miller BS, Ammori JB, Ganger PG, Broome JT, Hammer GD, Doherty GM. Laparoscopic resection is inappropriate in patients with known or suspected adrenocortical carcinoma. [published online ahead of print April 7, 2010] *World J Surg*. doi: 10.1007/s00268-010-0532-2.
11. Gill IS. The case for laparoscopic adrenalectomy. *J Urol*. 2001;166:429-436.
12. Soon PS, Yeh MW, Delbridge LW, et al. Laparoscopic surgery is safe for large adrenal lesions. *Eur J Surg Oncol*. 2008;34(1):67-70.
13. National Institutes of Health. NIH state-of-the-science-statement on management of clinically inapparent adrenal mass ("incidentaloma"). *NIH Consens State Sci Statements*. 2002; 19(2):1-25.
14. Sharma R, Ganpule A, Veermani M, Sabnis RB, Desai M. Laparoscopic management of adrenal lesions larger than 5 cm in diameter. *Urol. J* 2009;6(4):254-259.
15. Suzuki K, Ushiyama T, Mugiya S, Kageyama S, Saisu K, Fujita K. Hazards of laparoscopic adrenalectomy in patients with adrenal malignancy. *J Urol*. 1997;158(6):2227.
16. de Lagausie P, Berrebi D, Michon J, et al. Laparoscopic adrenal surgery for neuroblastomas in children. *J Urol*. 2003;170:932-935.
17. Greene FL, Kercher KW, Nelson H, Teigland CM, Boller AM. Minimal access cancer management. *CA Cancer J Clin*. 2007;57(3):130-146.

Difficulties in Laparoscopic Renal Cyst Removal and Giant Hydronephrosis Nephrectomy

13

Hamdy M. Ibrahim, Ahmed M. Al-Kandari, Hani S. Shaaban, and Inderbir S. Gill

Introduction

A giant kidney is a massively enlarged kidney having more than 1 L of fluid within the collecting system or is one that is the seat of large multiple cysts. It is defined radiographically when the enlarged kidney meets or crosses the midline, or spans more than five vertebral lengths.[1] The majority of giant hydronephrotic kidneys are nonfunctional and symptomatic, making nephrectomy the procedure of choice.[2] Because of the massive size and altered anatomic relationships of these kidneys, surgical excision is challenging. The other common cause of giant hydronephrotic kidney is the presence of large renal cysts, which may be simple or associated with other pathologies. Renal cystic disease is a common incidental, radiographic, and postmortem finding. It is estimated that evidence of renal cysts exists in 50% of the adult population.[3] The increased use of imaging modalities, such as ultrasonography and computed tomography (CT), has produced a corresponding increase in the detection of renal cystic disease. Simple renal cysts occur with an incidence of at least 20% by age 40 and 33% at age 60.[4] Most of these lesions are asymptomatic. At times, the lesions may be associated with dull renal angle pain, flank pain, hypertension, a palpable mass, hematuria, infection, and collecting system obstruction.[5,6] Certain renal cysts can be associated with other pathologic conditions, such as autosomal dominant polycystic kidney disease (ADPKD) and acquired cystic disease in chronic dialysis. ADPKD is an important cause of renal failure, accounting for approximately 9–10% of patients on chronic hemodialysis. Other clinical manifestations include hypertension, chronic pain, hematuria, urinary tract infection, stone formation, and cyst infection. Symptomatic renal cysts can be treated by percutaneous aspiration with or without injection of sclerosants,[7] percutaneous marsupialization, open surgery, and, currently, by laparoscopic surgery by transperitoneal and retroperitoneal access with similar efficacy to open surgery and less morbidity.[5,7,8] The excellent

A.M. Al-Kandari (✉)

Department of Surgery (Urology), Faculty of Medicine, Kuwait University, Jabriyah, Kuwait

e-mail: drakandari@hotmail.com

A.M. Al-Kandari and I.S. Gill (eds.), *Difficult Conditions in Laparoscopic Urologic Surgery*,   **149**

DOI: 10.1007/978-1-84882-105-7_13, © Springer-Verlag London Limited 2011

results achieved with laparoscopic decortication of symptomatic simple renal cysts, first described by Hulbert et al. in 1992, have prompted its acceptance.[9] In this chapter, the authors present the laparoscopic approaches for giant kidneys of varied pathology with an emphasis on the surgical options used in their management.

Evaluation

Evaluation of Renal Cystic Disease

Renal cystic disease can be adequately evaluated with ultrasonographic techniques. For more complicated lesions, renal CT is the cornerstone of diagnosis. Based on CT scan, renal cysts have been classified into four categories by Bosniak[10]:

Type I: This simple cyst is the most common and generally requires no treatment. A large simple cyst will rarely cause symptoms or obstruction, which would require intervention.

Type II: This homogenous, hyperdense cyst has thin septations and fine calcifications that do not enhance after intravenous injection of contrast medium. Cysts that contain multiple hairline thin septa and/or walls or smooth, minimally thicker septa and/or walls may contain perceived enhancement and/or coarser calcification but no measurable enhancement. Also included are uniformly high attenuation lesions greater than 3 cm that may be totally intrarenal.[11]

Type III: This multiloculated cystic mass or cyst has thick, irregular calcifications, a thick wall, or nodularity.

Type IV: A cyst associated with a solid component; such lesions are considered to be cystic malignancies and should be managed with radical nephrectomy.

Ultrasound is the recommended imaging modality for reliable identification and follow-up of cystic lesions. Adding the IIF category increases the accuracy and, thus, the clinical impact of the categorization system, as evidenced by a low rate of progression in category IIF cysts and an increased malignancy rate in surgically treated category III lesions. Progression in complexity but not in size appears to be the most important indication of malignancy. The high malignancy rate suggests that all category III cysts should undergo definitive treatment when clinically feasible.[12] For complicated cysts that are more likely benign (category II), but have some worrisome findings, follow-up CT should be performed to establish the benign behavior of the lesion (category IIF). An initial follow-up CT is performed at 6 months and 1 year, and then again after one more year. If the lesion has not changed in appearance during this period, a benign nature is established.[13] Equivocal cysts raising the possibility of malignancy can be further evaluated with CT, but, if any doubts remain regarding the nature of the lesion, percutaneous aspiration or biopsy is advocated to provide a definitive answer. The sensitivity for the detection of malignancy using percutaneous techniques is 90%. The specificity for the determination of benign disease is 92%.[14]

Indications

Depending on the symptoms, size, site, locations, number, presence of infection, suspicion of malignancy, and other associated pathologic conditions, the following renal cystic disorders can be managed by laparoscopic intervention:

1. Bosniak type I and II renal cysts – large symptomatic renal cysts (≥10 cm in size) may be directly taken up for laparoscopic management. Smaller symptomatic renal cysts may be treated by percutaneous aspiration alone or with a sclerosing agent, and, failing that, a laparoscopic resection can be undertaken.[8]
2. Renal cystic masses with malignancy should be treated by laparoscopic radical nephrectomy.[10]
3. Peripelvic or parapelvic cysts,[15] ADPKD, renal hydatid cysts.

Laparoscopic evaluation, marsupialization, excision, and radical nephrectomy for a cystic mass harboring malignancy offer a definitive treatment for patients who have renal cystic diseases and can obviate open surgery.[16]

Evaluation of Giant Hydronephrosis

Giant hydronephrosis can be adequately evaluated with ultrasonographic scanning. It is very important to delineate the extent of the dilated hydronephrotic kidney and its relationship to surrounding organs. The addition of coronal views on a CT scan is very helpful (Fig. 13.1). Magnetic resonance imaging (MRI) is also useful in delineating the intraabdominal anatomy in these challenging cases. Renal dynamic scintigraphy is used to determine the split function (split GFR mL/min) of the hydronephrotic units. Kidneys with a split glomerular filtration rate (GFR) of less than 10 mL/min are considered unsalvageable. Most giant hydronephrotic kidneys are almost nonfunctioning and any indication for retrograde ureteropyelography is rare. Routine blood work ups, including complete blood cell count (CBC), renal function tests, and urine tests, should be performed. If a patient is having respiratory difficulty due to the large hydronephrotic kidney compressing the diaphragm, nephrostomy drainage may be required for 3 days or longer until the patient's condition stabilizes. In case of significant laparoscopic difficulties, the patient should consent to a possible open conversion.

Operative Techniques

The authors have reported single stage decompression of giant hydronephrotic kidney. This is achieved under the same anesthesia with a percutaneous nephrostomy insertion and decompression until no further drainage is noted. Then transperitoneal trocars are inserted (as routine) and the procedure is continued.[17] Others have suggested a staged approach because of the possible effects of sudden abdominal decompression that results in a change

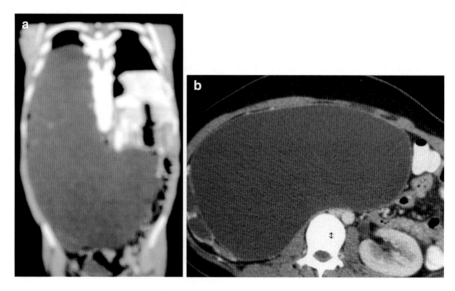

Fig. 13.1 (**a**) Preoperative CT with IV contrast showing right-sided giant hydronephrosis occupying the whole abdomen and displacing abdominal contents. (**b**) Right-sided giant hydronephrosis with no contrast excretion. Notice the normal average-sized left kidney

in the hemodynamic balance. The hydronephrotic kidney is first slowly decompressed with drainage, and nephrectomy is then performed after the patient's cardiorespiratory and alimentary systems have been stabilized. Therefore, a two-stage procedure with slow decompression by percutaneous nephrostomy before the nephrectomy is preferred in the compromised patient.[15,17–19] Recently Harper et al. claimed that, prior to laparoscopic nephrectomy, renal decompression via ureteral catheters is helpful to achieve adequate working space.[19] Retrograde ureteral decompression is an important consideration to reduce spillage of potentially infected urine into the peritoneum or retroperitoneum. Also, partial decompression of the kidney to 25–50% turgidity allowed adequate space for dissection and visualization while preserving enough turgidity to allow easier identification of surgical structures.

Retroperitoneal Approach

Laparoscopic Nephrectomy Technique

General anesthesia was given via a cuffed endotracheal tube and the patient was catheterized preoperatively. The patient was placed in the kidney position with a minimal kidney bridge – enough to increase the space between the costal margin and iliac crest without compromising the retroperitoneal space. A 1.5-cm to 2-cm transverse skin incision was made 1–2 cm below and posterior to the tip of the 12th rib in the lumbar (Petit's) triangle between the 12th rib and the iliac crest, bounded by the lateral edges of the latissimus dorsum and external oblique muscles. A tunnel is created down to the retroperitoneal space by blunt dissection using Overhold or Kocher forceps. This tunnel is dilated until an index finger can be inserted to push the peritoneum forward, thus creating a retroperitoneal cavity. Three dissection techniques of the retroperitoneum are used. The first technique uses a modification of the Gaur balloon technique by ligating a latex balloon using the middle finger of a powder-free surgical glove on an 18 F Mercier catheter. The second technique employs a balloon trocar system consisting of a latex balloon ligated to an 11 mm metal trocar sheath. During instillation of 500–1,000 cc warm normal saline through the insufflation channel of the trocar, dissection was monitored with the telescope inserted into the trocar sheath. In the last technique, dissection of the space between the lumbar aponeurosis and renal (Gerota's) fascia is performed exclusively with the index finger.[20]

Two secondary trocars (ports II and III) were inserted to one side of an index finger introduced through the primary access site. To avoid injury to the finger, a track was dilated first, using forceps. The initial incision (port I) was closed around the port using a mattress suture to prevent gas leakage. After establishing pneumoretroperitoneum (maximum carbon dioxide pressure 15 mmHg), residual minor adhesions were lysed easily and the renal fascia was opened longitudinally for exposure of the psoas muscle, representing the most important anatomical landmark of retroperitoneoscopy. If necessary, an additional 5 mm trocar (port IV) was inserted under endoscopic view to retract the kidney during the dissection.

Independent of the individual retroperitoneoscopic procedure, it is important to incise Gerota's fascia completely. The wide longitudinal incision opens the retroperitoneal space, thereby adding to the effect of the carbon dioxide insufflation, allowing retraction of the peritoneum and exposing all further anatomical landmarks. The usual technique of identifying the upper ureter first and then tracing it up to the renal pelvis and vessels has been modified as the hugely dilated kidneys restrict exposure of the upper ureter. The kidney was dissected posterior and then along the lateral surface as far medial as possible, and along the upper and lower poles. Inadvertent injury to the renal sac with early deflation of the kidney before the initial mobilization causes considerable difficulty in the subsequent dissection as the sac collapses, and thus special care should be taken to prevent this complication.[2]

Once vision and available space limit further dissection, the hydronephrotic sac was deflated by percutaneous aspiration using a Veress needle along the anterior axillary line, while simultaneously monitoring the insertion and deflation laparoscopically. The aspirated fluid was measured to determine the volume of the hydronephrotic kidney. Further posterior dissection was performed after retracting the kidney anterior using a tri-flange retractor.

Once adequately dissected, the collapsed renal sac was brought out through the anterior port (extracorporeal retraction) as intracorporeal retraction of the large renal sac does not provide adequate countertraction to aid dissection. This procedure stretched the hilar structures and further dissection around the hilar region was performed with relative ease, allowing for individual clipping of the renal vessels. The ureter was then clipped and divided between clips.[2]

The kidney, partly freed extracorporeally with the rest in the retroperitoneal space, was delivered after suitably enlarging the anterior port used for extracorporeal retraction. The retroperitoneum was then irrigated with saline and inspected for hemostasis, and a drain was placed. Finally, the port sites were closed with muscle and skin sutures.

Laparoscopic Management of Renal Cysts

If the retroperitoneal space is created underneath Gerota's fascia, the kidney lies directly in front; otherwise, the overlying fascia of Gerota is usually thinned out and the blue-domed cysts are easily recognized. Gerota's fascia is divided in relation to the location of the cyst. If the cyst is located anteriorly, medially, or anteromedially, the kidney is mobilized on the lateral border and retracted posteriorly with the help of a triflanged retractor to delineate the anterior surface of kidney.

A combination of blunt and sharp dissection using a dissector and scissor permits rapid and complete mobilization of the cyst surface. If the cyst is very tense after initial exposure, it can be punctured and grasped with the help of an atraumatic dissector that provides countertraction for further dissection. The renal cyst can be further treated in the following ways.

- The renal cyst can be completely excised when a good plane of cleavage can be developed between the cyst and the underlying parenchyma.
- If the previous maneuver is not possible, near total excision of the cyst wall is performed to avoid damage to the underlying collecting system or renal parenchyma.
- The renal cyst can be marsupialized by excising the wall.

In cases of peripelvic cysts, the presence of a ureteral catheter is of great help in identifying the compressed and distorted collecting system. Because the cysts are deeply placed in the renal sinus, aggressive resection of the cyst wall should not be attempted; instead, marsupialization must be performed. At the end of the procedure, sterile methylene blue is injected through the preplaced ureteral catheter to identify any leak from the pelvicaliceal system.

When the cyst wall is excised, the edges and base of the residual cyst wall are fulgurated. The surgeon should be extremely cautious while fulgurating the base because it overlies renal parenchyma and is in close proximity to the pelvicaliceal system. To prevent recurrence, a pedicle of perirenal fat is placed in the residual cavity subsequent to excision or marsupialization and finally a drain is placed.

Transperitoneal Approach

Laparoscopic Nephrectomy Techniques

This approach was the preferred access for cases with unilateral giant kidney as it provides a better space and orientation, otherwise preoperative drainage of the hugely dilated kidney (Fig. 13.1) or intraoperative deflation using a percutaneous needle are needed to gain access to the retroperitoneum (Fig. 13.2).[17] One needs to compress the flank until no more

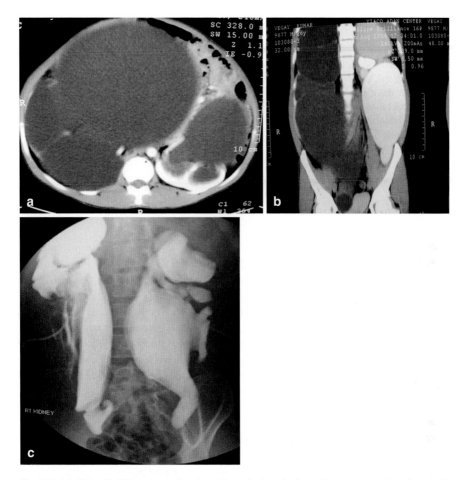

Fig. 13.2 (**a**) CT with IV contrast showing bilateral giant hydronephrosis occupying the whole abdomen and displacing abdominal contents. (**b, c**) Antegrade pyelography showing arrest of the contrast at the pelviureteric junction (PUJ). Note the difference in the volume after insertion of the percutaneous nephrostomy (PCN). Right-sided nephrectomy was performed on the poorly functioning right kidney

drainage noticed. The patient is placed in a shallow flank position (30 degrees ipsilateral side up), and Veress needle insufflation is performed at the superior aspect of the umbilicus. A 12-mm laparoscopic port is placed at the umbilicus, and the remaining ports are placed under laparoscopic vision.

For the left side, a 10-mm to 12-mm port is placed just below the umbilicus along the midclavicular line, and a 5-mm port is placed in the midline between the xiphoid and the umbilicus. On the right side, a 12-mm upper midline and a 5-mm midclavicular line port are placed. An optional 5-mm port is placed along the anterior axillary line between the iliac crest and the costal margin to facilitate retraction of the liver or spleen.

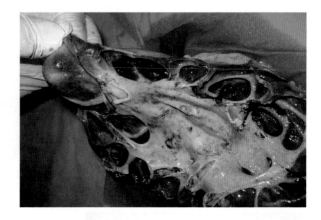

Fig. 13.3 Gross specimen of a giant hydronephrotic kidney removed laparoscopically. Since the parenchyma was very thinned out, there was no need for morcellation as it was removed intact through one of the ports

Because of the large kidney underneath, care must be taken during trocar placement to prevent injury to the renal sac and other abdominal viscera. Once the colon is dissected off the kidney, the kidney is mobilized as far as possible before percutaneous deflation of the renal sac. During deflation, especially in a transperitoneal procedure, spillage of the renal contents into the peritoneum must be minimized. Traction on the renal sac extracorporeally facilitates further dissection at the renal hilum. In the transperitoneal approach, the renal sac is delivered through the lateral port near the more mobilized pole (generally the inferior pole). The remaining steps are similar to conventional transperitoneal laparoscopic nephrectomy. The kidney, once completely mobilized, can be delivered through the port used for retraction (Fig. 13.3).[2]

Transperitoneal Laparoscopic Renal Cyst Decortication

Although the risk of collecting system injury is rare for peripheral cysts, peripelvic cysts and cysts associated with adult polycystic kidney disease may impinge on the collecting system, thereby increasing the risk for injury. The optional placement of a ureteral catheter provides a route for injection of indigo carmine or methylene blue to facilitate identification of inadvertent collecting system injury. If the injury is identified intraoperatively and is large, then laparoscopic repair is advised. If the injury is small, then the ureteral catheter can be converted to an internal ureteral stent after completion of the laparoscopic procedure.[21] Initially, the procedure was performed using four ports, although simple cysts can be treated using three ports. In cases of ADPKD, four ports are invariably needed. The technique is similar to that previously described.

After incising the line of Toldt from the iliac vessels to the splenic or hepatic flexure, the colon is mobilized medially and Gerota's fascia is opened. The kidney does not need to be mobilized in its entirety for unroofing of a solitary cyst. In contrast, for ADPKD, the kidney is mobilized completely and the hilum exposed to provide optimal access to the maximum number of cysts.

The surface of the kidney overlying the cyst is dissected until a rim of normal renal parenchyma surrounding the cyst is exposed. For large cysts, dissection may be facilitated by partially decompressing the cyst using an 18-gauge spinal needle placed percutaneously and guided by laparoscopic vision. The cyst wall is grasped and excised using electrocoagulating scissors until it is flush with the renal capsule. The cyst is then sent for histopathologic evaluation. Other energy devices, like an ultrasonic activated device such as the Ultracision® Harmonic Scalpel® (Ethicon Endo-Surgery, Inc., Cincinnati, OH) or an electrocautery device like LigaSure™ (ValleyLab, Boulder, CO) can be used. The base of the cyst is inspected for suspicious nodules or irregularities that are excised for biopsy with cup biopsy forceps.

Hemostasis is secured at the biopsy site and along the incised cyst wall with cautious use of electrocautery or the argon beam coagulator. Routine coagulation of the base of the cyst is discouraged because of the risk of collecting system injury. Perirenal fat or a tongue of omentum may be mobilized and placed into the cyst cavity to act as a wick to divert cyst fluid and prevent reaccumulation. For large cysts, a 7-mm suction drain is placed through a lateral port and is left in place for 1–2 days. As an alternative to mobilizing the colon to expose the kidney, some authors describe accessing a right renal cyst directly through a window in the mesocolon.[22] This approach, however, risks ischemic bowel injury, and the authors advise caution to avoid injury to the ileocolic and right colic arteries.

For peripelvic cysts, the renal hilum and pelvis are exposed. Identification of the cyst is facilitated by injection of indigo carmine stained saline into the renal pelvis through a ureteral catheter, with alternating filling and draining of the pelvis to distinguish it from the cyst. The cyst wall is incised without the use of electrocautery because of the close proximity to the renal vessels and collecting system. The use of laparoscopic ultrasound may help distinguish the cyst from the renal vein.[23] It is essential to fill the residual cavity by fixing perinephric fat or a polytetrafluoroethylene wick. In contrast to a simple renal cyst, a peripelvic cyst is considered a contraindication to percutaneous sclerosis. These cysts can be managed effectively, although the procedure is more complex than decortication of simple renal cysts. The peripelvic cyst located near the hilum and pelvis requires more complicated, skillful, and challenging dissection.[16]

For ADPKD, the objective is to unroof as many cysts as possible, or to be aspirated if excision of the cyst wall is precluded by the presence of surrounding renal parenchyma. A 7 mm suction drain is placed through a lateral port for 1–2 days. Because of extensive mobilization of the kidney, Elashry et al. advocate performing a nephropexy at the conclusion of the procedure.[24]

Conclusion

Laparoscopic surgery has almost replaced open surgery in benign nephrectomy as in hydronephrotic kidneys. But this subset of unusually and massively enlarged hydronephrotic kidneys are really challenging cases that need laparoscopic experience. Typically, a transperitoneal approach is more efficient. The key to success is to create enough space by decompressing the massively dilated kidney and respecting other organ anatomy. In regards to laparoscopic cyst removal, the authors prefer the transperitoneal approach (although both approaches can be performed), and cyst wall excision with different energy devices is mostly curative.

References

1. Crooks KK, Hendren WH, Pfister RC. Giant hydronephrosis in children. *J Pediatr Surg.* 1979;14:844-850.
2. Hemal AK, Wadhwa SN, Kumar M, Gupta NP. Transperitoneal and retroperitoneal laparoscopic nephrectomy for giant hydronephrosis. *J Urol.* 1999;162:35-39.
3. Kissane JM. The morphology of renal cystic disease. In: Gardner KD Jr, ed. *Cystic Diseases of the Kidney.* New York: Wiley; 1976:31-63.
4. Laucks SP Jr, McLachlen MS. Aging and simple cysts of the kidney. *Br J Radiol.* 1981;54: 12-14.
5. Holmberg G, Hietala SO. Treatment of simple renal cysts by percutaneous puncture and instillation of bismuth-phosphate. *Scand J Urol Nephrol.* 1989;23:207-212.
6. Rubenstein CS, Hulbert JC, Pharand D, Schuessler WW, Vancaille TG, Kavoussi LR. Laparoscopic ablation of symptomatic renal cysts. *J Urol.* 1993;150:1103-1106.
7. Fontana D, Porpiglia F, Morra I, Destefanis P. Treatment of simple renal cysts by percutaneous drainage with three repeated alcohol injections. *Urology.* 1999;53:904-907.
8. Hemal AK, Aron M, Gupta NP, Seth A, Wadhwa SN. The role of retroperitoneoscopy in the management of renal and adrenal pathology. *BJU Int.* 1999;83:929-936.
9. Hulbert JC, Shepard TG, Evans RM. Laparoscopic surgery for renal cystic disease. *J Urol.* 1992;147(suppl):443 [abstract 882].
10. Bosniak MA. The current radiological approach to renal cysts. *Radiology.* 1986;158:1-10.
11. Israel GM, Bosniak MA. An update of the Bosniak renal cyst classification system. *Urology.* 2005;66:484.
12. O'Malley RL, Godoy G, Hecht EM, Stifelman MD, Taneja SS. Bosniak category IIF designation and surgery for complex renal cysts. *J Urol.* 2009;182:1091-1095.
13. Bosniak MA. The use of the Bosniak classification system for renal cysts and cystic tumors. *J Urol.* 1997;157:1852.
14. Wolf JS. Evaluation and management of solid and cystic renal masses. *J Urol.* 1998;159: 1120-1133.
15. Talukder BC, Chatterjee SC, Agarwal TN, De PP. Giant hydronephrosis. *Br J Urol.* 1979;51(4):322-323.
16. Hemal AK. Laparoscopic management of renal cystic disease. *Urol Clin North Am.* 2001;28:115-126.
17. Ibrahim HM, Al-Kandari AM, Taqi A, et al. Etiology and management of adult giant hydronephrosis. *Arab J Urol.* 2008;6(2):21-25.
18. Chiang PH, Chen MT, Chou YH, Chiang CP, Huang CH, Chien CH. Giant hydronephrosis: report of 4 cases with review of the literature. *J Formos Med Assoc.* 1990;89:811-817.
19. Harper JD, Shah SK, Baldwin DD, Moorhead JD. Laparoscopic nephrectomy for pediatric giant hydronephrosis. *Urology.* 2007;70:153-156.
20. Rassweiler JJ, Seemann O, Frede T, Henkel TO, Aiken P. Retroperitoneoscopy: experiences with 200 cases. *J Urol.* 1998;160:1265-1269.

21. Pearle MS, Traxer O, Cadeddu JA. Renal cystic disease: laparoscopic management. *Urol Clin North Am*. 2000;27:661-673.
22. Leveillee RJ, Amaral J, Stein BS. Laparoscopic unroofing of a renal cyst via a mesocolonic window: a different approach. *J Laparoendosc Surg*. 1994;4:227-232.
23. Hoenig DM, McDougall EM, Shalhav AL, Elbahnasy AM, Clayman RV. Laparoscopic ablation of peripelvic renal cysts. *J Urol*. 1997;158:1345-1348.
24. Elashry OM, Nakada SY, Wolf JS Jr, McDougall EM, Clayman RV. Laparoscopy for adult polycystic kidney disease: a promising alternative. *Am J Kidney Dis*. 1996;27:224-233.

Difficulties in Laparoscopic Simple Prostatectomy

14

Rene J. Sotelo Noguera, Juan C. Astigueta Pérez, and David Canes

Introduction

Open surgical simple prostatectomy has traditionally been the treatment of choice for symptomatic benign enlargement of the prostate.[1] In 1894, Eugene Fuller performed a series of suprapubic prostatic adenomectomies in New York city. Eleven years later, he published an investigative work entitled "The question of priority in the adoption of the method of total enucleation suprapubically of the hypertrophied prostate."[2] However, it was not until 1912 that, thanks to the results obtained by Peter Freyer, this approach was popularized using a technique consisting of enucleation of the prostatic adenoma through an extraperitoneal incision in the wall of the bladder. This surgical technique did not change until 30 years later when Terence Millin described his technique for a retropubic simple prostatectomy in 1945. Millin developed the innovative trans-capsular approach, which spared the bladder from unnecessary incisions. This avoided the morbidity and complications associated with the vesicotomy.[3]

Later, endoscopic transurethral techniques superseded open surgery for the majority of cases of benign prostatic hyperplasia (BPH).[4-6] Modifications of the standard transurethral resection, such as the bipolar transurethral resection, holmium laser resection, or potassium-titanyl-phosphate (KTP) laser vaporization have successively been incorporated into clinical practice. These and other minimally invasive techniques are becoming increasingly popular, including transurethral needle ablation and thermotherapy, although the latter are typically reserved for small volume glands.[7]

The choice of technique depends on various factors unique to a given patient, including gland volume, patient age, patient preference, particular glandular anatomy (e.g. presence of median lobe), and institutional access to technology (e.g. availability of holmium laser). Gland volume is far and away the main driving force in the decision process. For instance, transurethral incision of the prostate (TUIP) is effective for small glands (≤ 30cc). For moderate-sized adenomas, transurethral resection of the prostate (TURP) is the gold standard.[8]

R.J.S. Noguera (✉)
Department of Urology, Centro de Cirugía Robotica y de Invasion, Minima, Instituto Médico la Floresta, Caracas, Venezuela
e-mail: renesotelo@cantv.net

A.M. Al-Kandari and I.S. Gill (eds.), *Difficult Conditions in Laparoscopic Urologic Surgery*,
DOI: 10.1007/978-1-84882-105-7_14, © Springer-Verlag London Limited 2011

Minimally invasive techniques have also been developed in an effort to offer ambulatory alternatives to the traditional TURP, including transurethral ablation by microwave thermotherapy (TUMT), and interstitial laser coagulation. Both have resulted in symptomatic improvement in properly selected patients. However, the persistence of irritative symptoms form thermal changes in residual prostatic tissue is not an infrequent occurrence after TUMT. These symptoms, as well as the greater time required with catheterization, unpredictable results, and high rates of secondary procedures, have restricted the use of these techniques.[9–11]

In general, open surgery is indicated for prostates that are larger than 100 g, especially if they coexist with other pathologies such as large bladder diverticula, multiple bladder stones, musculoskeletal restrictions that preclude lithotomy positioning. The advantages of the retropubic technique over the suprapubic approach include better exposure of the prostatic anatomy, visualization of the adenoma during the enucleation with the subsequent assurance of complete removal, direct view of the proximal urethra, direct access to the prostatic fossa for post-nucleation hamostasis, and minimal trauma to the bladder. The suprapubic approach offers the basic advantage of excellent exposure to the bladder neck. Finally, the transperineal approach, by which access to the retroperitoneum is avoided, is useful for patients with extensive prior abdominal or retroperitoneal surgery.[12,13]

The use of laparoscopy in urologic surgery continues to expand. High volume centers are exploring new techniques, including outcomes research, with laparoscopic simple prostatectomy, which attempts to duplicate the open approach in a minimally invasive fashion. The laparoscopic technique appears to have decreased morbidity, less pain, shorter hospital stay, and quicker return to regular activities. Laparoscopy combines the advantages of minimally invasive techniques with the favorable results of open surgery.[14]

In 2002, Mariano and coworkers performed the first laparoscopic simple prostatectomy for BPH. Final pathology revealed a prostatic adenoma weighing 120 g removed through a longitudinal vesical-capsular incision.[15] Four years later, the same authors published a report on a series of 60 patients treated with the same technique, with average specimen weight of 144.5 g.[16]

Other urologists, like Baumert and van Velthoven, have also reported their initial experiences in series with 20 and 18 cases, respectively.[17,18] Recently, Sotelo and colleagues described their technique for laparoscopic retropubic simple prostatectomy on 17 patients with obstructive BPH for large (>60 cc) glands by TRUS estimate, averaging 93 g on final pathology. The same authors have described the extraperitoneal technique in 71 patients with mean estimated blood loss of 275 mL, operating times of 140. min, and adenoma weights of 65 g.[19]

Various experiences with laparoscopic simple prostatectomy are reported in the literature, such as reports by Porpiglia et al., Blew et al., and Rehman et al., among others.[20–25] Laparoscopic techniques have their limitations when compared to open surgery, including difficult learning curves and the requirement for significant previous laparoscopic expertise. Nevertheless, preliminary reports from high volume centers are encouraging.[26–29] Robotic surgery, as an extension of laparoscopy, has recently been demonstrated to be a feasible approach to simple prostatectomy as well.[30,31]

In the following chapter, the authors describe the technique they have developed for laparoscopic simple prostatectomy, inculding tips and suggestions that they have found particularly useful in achieving an optimal result.

Equipment and Instruments Required

Equipment

- Olympus laparoscopic video tower (21-in. monitor, EXERA II image processor with light source; Olympus Medical Systems, Tokyo, Japan)
- High definition video laparoscope with chip on the tip (30° EndoEye, Olympus Medical Systems, Tokyo, Japan)
- UHI-3 high flow CO_2 Insufflator (up to 35 L/min) (Olympus Medical Systems, Tokyo, Japan)
- SonoSurg ultrasound generator (Olympus Medical Systems, Tokyo, Japan)
- Electro-surgical unit (monopolar/bipolar)
- Surgipump aspiration/irrigation pump (Olympus Medical Systems, Tokyo, Japan)

Instruments

- Trocars: three 5 mm one 10 mm, and one12 mm
- 5-mm surgical grasper (two crocodile fenestration, one with and one without ratchet; one surgical grasper with ratchet)
- 5-mm suction-irrigator
- Two needle drivers (Olympus Medical Systems, Tokyo, Japan)
- Metzenbaum reusable scissors (Olympus Medical Systems, Tokyo, Japan)
- 5-mm L-shape high frequency hook type monopolar electrode
- SonoSurg ultrasonic 5-mm scissor
- Metal urethral sound 24 Fr
- Carter-Thomason suture passer (CooperSurgical Inc., Trumbull, CT)
- Endopouch laparoscopic extraction pouch (Ethicon Endo-Surgery, Cincinnati, OH)
- Silicone Foley catheter 20 Fr
- Metal urethral catheter guide
- Sutures: 0-Monocryl™ with CT-1 needle (Ethicon, Inc., Somerville, New Jersey); 3-0 Catgut with SH needle (hemostasis); 2-0 Monocryl™ with UR 6 needle (Ethicon, Inc. Somerville, New Jersey) (trigonization); 0-Vicryl™ with CT-1 needle (Ethicon, Inc., Somerville, New Jersey) (capsulotomy closure)
- Blake drain 10 F
- Optional: Endoscopic GYNECARE type Morcellator (Ethicon, Inc., Somerville, NJ)

Preoperative Preparation

1. Routine preoperative testing (including urine culture), pulmonary exercises with incentive spirometer.
2. Bowel preparation, magnesium citrate
3. Preoperative antibiotics (1st generation cephalosporin covering skin flora)

4. Review the preoperative ultrasound (estimated volume and expected anatomy of the middle lobe)
5. Cystoscopy (in cases of hematuria, acute urinary retention, or urinary lithiasis)

Patient Positioning

The patient is treated with chemoprophylaxis for deep venous thrombosis or intermittent compression devices on the lower extremities, according to risk factors and institutional practice patterns. With the patient supine, the upper and lower extremities are in adduction with a support behind the shoulders to prevent slipping. A 20F silicone Foley catheter is inserted prior to initial access. Immediately after the first trocar is placed, steep Trendelenburg is initiated. Note that the foley balloon need not be inflated, as the catheter will be subsequently removed.

If there is difficulty in delineating the anatomical structures, the balloon can be inflated to 20 cc and moved back and forth, thus accentuating the prostatovesical junction.

Room Setup

The laparoscopic tower is placed near the patient's feet at a height that is comfortable for clear viewing of the monitor and inflation equipment. The principal surgeon is positioned to the left side near the patient's shoulder, the first assistant to the right side, and the second assistant to the left of the principal surgeon. The instrument technician is positioned diagonally from the principal surgeon (Fig. 14.1).

Approaches

Extraperitoneal

Advantages:

- In theory, operating time is shorter, considering that the dissection of the preperitoneal space is done digitally or with a balloon.
- Lower risk of bowel injury.
- Smaller probability of developing postoperative ileus in case of urine leakage.

Disadvantages:

- Small working space, collapses readily when suction is applied.
- Since the space is bluntly established, increased minor bleeding can diminish visibility.

Fig. 14.1 Distribution of the surgical equipment

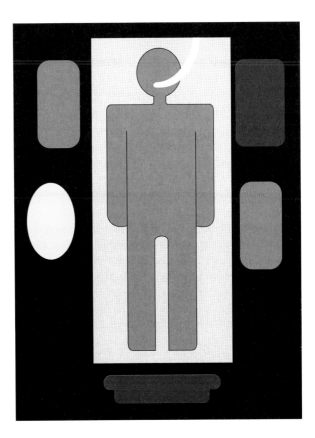

Transperitoneal

Advantages:

- Even when the bladder is released from the abdominal wall, entering the prevesical space, this is done with sharp dissection thereby limiting bleeding and improving optics (blood does not absorb the light).
- Large working space (useful with large adenomas), resulting in less collapse of the operating field with suction and less interruption of visibility from fluids such as blood or saline solution for irrigation, since gravity forces them into the upper abdomen.
- Allows for the placement of the surgical specimen outside of the work area.

Disadvantages:

- Greater risk of bowel injury
- Higher probability postoperative ileus.

Transperitoneal with Two Windows

This is an intermediate situation, a technique in which after initiation of the transperitoneal approach two lateral peritoneal windows are created, giving access to the prevesical space. Thus, the advantages of the extraperitoneal approach are obtained as well as the range of space inherent in the transperitoneal approach.

Trocar Placement

Extraperitoneal

The trocars are arranged in a "W," as this is the most correct and comfortable manner (Fig. 14.2). In the extraperitoneal approach, the first 10-mm trocar is placed immediately below the umbilicus. A vertical or horizontal incision is performed in the skin with a scalpel, followed by dissection of the subcutaneous tissue, a horizontal incision in the anterior layer of the abdominal rectus sheath, and lateral displacement of the rectus muscles.

Two ways to gain access to the extraperitoneal space will be described. The first is done by transverse incision of the anterior rectus fascia and then a longitudinal section of the entire midline with scissors, then dissecting the prevesical space digitally or with a

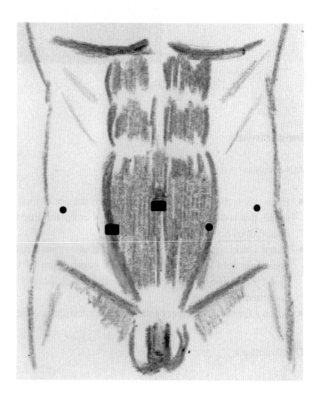

Fig. 14.2 Placement of the trocars

balloon. The second involves longitudinal division of the anterior and posterior layer of the rectus sheath, entering the space between the posterior rectus sheath and the peritoneum, dissecting with a lubricated finger in this preperitoneal space, advancing first to the direction of the pubis, and then laterally, being careful not to accidentally open the peritoneum or tear perforating vessels located principally in the epigastric zone.

Problem: It is important that no perforations are made while dissecting the peritoneum. If this happens, CO_2 will enter the peritoneal cavity, pushing the bladder into the potentialspace, causing difficulty with the surgery.

Solution: If this occurs, the solution is to expand the peritoneal continuity and create another window on the contralateral side, so that the CO_2 can circulate freely between the two cavities.

To create an airtight space, one may use a Hasson trocar. Alternatively, use a large needle and monofilament suture, and place a figure-of-eight stitch through the entire thickness of the abdominal wall (from the skin to the posterior rectus sheath). Loosen the stitch, introduce the trocar without its obdurator, and quickly tie a half hitch, adjusting it with a Kelly clamp to prevent the air leak.

The importance of this type of stitch to prevent the air leak is to easily and quickly reestablish pneumoperitoneum in the event that it is necessary to remove the specimen during the operation. This may be required when the specimen obstructs the working space and cannot be placed aside (e.g. extraperitoneal approach).

Next, inflate with CO_2 to a pressure of 15 mmHg, and complete the dissection, using the lens for dissection, with forward and fanning movements. This bluntly expands the extraperitoneal space cephalad.

Tip: The camera tip should be placed 1 cm inside the trocar to maintain a clear optic during blunt extension of the extraperitoneal space using the camera trocar.

The second 5-mm trocar is placed at the pararectal level on the left, slightly below the line that connects the umbilicus and the anterior superior iliac spine. The third 5-mm trocar is located 2 cm above and inside of the left anterior superior iliac spine. The fourth 12-mm trocar is placed contralateral to the left pararectal, and the fifth 5-mm trocar 3 cm above and inside of the right anterior superior iliac spine.

It is important to remember that an adequate dissection of the bladder and the extraperitoneal space must be made so that the trocars do not go across the peritoneal reflection, potentially out of sight, risking unrecognizable bowel injury.

Transperitoneal

The distribution of the trocars is similar to that in the extraperitoneal approach. This can be initiated by using a Veress needle or with the Hasson technique. Once created, the pneumoperitoneum is introduced in the first trocar, which has a safety system with a retractable sleeve. After inserting the laparoscope and exploring the peritoneal cavity, place the other trocars under direct vision.

The depth of the trocars as well as their fixation to the abdominal wall are extremely important to ensure that they do not move, either coming out or going in accidentally.

The tips of the more medial pararectal trocars should be 2 or 3 cm (from the inside) so that they do not interfere with the movement of the graspers. In contrast the lateral trocars may be introduced to almost their entire length. This helps to avoid inadvertent small bowel injury by the assistant during instrument insertion, which often occurs outside of the camera view. With both approaches, special attention should be made that the two pararectal trocars have a separation of 18–20 cm between them.

The first assistant uses the transumbilical trocar to introduce the 30° lens, which is manipulated with the left hand, and uses the right hand to introduce the suction-irrigation canula and other instruments in the fifth trocar. The second assistant uses the right hand for retraction of the bladder for countertraction during the adenoma mobilization, and the left hand to manipulate the metallic intraurethral sound.

It should be made clear that the authors use a 30° highdefinition laparoscopic video (EndoEye) for its multiple advantages, as it allows the first assistant to manipulate it just with one hand. Furthermore, the 30° optical allows for a lateral view and a depth perception that is not possible with the 0° angle.

Creation of the Lateral Transperitoneal Windows

In order to overcome the difficulty of peering around the corner as the lateral windows are created on either side of the bladder, take advantage of the angled lens. The 30° lens is introduced through the first trocar, with the camera shaft pointed towards the right lower quadrant, and the 30° lens looking to the left. The surgeon, with the grasper introduced through the left pararectal trocar, applies tension to the urachus and cuts the peritoneum in the external border of the right umbilical ligament with the L-shape hook type monopolar electrode, introducing it through the right pararectal trocar, creating a lateral window in the cranio-caudal direction that goes alongside the umbilical ligament towards the right vas deferens (Fig. 14.3a, b).

The surgeon proceeds in a similar manner on the left side until the two dissection planes meet. For the left lateral dissection, often working through the two left trocars is the optimal approach. The first assistant helps with counter-traction through any of the right ports. In this manner, the surgeon completes the dissection of the Retzius space arriving at the pubis, the avoiding surface of the bladder.

Access to the Adenoma

Using the grasper and the Ultrasonic scissor, the surgeon dissects the fat located from the anterior surface of the prostatic fascia, back to the expected location of the bladder neck. The procedure does not require opening of the endopelvic fascia, or the ligation of the dorsal venous complex, as in radical prostatectomy (Fig. 14.4a, b).

There are different techniques for gaining access to the prostatic adenoma: (1) through the prostatic capsule with a tranverse incision (Millin), (2) longitudinal transcervical-capsular

Fig. 14.3 (**a**) Umbilical ligaments and (**b**) prevesical dissection and creation of side windows

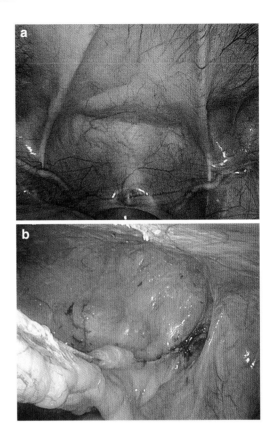

(Mirandolino), and (3) the technique which the authors favor, a transverse incision in the bladder neck at its junction with the prostate.

Aperture of the Bladder

Once the union between the bladder and the prostate has been identified, the surgeon makes a cut over the bladder using the 5-mm L-shape, high frequency hook type monopolar electrode, performing the initial section at a depth where the bladder mucosa is seen. Then, using the SonoSurg, laterally complete the transverse cystotomy wide enough to allow for the identification of the existence of a prominent middle lobe, visualizing the interior of the bladder and the ureteral orifices (Fig. 14.5).

One way to recognize the junction of the prostate and the bladder is by differentiating the characteristic of the fat on the prostatic surface (easily peeled away) and the the bladder (denser and adherent). Alternatively, place gentle traction on the foley catheter with the balloon inflated. The movement of the balloon will delineate the bladder neck.

Fig. 14.4 (**a**, **b**) Dissection of the
anterior face of the prostate

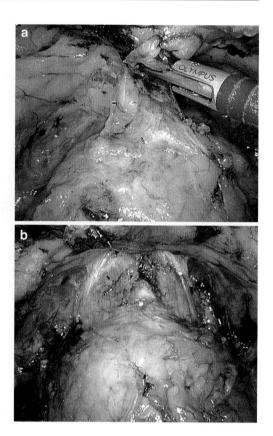

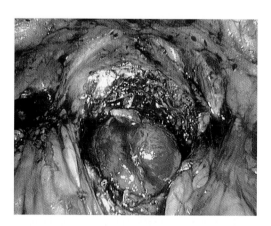

Fig. 14.5 Identification of the
bladder-prostate junction and
transverse cistotomy

*The reason for first using the monopolar electrode cut is the need to make a clean cut
that allows for distinguishing of the detrusor of the bladder until entering it, and the
SonoSurg is used on the lateral extension because it is a vascularized area and needs to be
kept as bloodless as possible.*

Dissection and Enucleation of the Prostatic Adenoma

Once the border between the prostatic adenoma and the posterior vesical mucosa has been recognized, the surgeon cuts with the hook type monopolar electrode and proceeds to outline the entire circumference, starting first in a posterior semicircle and slowly going deeper until reaching the adenoma and completing and the entire circumference.

At the border between the adenoma and the vesical mucosa where the incision should be made, a difference in mucosal color is normally observed. In most patients, an injected appearing strip of hypervascular mucosa can be identified. This serves as a reliable reference for the incision.

The whitened tissue of the prostatic adenoma is easily identifiable and the dissection plane between the surgical capsule and the adenoma is made using the monopolar type hook and the ultrasonic scissors, in addition to blunt with the suction cannula (Fig. 14.6).

If faced with a prostate with a prominent median lobe, before initiating the dissection and enucleation, place a figure-of-eight traction stitch into the median lobe with 1-0 Monocryl™ on a CT needle . Exteriorize the suture ends through the abdominal wall in the suprapubic region using a Carter-Thomason device, and secure them with a Kelly clamp at the skin surface. This will serve to expose the posterior vesical mucosa in the region of your initial incision.

In general, when the initial dissection of the adenoma is complete, proceed to place a figure-of-eight suture in the lateral lobes of adenoma with a 1-0 Monocryl™ suture on a CT-1 needle, leaving the ends of the suture long enough to serve as a source of traction (Fig. 14.7a, b).

The advantage of using the monofilament suture with a large needle such as the 1-0 Monocryl™, CT-1 is that it allows for deep introduction and easily passes through the adenoma, thus providing firm surfaces that do not come undone from the traction. A very important trick that the authors call "fishing" is to not cut the needle of the traction stitch. As more adenoma is exposed with further dissection, take another "bite" of the adenoma with the original stitch, and repeat as necessary. In this manner, countertraction remains effective as more tissue is exposed.

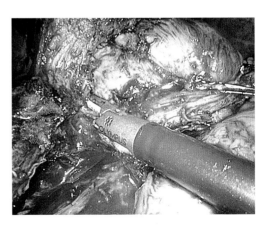

Fig. 14.6 Dissection of prostate adenoma with SonoSurge

Fig. 14.7 (**a, b**) Retraction of prostate
adenoma with monofilament suture

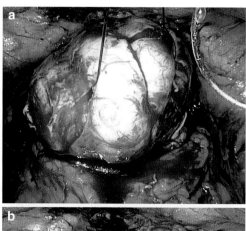

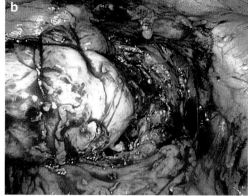

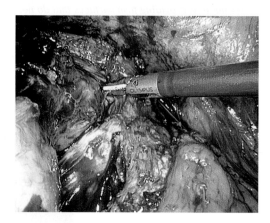

Fig. 14.8 Ligation of intracapsular
prostatic pedicles with the SonoSurg

While manipulating the traction stitch in all directions, small perforating branches will
appear; with the use of the monopolar coagulator or the ultrasonic shears, these perforators
can be controlled. This allows continued enucleation in a relatively avascular plane.

*More attention should be paid to the 4–5 and 7–8 o'clock areas, corresponding to the
zones of the lateral prostatic pedicles* (Fig. 14.8).

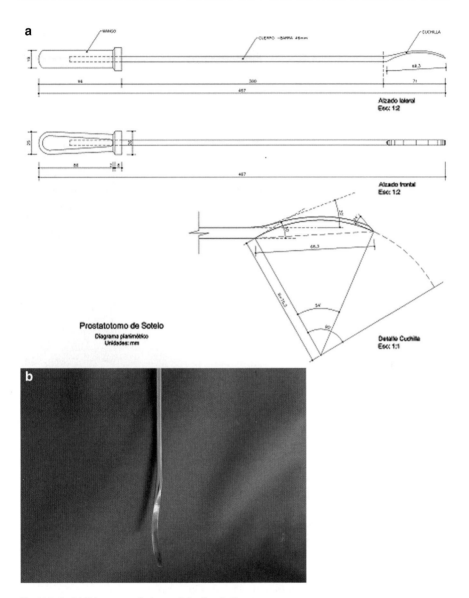

Fig. 14.9 (**a, b**) Diagram and photo of the Sotelo Prostatotomo

A useful instrument designed specifically for the dissection of the prostatic adenoma is the Sotelo Prostatotomo, which consists of three parts: a Teflon® sleeve, a stainless steel cylinder body, and a distal curve of the same material in a concave shape with sharp edges that aid in the enucleation (Fig. 14.9a, b). Using both its convex and its concave elements, develop the dissection plane. At the smallest sign of difficulty in advancing the dissection, which generally coincides with areas with perforating vessels or adhesions, this tool should be removed and the limiting band either cauterized or divided with ultrasonic shears (Fig. 14.10a, b).

Fig. 14.10 (**a**, **b**) Dissection of prostatic adenoma with the Sotelo Prostatotomo

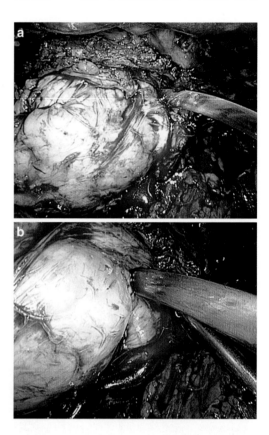

When retracting the adenoma from side to side, it is important not to do so directly with graspers because the adenoma will tear. Tearing the adenoma subsequently makes the dissection more difficult, and finding the correct plane problematic. At times, due to adenoma size obstructing the dissection view, one may deliberately fragment the adenoma. In general, avoid cutting the median lobe since this is what engages the lateral lobes and allows for their enucleation. Usually it is necessary to first enucleate one of the lateral lobes, then cut the urethra laterally and enucleate the other lobe.

The urethra can be clearly identified and should be divided sharply with scissors. The metal sound in the urethra can help to identify the borders of the urethra and help to compress it in case of bleeding from the dorsal vein complex.

Hemostasis, Trigonization, and closure of the Bladder

After completing the enucleation, hemostasis should be confirmed and the pneumoperitoneum pressure decreased. Any venous channels that have been compressed under pressure are typically revealed and can be addressed. Then move the lens 30° to see laterally inside the capsule and inspect very carefully, primarily in those areas where bleeding may be

Fig. 14.11 Entering with the Foley catheter guide

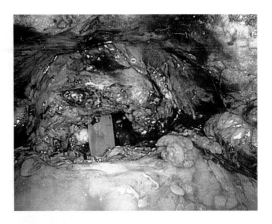

expected such as the lateral pedicles and the dorsal venous complex. If there is the slightest doubt, bipolar, ultrasonic shears or fixation sutures should be placed using Catgut 3-0 SH.

Trigonization should then be performed, bringing the vesical mucosa to the posterior prostatic capsule or posterior border of the urethra. This is normally done with two or three stitches, one central and two lateral, with absorbable sutures (2-0 Monocryl™, UR 6). The knots are tied intracorporeally.

Introduce a silicone three-way 24 Fr Foley catheter with a sound and, after finishing closure of the bladder, fill the balloon with 30–50 cc depending on the size of the prostatic fossa, leaving it inside the bladder and connecting to continuous irrigation (Fig. 14.11).

For closure of the bladder, 2-0 Vicryl™, CT1 is used in a running fashion from each corner of the opening, tied to each other in the midline (Fig. 14.12a–d).

It is very important to check for watertightness of the suture line at the end. Additional interrupted sutures must be placed at any focal point of leakage.

Drainage

It is important to provide drainage (Blake drain) to aid in the removal of any urine that leaked, exteriorizing it in any one of the lateral incision ports. This should be maintained until no more than 30 cc drains in a 24 h period, which, on average, should occur on the second or third day after the operation.

Extraction of the Operatory Clamp

The mouth of the specimen bag should be exteriorized, and the specimen fragmented (Fig. 14.13a, b). Usually there is no need to extend the umbilical incision.

Fig. 14.12 (**a**–**d**) Closure of bladder

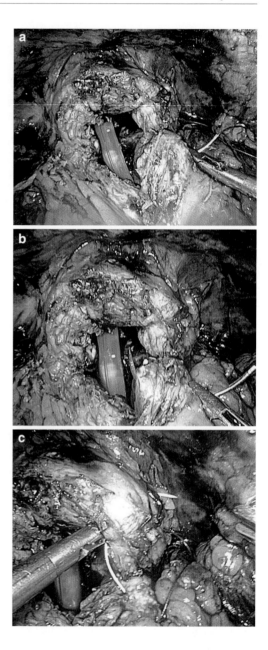

Fig. 14.12 (continued)

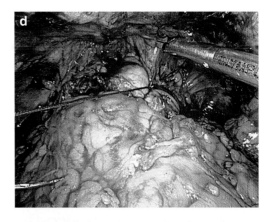

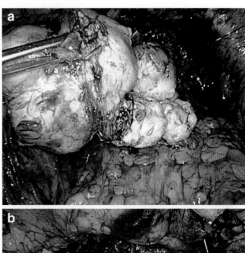

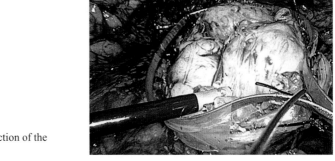

Fig. 14.13 (**a**, **b**) Extraction of the surgical specimen

Postoperative Care

- On average, continual irrigation is stopped within 12–24 hs if the urine is clear.
- On average, the drain is removed in 48 h once drainage falls below 30cc in an 8 h shift.
- The Foley catheter is removed in 5–7 days A cystogram is not mandatory but can be performed per the surgeon's discretion.

References

1. Roehrborn CG, Bartsch G, Kirby R, et al. Guidelines for the diagnosis and treatment of benign prostatic hyperplasia: a comparative, international overview. *Urology*. 2001;58(5):642-650.
2. Fuller E. The question of priority in the adoption of the method of total enucleation suprapubically of the hypertrophied prostate. *Ann Surg*. 1905;41:520-534.
3. Millin T. Retropubic prostatectomy: a new extravesical technique. *Lancet*. 1945;1:693-696. Report on 20 cases.
4. Lu-Yao GL, Barry MJ, Chang CH, Wasson JH, Wennberg JE, Prostate Patient Outcomes Research Team (PORT). Transurethral resection of the prostate among Medicare beneficiaries in the United States: time trends and outcomes. *Urology*. 1994;44(5):692-698.
5. McNicholas TA. Management of symptomatic BPH in the UK: who is treated and how? *Eur Urol*. 1999;36(Suppl 3):33-39.
6. Gordon N, Hadlow G, Knight E, Mohan P. Transurethral resection of the prostate: still the gold standard. *Aust N Z J Surg*. 1997;67:354-357.
7. Kuntz R, Lehrich K. Transurethral holmium laser enucleation versus transvesical open enucleation for prostate adenoma greater than 100 gm.: a randomized prospective trial of 120 patients. *J Urol*. 2002;168:1465-1469.
8. AUA Practice Guidelines Committee. AUA guideline on management of benign prostatic hyperplasia (2003). Chapter 1: diagnosis and treatment recommendations. *J Urol*. 2003; 170:530-547.
9. Tubaro A, Vicentini R, Renzetti R, Miano L. Invasive and minimally invasive treatment modalities for lower urinary tract symptoms: what are the relevant differences in randomised controlled trials? *Eur Urol*. 2000;38(Suppl 1):7-17.
10. Moody JA, Lingeman JE. Holmium laser enucleation for prostate adenoma greater than 100 gm.: comparison to open prostatectomy. *J Urol*. 2001;165:459-462.
11. Sandhu JS, Ng C, Vanderbrink BA, Egan C, Kaplan SA, Te AE. High-power potassium-titanyl-phosphate photoselective laser vaporization of prostate for treatment of benign prostatic hyperplasia in men with large prostates. *Urology*. 2004;64:1155-1159.
12. Oesterling J. Retropubic and suprapubic prostatectomy. In: Walsh PC, Retik AB, Vaughan ED Jr, Wein AJ, eds. *Campbell's Urology*, vol. 2. 7th ed. Philadelphia: W.B. Saunders; 1998: 1529-1540.
13. de la Rosette J, Alivizatos G, Madersbacher S, et al. Guidelines on Benign Prostatic Hyperplasia. European Association of Urology; 2004. Available at: http://www.uroweb.org/fileadmin/tx_eauguidelines/2004/Full/BPH_2004.pdf. Accessed May 16, 2010.
14. Sotelo R, Clavijo R. Open adenomectomy: past, present and future. *Curr Opin Urol*. 2008;18(1):34-40.
15. Mariano MB, Graziottin TM, Tefelli MV. Laparoscopic prostatectomy with vascular control for benign prostatic hyperplasia. *J Urol*. 2002;167:2528-2529.

16. Mariano MB, Tefilli MV, Graziottin TM, Pinto Morales CM, Goldraich IH. Laparoscopic prostatectomy for benign prostatic hyperplasia: a six year experience. *Eur Urol.* 2006;49: 127-132.

17. van Velthoven R, Peltier A, Laguna MP, Piechaud T. Laparoscopic extraperitoneal adenomectomy (Millin): pilot study on feasibility. *Eur Urol.* 2004;45:103-109.

18. Baumert H, Gholami SS, Bermúdez H, et al. Laparoscopic simple prostatectomy. *J Urol.* 2003;169(suppl):109 [abstract V423].

19. Sotelo R, Spaliviero M, Garcia-Segui A, et al. Laparoscopic retropubic simple prostatectomy. *J Urol.* 2005;17:757-760.

20. Porpiglia F, Renard J, Volpe A, et al. Laparoscopic transcapsular simple prostatectomy (Millin): an evolving procedure. *J Urol.* 2007;177(4 suppl):578 [abstract 1739].

21. Blew BD, Fazio LM, Pace K, D'A Honey RJ. Laparoscopic simple prostatectomy. *Can J Urol.* 2005;12:2891-2894.

22. Rehman J, Khan SA, Sukkarieh T, Chughtai B, Waltzer WC. Extraperitoneal laparoscopic prostatectomy (adenomectomy) for obstructing benign prostatic hyperplasia: transvesical and transcapsular (Millin) techniques. *J Endourol.* 2005;19:491-496.

23. Rey D, Ducarme G, Hoepffner JL, Staerman F. Laparoscopic adenectomy: a novel technique for managing benign prostatic hyperplasia. *BJU Int.* 2005;95:676-678.

24. Lufuma E, Gaston R, Piechaud T, et al. Finger assisted laparoscopic retropubic prostatectomy (Millin). *Eur Urol Suppl.* 2007;6(2):164.

25. Ngninkeu BN, de Fourmestreaux N, Lufuma E. Digitally-assisted laparoscopic prostatic adenomectomy: a preliminary report of 75 cases [abstract 1740]. *J Urol.* 2007;177(4 suppl):578.

26. Porpiglia F, Terrone C, Renard J, et al. Transcapsular adenomectomy (Millin): a comparative study, extraperitoneal laparoscopy versus open surgery. *Eur Urol.* 2006;49:120-126.

27. Barret E, Bracq A, Braud G, et al. The morbidity of laparoscopic versus open simple prostatectomy [abstract 1005]. *Eur Urol Suppl.* 2006;5(2):274.

28. Baumert H, Ballaro A, Dugardin F, Kaisary AV. Laparoscopic versus open simple prostatectomy: a comparative study. *J Urol.* 2006;175:1691-1694.

29. Peltier A, Hoffmann P, Hawaux E, Entezari K, Deneft F, van Velthoven R. Laparoscopic extraperitoneal Millin's adenomectomy versus open retropubic adenomectomy: a prospective comparison. *Eur Urol Suppl.* 2007;6(2):163 [abstract 564].

30. Sotelo R, Clavijo R, Carmona O. Robotic simple prostatectomy. *J Urol.* 2008;179:513-515.

31. Yuh B, Laungani R, Perlmutter A, et al. Robot-assisted Millin's retropubic prostatectomy: case series. *Can J Urol.* 2008;15(3):4101-4105.

Difficulties in Laparoscopic Radical Prostatectomy

15

Rene J. Sotelo Noguera, Juan C. Astigueta Pérez, and Camilo Giedelman

Necessary Equipment and Instruments

Equipment

- Olympus laparoscopic video tower (21-in. monitor, EXERA II image processor with light source) (Olympus Medical Systems, Tokyo, Japan)
- High-definition laparoscopic EndoEye 30° "chip-on-a-stick" laparoscope (Olympus Medical Systems, Tokyo, Japan)
- High flux UHI-3 CO_2 insufflator (up to 35 L/min) (Olympus Medical Systems, Tokyo, Japan)
- SonoSurg ultrasonic generator (Olympus Medical Systems, Tokyo, Japan)
- Electrosurgery unit (monopolar/bipolar)
- SurgiPump suction/irrigation pump (Olympus Medical Systems, Tokyo, Japan)

Instruments

- Trocars: Three 5-mm TroQ trocars (Olympus Medical Systems, Tokyo, Japan) and two disposables, 10 and 12 mm
- 5-mm graspers: Two fenestrated alligator clips, one with and the other without a locking handle; one alligator grasper
- 5-mm suction-irrigation cannula
- Two Olympus straight laparoscopic needle-holders (Olympus Medical Systems, Tokyo, Japan)
- Olympus reusable Metzenbaum scissors (Olympus Medical Systems, Tokyo, Japan)
- 5-mm high-frequency L-hook-type monopolar electrode
- 5-mm SonoSurg cutting and coagulation shears (Olympus Medical Systems, Tokyo, Japan)

R.J.S. Noguera (✉)
Department of Urology, Centro de Cirugía Robotica y de Invasion, Minima, Instituto Médico la Floresta, Caracas, Venezuela
e-mail: renesotelo@cantv.net

A.M. Al-Kandari and I.S. Gill (eds.), *Difficult Conditions in Laparoscopic Urologic Surgery*, 181
DOI: 10.1007/978-1-84882-105-7_15, © Springer-Verlag London Limited 2011

- 5-mm and 10-mm Weck Hem-o-lok® clip appliers (Teleflex Medical, Research Triangle Park, NC, USA)
- 5-mm Olympus titanium clip applier (Olympus Medical Systems, Tokyo, Japan)
- 24 F Urethral bougie (Beniqué)
- 10-cm Ethicon Endopouch laparoscopic extraction pouch (Ethicon Endo-Surgery, Cincinnati, OH)
- 20 F Foley silicone-coated catheter
- Metallic urethral catheter guide
- Sutures:

    - Dorsal vein complex ligation: 0-Vicryl™ on CT-1 needle (Ethicon, Inc., Somerville, NJ, USA)
    - Urethrovesical anastomosis: 2-0 Monocryl™ on UR-6 needle, or alternative 2-0 Biosyn™ on GU-46 needle (Covidien, Dublin, Ireland)

- Olympus fascia seal needle (to seal orifices or bleeding epigastric vessels) (Olympus Medical Systems, Tokyo, Japan)
- Storz 10-mm right angle dissector (Karl Storz, Tuttlingen, Germany)
- 10 F Blake drain with collection chamber.

Patient Preparation

- Routine preoperative studies (urine culture), respiratory exercises with incentive inspirometer
- Bowel preparation with magnesium citrate
- Preoperative antibiotics
- Detailed review of the preoperative ultrasound regarding the estimated volume, expected anatomy of the median lobe, and type of apex
- Consider performing cystoscopy in patients with symptoms of urinary obstructions and/or history of hematuria
- Digital rectal examination under anesthesia.

Patient Positioning

Antiembolic stockings or intermittent compression devices are placed on both legs. The patient is placed supine with the upper extremities in adduction and with the shoulder supported to prevent sliding. A 20 F silicone-coated Foley catheter is inserted without filling the balloon to evacuate the bladder. After application of the first trocar, the patient is placed in a steep Trendelenburg position.

When performing antegrade dissection and encountering difficulty in delineating the plane between the bladder and prostate, one may inflate the balloon with 10 cc and slide it distally, thus the junction between the two structures will be demonstrated.

Surgical Setup

The laparoscope tower is placed at the patient's feet at a height whereby the monitor and insufflation equipment are clearly visible. The main surgeon is positioned on the patient's left, the first assistant to the right and the second assistant to the left of the main surgeon. The surgical orderly is positioned diagonal to the second assistant (Fig. 15.1).

Approaches

Extraperitoneal

Advantages

- In theory, surgery duration is shorter, considering that the dissection of the preperitoneal space is done digitally or with a balloon.
- Decreased risk of bowel injury.

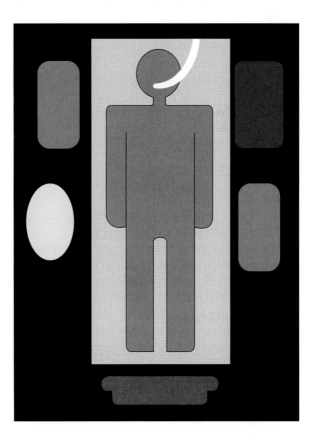

Fig. 15.1 Surgical setup. Surgeon (*blue*), first and second assistant (*sky blue*)

- Decreased likelihood of developing postoperative ileus in the event of urine leak.
- A shallower Trendelenburg position is required since the bowel is naturally retracted by the veil of the peritoneum.

Disadvantages

- Small working space
- Potentially increased tension on the urethrovesical anastomosis
- Occasional bloody dissection of the preperitoneal space, decreasing visibility.

Transperitoneal

Advantages

- The space created with direct-vision through an avascular plane allows for a "clean" work field, taking greater advantage of light, thus obtaining better image and color.
- Wider working space, with reduced incidence of collapse of the operating field during suction and less interruption of visibility by fluids like blood or saline solution when irrigating, since they escape into the upper abdomen due to gravity.
- Wide bladder mobilization allows it to be brought down to the anastomosis with less tension.
- Storage of the specimen away from the work area, especially when it is large, does not hinder the execution of the anastomosis.
- Proximal extended lymph node dissection is more readily achieved.

Disadvantages

- Greater risk of bowel injury
- Increased likelihood of developing postoperatory intestinal obstructions due to manipulation of the wall, and mainly because of leaked urine.

Transperitoneal with Two Windows

The authors have carried out an intermediate situation, in which after the transperitoneal approach, two lateral peritoneal windows are created to gain access to the prevesical space. This technique obtains some of the advantages of the extraperitoneal approach (bowel retraction) as well as the wider space of the transperitoneal approach.

Trocar Placement

Extraperitoneal

Placement of the trocars in a "W" tends to be the most correct and comfortable technique. In the extraperitoneal approach, the first trocar (10 mm) is placed immediately below the navel. A vertical or horizontal incision in the skin is performed with a scalpel, followed by dissection of the subcutaneous cellular tissue, and a horizontal incision into the anterior rectus abdominus sheath.

The authors will describe two ways of gaining access to the work space: the first method requires the surgeon to section the entire middle raphe of the rectus sheath with scissors and dissect the prevesical space digitally or with the balloon. The second method requires the surgeon to vertically section the posterior of the rectus sheath and gain access to the space between the posterior sheath of the rectus and peritoneal. The surgeon then dissects with a lubricated finger, heading first toward the pubis, the Retzius space and then moving laterally, taking care not to accidentally open the peritoneal or section the perforable vessels located mainly in the epigastric zone.

Problem: It is important that the dissection of the peritoneum cavity generates no perforations. If perforated, CO_2 will enter the peritoneal cavity and push the bladder towards the created space, making surgery difficult.

Solution: Should a perforation occur, the peritoneal continuity solution should be broadened and another should be created contralaterally so that the CO_2 can freely circulate between both cavities.

In order to cut costs, a Hasson trocar is not used. To maintain an airtight seal, a pulley stitch is placed using a retention needle through the entire width of the wall from the skin to the posterior aponeurosis of the rectus. The suture is loosened and the trocar is introduced without the obdurator. The surgeon then makes a half-knot and adjusts it with the Kelly forceps to avoid gas leakage.

The importance of this type of suture is to enable the operation to progress smoothly, as it is easy to quickly reestablish the pneumoperitoneum hermetically after removing the operatory piece to review the borders of the section or simply to create a greater work space.

Insufflation then proceeds at a pressure of 15–17 mmHg and the blunt dissection is completed under direct vision with the scope moving forward in a fanning motion.

Tip: The scope should be 1 cm within the trocar to prevent it from getting dirty and wasting time cleaning it. Alternatively, a bariatric trocar (which is much longer) may be employed.

The second trocar (5 mm) is placed at the left pararectal level, a little below the line that unites the navel and the anterior superior iliac spine; the third trocar (5 mm) is placed 2 cm above and within the left anterior superior iliac spine. The fourth trocar (12 mm) is placed contralaterally to the left pararectal and the fifth trocar (5 mm) is placed 3 cm above and within the right anterior superior iliac spine.

Tip: It is worth remembering that one should perform the dissection of the bladder and prevesical space adequately, so that the trocars may be placed in the appropriate position.

Transperitoneal

For the initial approach, the authors use a modified Veress needle entry with abdominal wall retraction. A vertical skin incision is made in the umbilicus with an 11 blade. The anterior rectus sheath is cleared off, and a 2–3 mm incision is made until preperitoneal fat is seen. Two holding sutures of 2/0 Vicryl™ (passed inside out on the fascia) are lifted for anterior traction on the abdominal wall. This serves to increase the distance between the abdominal wall and underlying structures and provides countertraction to the resistance of the peritoneum encountered by the Veress needle.

Once pneumoperitoneum is created, the first trocar is placed blindly using a safety trocar that has a retractible blade. After introduction of the optical scope and exploration of the cavity, the other trocars are placed under direct vision. The order is similar to that of the extraperitoneal approach, or in accordance with what is discovered during exploration (Fig. 15.2).

Tips: It is important that the depth and rigging of the trocars be in such a way that they do not move, to prevent them from entering or exiting accidentally.

The first assistant employs the transumbilical trocar to introduce the 30° optical scope (which is manipulated with the left hand), and the fifth trocar to introduce the suction-irrigation cannula and other instruments (which are manipulated using the right hand). The second assistant uses the right hand to retract the bladder or bowel with a grasper through the third trocar, and the left hand to manipulate the metallic intraurethral bougie.

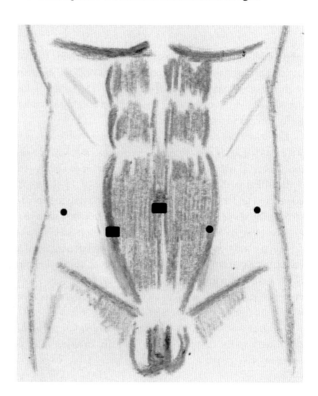

Fig. 15.2 Trocar placement. 10–12 mm (*square*), 5 mm (*circle*)

The authors use a high-definition 30° EndoEye laparoscopic video because of its multiple advantages. It allows the first assistant to manipulate it with one hand, and the 30° scope allows for lateral vision and a sense of depth not possible at with a 0° scope.

During dissection of the anterior wall of the prostate, bladder, and urethra, the bevel is pointed downwards and to the sides. In the lateral pedicles, the bevel is positioned upwards and to the middle. In the posterior wall of the prostate and the Denonvillier's fascia upwards, in the initial points of the anastomosis to the level of the urethra upwards, and in the rest it is downwards and to the side.

Transperitoneal Creation of Lateral Windows

With the 30° scope introduced in the peritoneal cavity through the first trocar (with the extreme distal located in the lower right quadrant and with the bevel pointed to the middle), the surgeon, with a grasper introduced by the left pararectal trocar, pulls on the urachus and presents the right umbilical ligament. Then using the 5-mm monopolar L-hook electrode introduced by the right pararectal trocar, the surgeon dissects the parietal peritoneum, creating a lateral window in the cephalo-caudal direction that proceeds laterally to the umbilical ligament down to the right vas deferens.

The surgeon proceeds in a similar manner on the left side until both dissection planes are united. The surgeon works using the two left 5-mm trocars and the first assistant performs counter-traction using the suction through the fourth trocar. Then, the second assistant introduces a grasper through the third trocar for cephalad retraction and posteriorly the peritoneal band made up of the urachus and the umbilical ligaments. In this manner, the surgeon completes dissection of the Retzius space reaching the pubis (Fig. 15.3).

Direction of Dissection

The laparoscopic dissection of the prostate was initially described in the antegrade direction, proceeding from base to apex. Other authors later presented the technique using retrograde dissection, similar to conventional open surgery.[1, 3] Nevertheless, both dissections have been combined with transperitoneal or extraperitoneal approaches. Technically, antegrade dissection is probably the most natural, in terms of the continuity of the prostate axis and taking into account the angle of the 0° scope. However, dissection of the lateral prostatic pedicle is difficult since the surgeon cannot spatially know the location of the distal point that he or she is heading towards.

Despite the use of the 30°scope and the ability to see the lateral border of the prostate, it is possible to lose the dissection plane of the lateral pedicle and head tangentially, sectioning the neurovascular bundles with consequent functional damage to the patient.

If difficulty is encountered in identifying the section's lateral line, the initial stitch (proximal) and the final one (distal), the authors first perform the retrograde dissection, which is possible due to the visibility obtained with the 30° scope. A proximal retraction

Fig. 15.3 (**a**, **b**) Umbilical ligaments and right lateral window

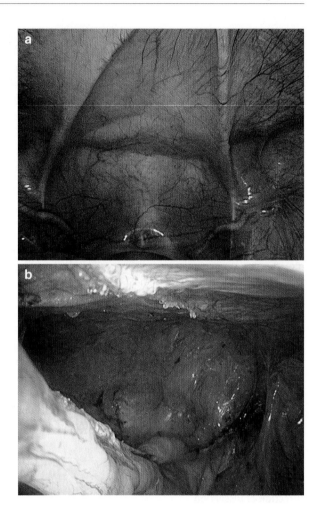

stitch in the prostate allows for it to be lifted, retracted, and for the apex to be turned, which makes dissection of the lateral bundles in a retrograde direction feasible. This approach makes the dissection safer as the stitch reached in the antegrade approach can be simply connected to the stitch where the retrograde approach ends.

Dissection of the Anterior Wall of the Prostate

The surgeon employs the grasper, SonoSurg and laparoscopic swab to remove the fat located in the anterior wall of the prostate. Dissection proceeds in a distal to the proximal direction; adipose tissue is removed as a continuous flap from the pubic bone back to the prostatovesical junction (Fig. 15.4).

Fig. 15.4 Dissection of fat in the anterior wall of the prostate

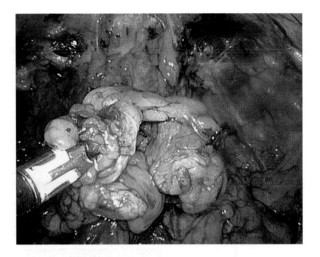

It is important to take care when sectioning the fat in the median distal line, because easy-to-bleed, superficial veins flow through this fat.

The presence of lymphatic ganglions in this tissue has been reported in some works, which is a reason to send it to anatomopathologic study.

Opening Endopelvic Fascia and Dividing the Prostatic Component of the Puboprostatic Ligament

The surgeon opens the endopelvic fascia, lateral periprostatic fascia and partial separation of the neurovascular bundles (from apex to base) with the scissors and the swab, sectioning the prostatic component of the puboprostatic ligament while respecting the fibers leading to the urethra.

On the right side, with the 30° scope bevel aimed to the left, the surgeon retracts the prostate to the contralateral side with a left hand grasper, and sections the endopelvic fascia with the scissors in the right hand. Then, the surgeon deepens the dissection of the fascia with the grasper in the left hand, retracts the medial cut edge of endopelvic fascia, exposing the posterolateral zone of the periprostatic fascia. The surgeon sections with the scissors in the right hand and dissects with a swab, cleaning the apex with in a clockwise motion (Fig. 15.5). The procedure on the left side is similar, but dissection of the apex with the torund requires counterclockwise movements.

Ligation and Division of the Dorsal Venous Complex

Prior to ligature of the vein complex, a proximal stitch is placed at the apex to group and unite the entire area of the complex along the median line for better definition, thus allowing for improved ligature. Furthermore, the stitch allows the application of traction and

Fig. 15.5 (**a**, **b**) Opening of
the endopelvic fascia

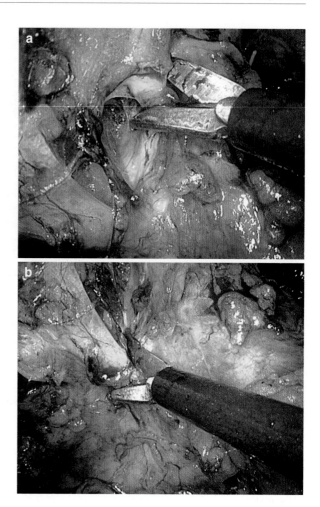

flection of the prostate to view the posterior component of the apex and thus facilitate retrograde dissection. Afterwards a second stitch is placed, which is the true distal stitch that encompasses the dorsal vein complex. Finally, with the Metzenbaum scissors, the dorsal vein complex is sectioned (Fig. 15.6).

Tip: To make proper placement of the needle used to ligate the vein complex easier, upon taking it with the needle-holder, press it against the anterior wall of the prostate and grasp it by its distal third. During its insertion it should be held straight; only after it has gone through nearly the entire complex should it be turned. If the needle is turned too quickly it may enter the complex.

Tip: When inserting the needle to ligate the vein complex, the first assistant should push the apex to the right with the suction device to see where the stitch exits. The second assistant should then go down with the Benique in the urethra, thus assuring that the needle enters between the area of the dorsal vein complex and the urethra.

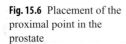

Fig. 15.6 Placement of the proximal point in the prostate

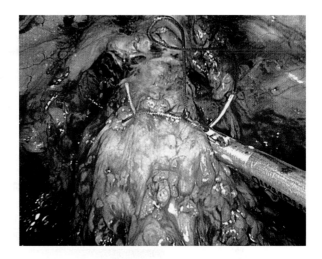

Problem: The dorsal vein complex bleeds after being ligated and sectioned.

Solution: The bleeding can be controlled with the Benique; compression should be applied beforehand against the arc of the pubis.

The placement of a linear stapling device is an alternative way to ligate the dorsal vein complex; it should be 30 mm in width, vascular, and placed with a TYCO clip that articulates and roticulates.

Tip: The placement of the linear device should be done in three movements: (1) articulation, (2) reticulation, and (3) another articulation. Keep the stapler closed for approximately 1 min to compress the tissue, expel edema, and improve tissue coaptation.

Some surgeons perform the antegrade dissection before ligating the vein complex and opening the endopelvic fascia. This technique was described by Gaston, who does not ligate the complex or open the fascia, but goes directly to open the vesicle neck, then advances laterally interfascial or intrafascial and finally ligates the dorsal vein complex. In the authors' case, they first connect the dorsal vein complex and proceed to the dissection of the urethra, performing the retrograde dissection of the prostate and then the antegrade dissection to communicate both dissections. Their technique will be further described in the following sections (Fig. 15.7).

Apical Dissection, Division of the Urethra

The laparoscopic nondisposable scissors are used to dissect the urethra; with lateral movements, proper identification the structures is possible with 30° of vision and the neurovascular bundles can be dissected laterally. The Benique is gently removed and sectioning of the anterior circumference of the urethra is performed with a single cut, if possible.

Tip: The urethral stump should be kept as long as possible, requiring dissection very close to the prostate, but without risking margin safety.

Fig. 15.7 (**a**–**d**) Ligation of
the dorsal venous complex
and point of suspension

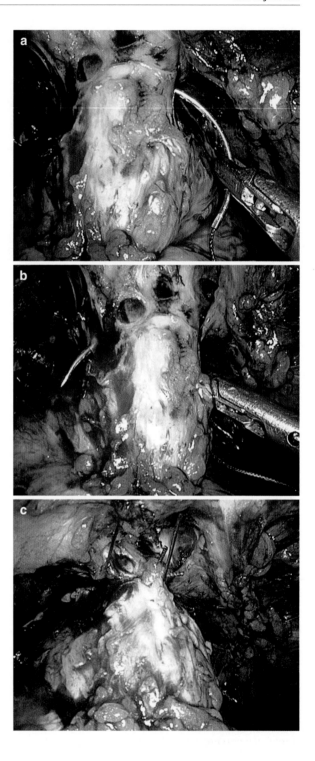

Fig. 15.7 (continued)

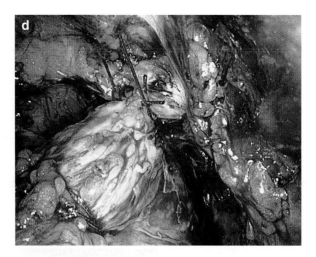

Tip: The opening angle of nondisposable scissors are greater than disposable ones, so transection of the urethra with regular continuous edges can be performed with fewer cuts.

With the help of the 10-mm right-angle dissector, the posterior plane of the urethra and the posterior rhabdosphincter are dissected. Before sectioning the posterior lip of urethra, the anatomy of the posterior lip of the prostate's apex is identified laterally using the 30° scope. This identification guarantees a correct cutting plane, since the posterior prostatic apex may extend distally beneath the urethra (Fig. 15.8).

Retrograde Dissection of the Prostatic Apex

Once the dorsal vein complex and the urethra are sectioned, the surgeon proceeds with retrograde dissection of the prostatic apex, sectioning the posterior rhabdosphincter, laterally dissecting the bundles, and reaching as far as the Denonvilliere fascia. Positioning the bevel of the 30° scope with downward and applying traction with the proximal stitch will help facilitate this dissection (Fig. 15.9).

Tip: For a better view during the retrograde dissection, the second assistant pulls from the proximal stitch and the surgeon, with a grasper in the left hand, pulls and bends the posterior lip of the apex.

Anterior Bladder Neck Dissection

Once retrograde dissection of the apex has been completed, the surgeon takes the prostate from the point of proximal traction. While performing lateral movements and with the posterior traction of the bladder, the cleavage plane between both structures can be clearly identified by observing the differences in mobility between a hollow organ (bladder) and a

Fig. 15.8 (**a**, **b**) Dissection
and division of the urethra

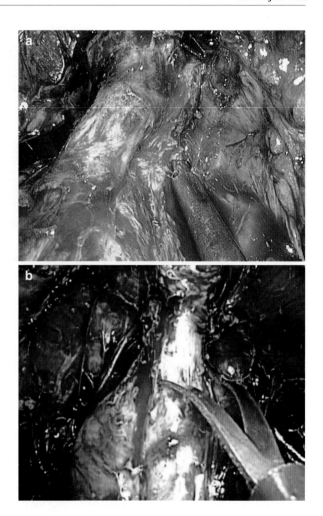

solid one (prostate). After identifying the line where the bladder and prostate meet, a transverse incision is performed using a 5-mm L-hook monopolar electrode until the bladder is
opened (Fig. 15.10).

*Another way to recognize the boundaries of the prostatic-vesicle is to differentiate the
fat on the prostatic surface (easily removable) and the bladder (denser and adheres to the
organ). It also helps to laterally follow the curvature of the prostate. A combination of
these maneuvers will aid in correctly identifying the limits for the cut.*

*A large median lobe may lead to confusion since the prostate and bladder may appear
to meet farther back. This may result in the surgeon sectioning in the wrong place, so care
should be taken in patients with large median lobes.*

*When cutting the anterior wall of the bladder, do not attempt to preserve the vesicle
neck since there is no evidence of improvement in continence by doing so. Performing the
anastomosis is difficult when the orifice is small, and at times it is impossible to determine*

Fig. 15.9 (**a**, **b**) Retrograde dissection of the prostatic apex

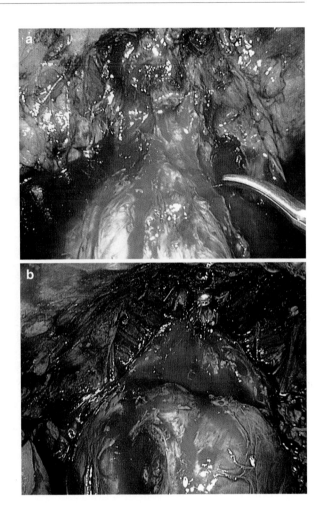

precisely whether there is or is not a median lobe. There is also the risk of cutting the posterior wall and leaving the lobe semidetached from the bladder.

With the anterior surface of the bladder sectioned, the authors release the traction of the prostate's proximal stitch and take the rim of the bladder that drops off, grabbing the prostate with a locking alligator grasper. The prostate is raised and bent, and the vesicle neck is laterally sectioned until the trigone is visible, which exposes the posterior mucous ending. (Fig. 15.11).

Posterior Bladder Neck Dissection

After sectioning the bladder's anterior wall and exposing the trigone, the authors section the lateral walls of the bladder, allowing the prostate to bend completely, separating it from the bladder. The authors then make a transversal incision with the electrocautery shears,

Fig. 15.10 (**a, b**) Anterior
bladder neck dissection

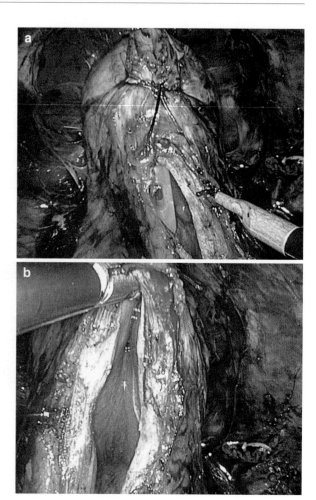

Fig. 15.10 (**a, b**) Anterior
bladder neck dissection

starting at the medial line and moving towards the entire depth of 4–5 mm along the shears
(which is the thickness of the wall), and then moving to the sides.

*Tip: If the median lobe appears, it can be retracted with suture. The posterior mucous
vesicle should be cut where the median lobe ends; generally it has hypervascularized, beefy
red mucosa that defines the border of the lobe and helps delineate the line of incision.*

Once the posterior wall of the bladder has been sectioned, the surgeon should pay careful attention to anatomic detail and identify the vertical vesicle fibers. This continues until
the areolar fat tissue is encountered and the deferential ducts appear.

*Tip: During dissection of the posterior wall of the bladder, once the vesicle fibers have
been visualized, the direction of dissection should change from frontal to posterior to finish
sectioning the posterior vesicle wall and reach the deferential plane and seminal vesicles.*

Once the adipose areolar tissue has been exposed, the second assistant changes the
grasper and takes the vesicle neck tissue stuck to the prostate, lifting it upwards and distal
to expose and bring the deferential ducts to the surface (Fig. 15.12).

Fig. 15.11 (**a, b**) Bladder trigone

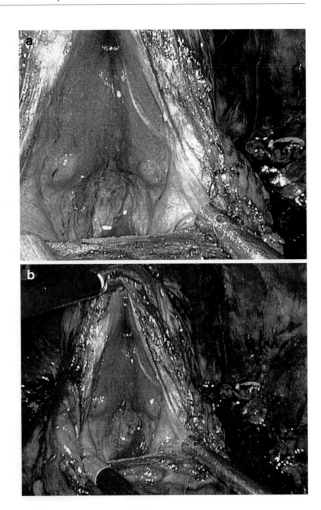

As the surgeon completes dissection of the posterior vesicle wall, the window is widened laterally before proceeding with the seminal vesicle to avoid working in a small cavity. As the prostate is freed from the lateral pedicles, the surgeon should finish releasing the bladder neck as it bends back and exhibits the deferential ducts and seminal vesicles.

Dissection of the Vas Deferens and Seminal Vesicles

Approaching the precise plane to dissect the deferential ducts and seminal vesicles requires meticulousness and care to gain adequate access to the area. Once the deferential ducts are visible, the surgeon begins pulling the planes apart. The assistant uses the grasper to retract the bladder backwards and the surgeon uses a hand to retract the duct, dissecting it as wide as possible.

Fig. 15.12 (**a–c**) Trigone and posterior bladder neck dissection with electrocautery

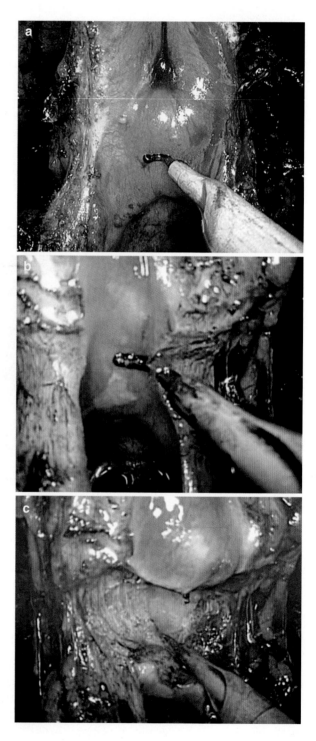

Fig. 15.13 (**a**, **b**) Dissection of the seminal vesicles

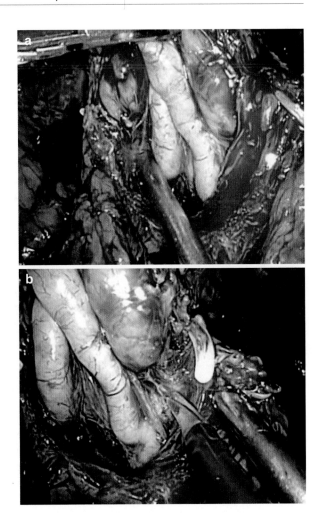

Tip: When performing the dissection of the deferential ducts (which form a rigid and easy-to-grab structure), do not be separate them from the vesicles. Instead, use the natural attachments of the vas to the seminal vesicles to deliver the seminal vesicles up.

Once dissection has progressed, the deferential ducts should be separated in order to dissect the seminal vesicles from within the duct. The surgeon begins with the internal wall of the seminal vesicles, which is under and within the duct, and ends with the outer wall. Generally, there is a vessel parallel to the deferential and seminal vesicle which is then directed to the external wall of the seminal vesicles (Fig. 15.13).

Dissection is performed with a swab or a swab-shaped piece of gauze to turn down the tissue that sticks to the seminal vesicles, only using clips and scissors to separate them. Once the seminal vesicles have been dissected, both should be lifted; it is recommended that the second assistant lift them, or the first assistant can lift one while the surgeon lifts the other. To dissect on the right side, the first assistant retracts the bladder and the surgeon takes the seminal vesicle. On the left side, the assistant should lift the vesicle while the surgeon retracts the bladder. It is also possible to insert a suprapubic 5-mm trocar to help to hold up the seminal vesicles.

Dissection of Denonvillier's Fascia

When the prostate is lifted upwards with a grasper applied over the seminal vesicles, Denonvillier's fascia is exposed. Downward retraction with the suction cannula over the rectum is applied. An incision is made using the scissors, with a cold transversal cut 2 mm below the prostate. A counter-traction maneuver is applied from the rectum downwards, exposing the yellowish tissue of the prerectal fat and separating it from the posterior wall of the prostate.

Tip: Once the transversal cut has been made, the 30° optical scope can be placed upwards to provide a better view of the posterior surface of the prostate during its dissection.

Tip: If there is a suspected injury to the rectum, fill the pelvic cavity with liquid and introduce a Foley catheter through the rectum to inject air. Air bubbles will indicate a rectal injury.

Ligation of Prostate Vascular Pedicles

Once Denonvillier's fascia and the rectum have been dissected, the surgeon and assistant should coordinate to dissect the lateral pedicle, keeping the prostate in upward traction. With the lateral walls of the prostate and the dissection line of the lateral periprostatic fascia in evidence, the surgeon proceeds to ligate the prostatic pedicles. This maneuver can be performed with 5- to 10-mm Hem-o-lok® clips, or alternatively, the SonoSurg can be employed during this step.

Once the prostate has been freed upon communicating the antegrade and retrograde dissection, the assistant should retract the bladder backwards and observe if there is any bleeding, particularly in the lateral pedicles. In case of bleeding, chromic cat gut figure-of-eight sutures can be placed (Fig. 15.14).

Tip: To perform ligature of the lateral pedicles, trace an imaginary line between the external lateral surface of the prostate and the medial surface. This will indicate which direction the surgeon should move. To ascertain depth, raise the prostate and search for the point of retrograde dissection that was previously reached.

Specimen Extraction

The prostate and seminal vesicles are placed in an extraction pouch (Endopouch). To shorten operative time in a transperitoneal approach, the specimen is placed in the cavity to be extracted at the end of the surgery. The thread fastening the extraction pouch (with

Fig. 15.14 (a–c) Dissection and ligature of the lateral pedicles

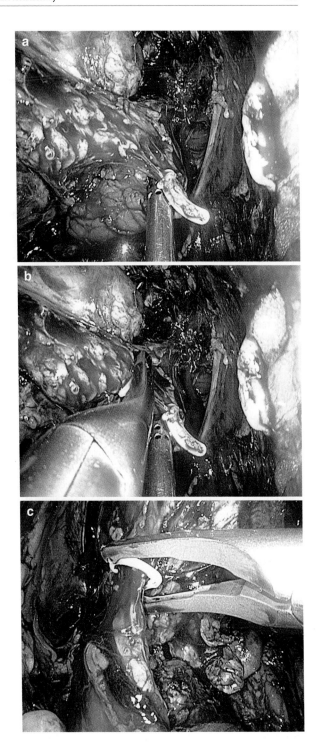

Fig. 15.15 Prostate and seminal vesicles in the extraction pouch

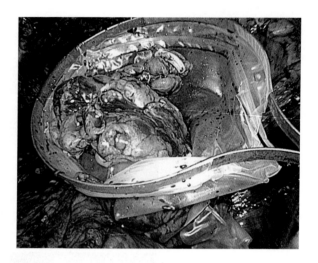

the specimen inside) is exteriorized with the umbilical trocar. This easily extracts the specimen once the surgery is complete (Fig. 15.15).

Urethrovesical Anastomosis

Generalities

Urethrovesical anastomosis is the reconstructive stage of this surgery, requiring experience and dedicated laparoscopic training. It represents a fundamental step in the results of a laparoscopic radical prostatectomy, and poor technique can have short- and long-term consequences, not just regarding morbidity (urine leak, duration of catheterization), but also functional outcomes (bladder neck contractures).

Instruments

There are some needle-holder models that automatically align or rectify the needle with the axis of the instrument to maintain a 90° angle. These types of needle-holders are not recommended for performing anastomosis as the needle needs to be at different angles to the needle holder axis during this part of the procedure.

Suturing Tips

1. *If possible, manipulate the target tissue into a favorable position for an easy forehand or backhand stitch.*
2. *If the target tissue is rigid or cannot be manipulated (e.g., the urethral stump), change the angle of the needle in the driver.*

3. *Simulate the movement of the needle (in the "air") before placing the stitch to ensure that the desired path will be accomplished.*
4. *If the previous suggestions do not achieve the optimal path, place the needle driver in a different trocar.*
5. *Try using the nondominant hand to achieve the best angle of approach.*

There are needle-holders made for the right hand and others for the left with curved points; the authors prefer the straight needle-holders that can be used in either hand. The Olympus brand is recommended as the distal extreme is slightly thicker, its jaws stronger and more robust, which prevents the needle from sliding and changing angles when held. Another benefit is that when the insert in the needle-holder wears out, only the insert needs to be changed and not the whole instrument.

The use of an absorbable monofilament such as Monocryl™ or Biosyn™ suture is recommended since it easily slides without tearing the tissues, mainly of the urethra. It is fundamental that there be a UR-6 type (Monocryl™) or GU-46 (Biosyn™) needle, as its curvature allows for optimal passage over the urethral stump.

For anastomosis, some use a Benique with a hole in the tip; the needle is inserted into the Benique orifice and when it is removed, the point of the needle falls into the urethra. Instead of this maneuver, the authors torque the sound to the side opposite the needle path. The needle tip passes in the space between the metal and the mucosa, rather than in the hollow bore of the sound itself. However, either technique is acceptable. Alternatively, an assistant can pass the Foley catheter tip in and out, coordinating with the needle movement to avoid incorporating the Foley catheter in the stitch.

Type of Anastomosis

Urethra-bladder anastomosis is described in several ways: with interrupted stitches, continuous stitches or a combination of the two. The advantage of anastomosis with continuous sutures is that it guarantees a superior water-tightness to results obtained using separate stitches. Anastomosis with continuous stitches may be performed in several ways; some surgeons perform it with a single suture, others with two sutures knotted together beforehand in their distal threads. These sutures go from outside to inside in the posterior wall of the bladder in such a way that the knot is in the outer wall (van Velthoven).[2]

In the authors' case, they employ individual sutures knotted separately in each initial stitch. The stitches advance circumferentially from the posterior plane to the anterior, the left going clockwise and the right counter-clockwise. The sutures meet around the back, one ending in the urethra and the other in the bladder and are finally tied together.

There are two reasosn to not use two prewoven sutures, the first being that there is a risk of stenosis of the anastomosis in a purse-string fashion, which can be avoided by using two separate sutures. The second reason is that when the stitches pass through the posterior urethral wall, the maneuver becomes difficult as posterior gaps may occur when pulling the posterior plate together, particularly when there is tension. For these reasons, the authors prefer to use separate sutures that allows each closure of the posterior wall to be checked.[4] As an alternative, the van Velthoven approach can be used with care to ensure that the posterior plate comes together completely. With either approach, a monofilament suture should be used.

Anastomosis with Two Separate Sutures with Continuous Stitches

With the 30° scope guided upwards, the first stitch is placed into the urethra at the 5 o'clock position with the right needle-holder, with the needle introduced from the outside in. When the needle goes in from outside, it is more posterior and takes up a greater quantity of the rhabdosphincter and urethral muscle (external circle and internal longitudinal). Then, upon turning the hand, the point of the needle enters the urethral lumen, perforating the cylindric epithelium very near the edge. This maneuver guarantees a greater consistency and solidity of the anchoring tissue, keeping the urethra from coming loose when tying the knot, and assures approximation of the bladder and urethra.

Once the suture is through the urethra, the surgeon proceeds to the bladder stitch. With the help of the left needle-holder to grip and retract the bladder from its anterior wall, allowing a downward view with the 30° scope, the posterior wall of the bladder and the passage of the needle with the right needle-holder from inside out in radio five.

The knot is placed outside of the anastomosis, towards the right. The first semi-knot loops around three times to maintain the tension and prevent slippage, while the second and third knot loop around twice.

Problem: Tension when lowering the bladder when tying the first knot.

Solution: After verifying that the second assistant has removed the traction on the bladder, the first assistant applies suction at the level of the trigone, which helps lower the bladder and reduce tension so that the first semi-knot can be adjusted. If tension persists, it causes difficulty in approaching the vesicle neck, impeding coaptation of the anastomosis knot. This generally occurs because the bladder has not been well dissected laterally and is solved by completing the dissection. A few additional millimeters can be gained by reducing the pneumoperitoneum pressure to <5 mm by having the assistant apply suction.

Once the first stitch is in and the knot is on the outside and the needle is on the right, there are two ways to continue with anastomosis: (1) pass the entire suture with the needle behind the knot (in order to be on the left side) and continue with a ipsilateral semicircle, or (2) take it with the right needle-holder and pass it diagonally from outside in, moving right to left throughout the entire length of the bladder so that it comes out from within on the left side. The second maneuver saves time and is the authors' preferred method.

Tip: Before putting the first stitch in the urethra, the perineum can be compressed, allowing for better exposure and visualization of the urethral stump.

Tip: As much for placing the stitches in the bladder, as for those in the lateral and anterior urethra walls, the bevel of the 30° scope is pointed downward, allowing for optimum visualization of the place where the needle goes in and/or comes out.

Now with the needle within the bladder, the authors end by putting the second stitch in the urethra with the right hand, from the inside out, with the 30° scope positioned upwards (Fig. 15.16).

Fig. 15.16 (a–b) First stitch in the urethra and passage of the needle in the posterior wall of the bladder

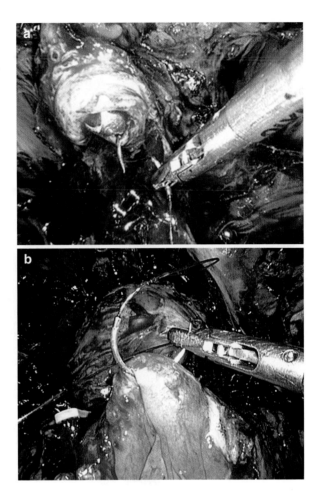

Tip: Before putting in the anastomosis stitch, make a separation with the Beniqué in the direction opposite to the needle's point of entry, leaving space between the Benique and the urethral wall. Once the point of the needle is in this space, remove the Benique to allow for the turn and exit of the needle outside the urethra.

The following two or three stitches of the left posterior quadrant of the urethra are placed with the left hand, moving clockwise, from inside out. Then in the left anterior quadrant, the needle-holder is switched to the right hand. With the bevel of the 30° scope positioned downwards to show the zone where the needle will pass with the free hand, stitches are placed in the bladder from the outside in with the left needle-holder in the posterior quadrant and with the right needle-holder in the anterior quadrant (Fig. 15.17).

To complete the urethrovesical anastomosis, the surgeon begins with a stitch at the 5 o'clock position in the right semicircle, using the right needle-holder. The stitch goes from inside out in the urethra and then, from outside in the bladder, and a double knot is tied on the outside. The stitches of the urethra are placed with the right hand in the poste-

Fig. 15.17 (**a**, **b**) Stitches of
the left semicircle

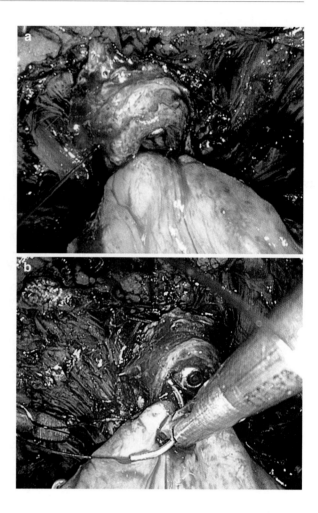

rior quadrant and with the left hand in the anterior quadrant; the stitches in the
bladder are done with the right hand (Fig. 15.18).

*Tip: Before passing the needle in the needle-holder through the tissue, simulate the
movement externally. This ensures that the needle will go in the direction that is mentally
expected, as the view is two-dimensional and without depth; potentially the point of the
needle can pass closer or farther away than intended.*

It is important to keep the ureteral orifices in sight during anastomosis. As this maneuver is complex, it is recommended that diuresis be forced to make the ejaculated urethral
evident or for intravenous carmine indigo be administered to mark the orifices. If the
bladder neck has been preserved and the ureteral orifices are well away from harm, no
additional attempt to expose them must be undertaken.

Upon finishing both semi-circles, the two suture threads are in the exterior of the urethra. The surgeon then passes into the bladder with the needle on the right side, first from

Fig. 15.18 Stitches of the
right semicircle

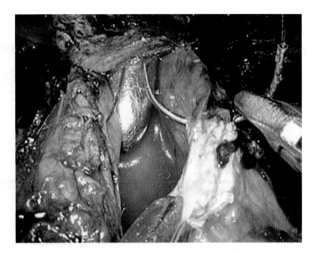

outside in and finally from inside out. This positions the sutures one in front of the other
before they are tied together.

Before tying the threads, the transurethral vesicle catheter should be introduced with a
metal guide. It is fundamental to visualize clearly that the catheter is ahead of the mucous
of the posterior vesicle wall to guarantee proper placement.

*Tip: Once the catheter has been placed within the bladder using the guide, the curve
will tent up the anterior bladder wall. Moving the guide from side to side will clearly
indicate its position.*

In cases where the size of the mouth of the bladder proportionally exceeds the dimen-
sions of the diameter of the urethral stump, the anastomosis must be remodeled using the
stitches in the urethra that are closest to each other and the stitches in the bladder that are
farthest apart. Nevertheless, if there is one too many in the bladder, it should be closed off
with another continuous suture after the threads are tied.

Drainage

It is important to put in drainage in the form of a Blake drain to help guide any leaked
urine. It is recommended that one of the most lateral ports be employed for that purpose
(Fig. 15.19). According to how it wears out it is maintained up to 24 h when it is less than
25 cc, this is on average between 2 and 5 days.

Specimen Extraction

The specimen is finally extracted through the umbilical orifice which can be progressively
extended to adapt to the size of the specimen. Care should be taken not to incorporate
bowel into the fascial closure.

Fig. 15.19 Blake drain

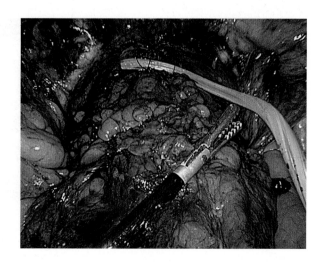

References

1. Gill IS, Zippe CD. Laparoscopic radical prostatectomy: technique. *Urol Clin North Am.* 2001;28:423-436.
2. van Velthoven RF, Ahleving TE, Clayman RU, et al. Technique for laparoscopic running ureterovesical anastomosis: the single knot method. *Urology.* 2003;161:699-702.
3. Rassweiler J, Marrero R, Hammady A, et al. Transperitoneal laparoscopic radical prostatectomy: ascending technique. *J Endourol.* 2004;18(7):593-600.
4. Branco AW, Kondo W, De Camargo A, et al. Laparoscopic running urethrovesical anastomosis with posterior fixation. *Urology.* 2007;70(4):799-802.

Difficulties in Robotic Radical Prostatectomy

16

Manoj B. Patel, Sanket Chauhan, Kenneth J. Palmer, and Vipul R. Patel

Introduction

The task of learning robotic-assisted laparoscopic prostatectomy (RALP) can be quite challenging for both novice and experienced open or laparoscopic surgeons alike. Therefore, prior to the first procedure, adequate training and planning is required as the entire surgical team prepares for the upcoming challenge. The learning curve to achieve basic competency has been estimated to be between 20 and 25 cases.[1, 2] However, during the initial stage of the learning curve, the surgeon should screen potential operative candidates cautiously to minimize the technical challenges of the procedure by selecting "ideal candidates" so that the surgical team can ease into the experience. As the experience of the surgeon and robotic team develops, one can begin to entertain the idea of tackling more challenging clinical scenarios, as studies have shown that difficult cases were attempted after performing a median of 50 procedures.[3]

After performing over 3,000 cases, it is the authors' opinion that no single learning curve exists and that there is a continual process of education and refinement. It is the authors' belief that after the initial learning curve, one naturally transitions to more challenging cases, often leading to longer surgical times and increased difficulty during surgery. This stepladder approach allows the surgeon to continually develop the skills to deal with even the most challenging patients. However, during the initial learning period, the authors recommend excluding obese patients and patients with prior abdominal surgery. The authors also advocate initially screening all patients with either flexible cystoscopy or transrectal ultrasound to detect and avoid patients with prominent median lobes, prior history of transurethral resection of the prostate (TURP) defects or large prostate gland size. In this chapter, various challenging scenarios during the RALP procedure will be entertained, followed by a discussion of the authors' approach to these various challenges.

M.B. Patel (✉)
Department of Urologic Surgery, Global Robotics Institute, Florida Hospital-Celebration Health, Celebration, FL, USA
e-mail: manojbpatel@msn.com

A.M. Al-Kandari and I.S. Gill (eds.), *Difficult Conditions in Laparoscopic Urologic Surgery*,
DOI: 10.1007/978-1-84882-105-7_16, © Springer-Verlag London Limited 2011

The Challenges of the Complex Patient

Management of Difficult Anesthesia Cases

The risk of anesthetic complications related to the pneumoperitoneum during robotic surgery is similar to other reported laparoscopic procedures. One major fatal complication is a gas embolism, which can cause severe cardiovascular failure and death if not detected promptly. It is believed to occur from carbon dioxide (CO_2) gas entering the venous vascular system and therefore is trapped in the right ventricle, causing outflow obstruction from the right ventricle into the pulmonary artery. The initial characteristic clinical findings are mill-wheel cardiac murmur, hypoxia, decreased end-tidal CO_2 concentration through the ET tube, and cyanosis. Intra-operative transesophageal echocardiography may confirm the diagnosis. Treatment protocol involves rapid release of pneumoperitoneum followed by hyperventilation with 100% oxygen and placing the patient in the left lateral decubitus and Trendelenburg position (to mobilize the gas bubbles from the right ventricle) and aspirating the gas embolus via a central venous catheter.

Patients with a significant history for emphysema or chronic obstructive pulmonary disease COPD present with an anesthesia challenge during RALP. Due to its high diffusion coefficient and soluble characteristics, CO_2 is the ideal gas for establishing pneumoperitoneum while minimizing the risks of gas emboli. Carbon dioxide levels are easily measured at the end of exhalation. The anesthesiologist should be adamant, especially in COPD cases, to monitor the CO_2 levels and to adjust the ventilator accordingly to remove excess CO_2, preventing hypercarbia and acidosis. Furthermore, the functional residual capacity is reduced during laparoscopy due to the limited expansion of the diaphragm from the pneumoperitoneum and patient positioning, resulting in decreased pulmonary compliance and ventilation/perfusion mismatching – further exaggerating the acidosis state. Increasing the minute volume may correct this, but patients with pulmonary dysfunction may present a particular challenge. This illustrates the need for careful selection of patients undergoing robotic surgery as well as preoperative pulmonary and cardiac clearance.

Difficult Access and Port Placement in Patients with Midline Laparotomies

There are many safe and effective methods of obtaining peritoneal access. Individual surgeon preference leads to the development of a technique that is comfortable and reproducible. It may be advantageous to know more than one technique, especially in cases where there is a history of prior abdominal surgery or a significant amount of subcutaneous fat. Veress needle access can achieve pneumoperitoneum quickly, though it is a blind procedure relying on the feel of the needle popping into the peritoneum. The reported rates of vascular and bowel injuries vary from 0.03% to 0.3%.[4] If a Veress needle is used, it is important to be cognitive of the location of the aorta and iliac vessels near the umbilicus, which can be injured with overzealous needle entry. The needle should be aspirated to ensure no return of blood or gastric content, followed by injection of saline. The "drop test" should be performed to confirm that saline flows freely into the peritoneum. If there is any doubt, the sequence should be repeated or the needle replaced. Once insufflation is started, a low intraperitoneal pressure (<5 mmHg) suggests correct needle placement. After insufflation is completed, the initial port can be placed blindly or with an optical access trocar. The optical access trocar allows visualization of tissue planes and may prevent bowel perforation.

An open or modified Hasson technique may used in patients with prior abdominal surgery to reduce the risk of inadvertent injury to the bowel or vascular structures by allowing direct visual placement of the trocar into the peritoneum. However, this approach can create leakage of gas from the established pneumoperitoneum. The authors' modified Hasson technique consists of making a 2-cm to 3-cm vertical incision supraumbilically, entering the peritoneal cavity under direct vision. More specifically, with the rectus fascia is exposed, anchoring sutures are placed on either end of the fascia; the fascia is incised through the midline linea alba while the fascia is tented up with the anchor sutures. These anchoring sutures will also facilitate closure of the rectus fascia at the conclusion of the procedure. After additional blunt dissection, a finger is then used to navigate an entry to the peritoneum. The extent of intra-peritoneal adhesions is assessed with the 5-mm laparoscopic camera. If extensive adhesions are noted, the incision is lengthened to a small mini-laparotomy incision of 2–3 in. This limited but spacious access allows for open lysis of adhesions until enough space is developed for the placement of at least two other trocars in their regular position. The mini-laparotomy incision is reapproximated around the camera port and pneumoperitoneum is established. Once the robot is docked, adhesions in the lower abdomen and pelvis can be efficiently released with the assistance of the 3D vision and wrist articulation of the robot.

The Obese Patient

Patients that are of an abnormal body habitus can provide a technical challenge for any type of surgical approach, including open, laparoscopic, or robotic. Abnormal body configurations often require the entire operative team, including anesthesia, nursing, and surgical staff, to deviate from their normal routines. This is particularly true for obese (body mass index or BMI>30) and morbidly obese patients (BMI>40), as they often have a large girth and breadth. The increased amount of internal and external body fat, along with their medical co-morbidities, often provides a challenge with anesthesia, positioning, and the surgical approach. However, understanding and adapting to the intricacies presented by these patients, in addition to the nuances of robotic surgery, will allow the surgical team to optimize the chances of success.

In preparation for robotic prostatectomy, patients are placed supine, in low lithotomy with a moderate Trendelenburg position. A study using the cadaveric model showed that hip abduction greater than 30° can cause significant strain on the obturator nerve to cause neural damage.[5] This strain is alleviated by flexing the hip by 45° or more. Therefore, during RALP, the authors attempt to minimize the amount of hip abduction and maximize the degree of hip flexion that still accommodates the robotic arms. It is extremely important that these patients be positioned properly, with adequate padding on the extremities, and stabilized to prevent unwanted movement during surgery. The authors recommend that the patient be placed centered on the table in low lithotomy with all pressure points padded on a desufflated bean bag that is strapped to the table. The authors' standard patient positioning is shown in Fig. 16.1. The desufflated bean bag will cradle the patient and prevent movement while the patient is in the Trendelenburg position. Once the robot has been docked, there can be no adjustment in the robotic surgical cart as it is locked in a fixed position adjacent to the patient. However, the operating room bed can be unlocked and moved into the optimal position for fine adjustments.

Once the patient is positioned, the next step is in determining optimal trocar selection and placement. One must be cognitive of the fact that the robotic arms have a maximum working length of 25 cm and complications can arise from placing the ports too near or too distant from the camera port. The working arm ports should be placed 8–10 cm from the camera port to not only avoid clashing of the instruments within the abdomen, but also with the arm collisions on the outside of the patient. For obese patients, the authors recommend using the extra long *da Vinci*® S robotic system (Intuitive Surgical Inc., Sunnyvale, CA) trocars and accessory instrumentation. This will allow the center point of the trocars to stay at the fascia level, facilitating optimal movement; in addition it will prevent the tips of the trocars from slipping out of the abdominal wall should there be an inadvertent drop in pneumoperitoneal pressure.

Even in obese patients, the authors tend to keep their trocar placement constant to optimize the movement of the robotic instruments and that of the assistant. The authors employ

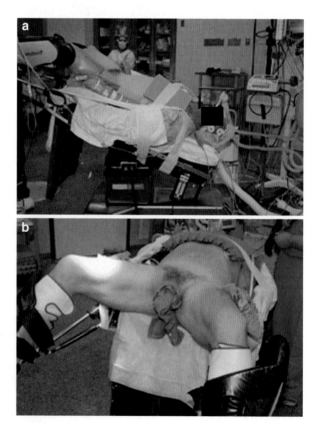

Fig. 16.1 (**a, b**) Patient positioning in steep Trendelenburg prior to draping

a 6-port transperitoneal approach for RALP, in which trocar placement has stayed constant over the last 1,500 cases. The authors' standard trocar placement is shown in Fig. 16.2. The assistant ports are positioned more cranially to allow maximum maneuverability without obstruction by the robot. The pubic bone to umbilicus length is not measured, as this is not the main issue in these patients; the issue is the challenging angles created by their body habitus. Many obese patients have an abdominal wall that is quite lax and inflates like a dome, moving the trocars further up and out (Fig. 16.3). In addition, the trocars are elevated well above the level of the pubic bone, often providing a challenging angle for the

Fig. 16.2 Trocar placement. With the exception of the 5 mm assistant port, each port should be placed 8–10 cm from each other. The 5 mm port is placed just cranial to the umbilical port and midway between the right robotic trocar and the umbilical camera port

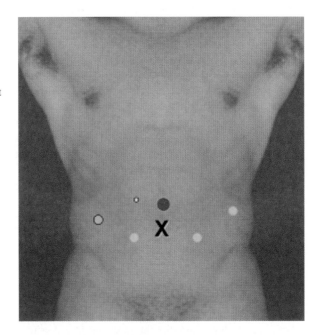

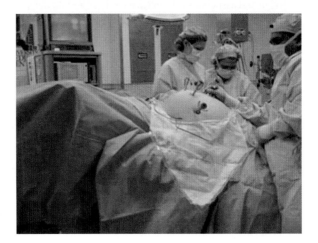

Fig. 16.3 Ballooning of trocars in an obese patient with rotund abdomen

robotic instruments as they try to tackle the apical area of the prostate. In this situation, instruments are often obstructed by the pubic bones. This will often require readjustment of the angles of the robotic arms by tucking them in lower on the abdominal wall. Even with these adjustments, it is possible that during the operation the instruments may have difficulty reaching the apex. In this scenario, the trocars can be advanced further by pressing the setup-joint button and inserting the trocar further into the abdomen under direct vision. It should be noted that this will often offset the center point of the trocar and should only be performed under necessitating circumstances. The newer version of the robot, the *da Vinci*® S system, is equipped with instruments that have a longer reach by 2 in., and therefore adjustment of trocar placement has not been necessary.

Another essential point that cannot be overemphasized is the importance of correct technique during trocar insertion in patients with thick abdominal walls secondary to fatty tissue. Due to the large distance between the skin and the fascia in these patients, an incorrect angulation of the trocar during insertion through the skin can be exaggerated significantly by the time it pierces the fascia. Optimally, the trocar should be inserted into the abdomen at a 90° angle to the fascia and skin. In obese patients, an oblique insertion will lead to the trocar entering the fascia at a location distant to that of the entry through the skin. This will alter the center point of the trocar and require it to pivot at two widely placed points of resistance at the skin and the fascia, potentially interfering with optimal instrument movement. An easy way to check whether a port is placed in the proper fashion is to view the exterior of the trocar after placement. If properly placed, it will project at a nearly perpendicular direction from the skin. On the other hand, a trocar that appears to be at an acute angle may indeed have a hole in the fascia distant from that in the skin, causing limited range of motion of the robotic instruments.

Once the operation has begun, obese patients often provide the additional challenge of increased intra-abdominal fat that obscures the vision of the surgical field. It is essential that the patient has been placed in Trendelenburg position and that adequate insufflation pressures (12–15 mmHg) be maintained. In addition, adequate retraction of the intra-abdominal contents will be necessary. The authors have found it beneficial to use the fourth robotic arm to hold back the fat and provide exposure. Another option employed by Ahlering and associates is to place a 0-silk suture on the urachus after the retropubic space has been developed. This suture is grasped and exited through the 5-mm trocar port with the end snapped to a clamp. This clamp is placed on traction by the assistant to allow the intestinal segments and fat to be pushed cranially by the retracted bladder (T. E. Ahlering, oral communication, May 2009). In obese patients, the anastomosis can be a challenge as the angles of the instrumentation and the working space is less than optimal. The key is to maintain adequate retraction and exposure while optimally using the wristed instrumentations to compensate for the lack of space and agility.

Patients with Prior Inguinal Hernia Repair

Open or laparoscopic radical prostatectomy performed after the prior repair of an inguinal hernia, especially with the placement of mesh products, can be challenging for a surgeon. The key issue is distortion of the planes in the retropubic space secondary to scarring from the prior dissection or placement of mesh. This problem can be similar after open or laparoscopic inguinal hernia repair surgery, however, the most difficult dissection is considered to be after a laparoscopic pre-peritoneal hernia repair. This is due to the fact that the exact space that needs to be entered during the robotic prostatectomy has been violated.

While hernia repair does distort the surgical anatomy, the authors have not found it to significantly deviate the surgical approach. The key has been identification of the surgical landmarks and precise dissection below the level of the hernia repair. Via the transperitoneal approach, it is usually quite apparent that a hernia repair has been performed as the mesh, sutures, or tacks are quite prominent laterally on the pubic bone. The authors' recommended approach is to first visualize the normal anatomy: the urachus, median umbilical ligaments, vas deferens, and, if possible, the pubic bone. The initial incision is best made in the midline above the bladder and then carried laterally. If one has difficulty visualizing the boundaries of the bladder, it can be filled externally via the urinary catheter with 200 cc of fluid to provide a more distinct anatomy. It is important to enter the retropubic space in the midline to localize the posterior aspect of the pubic symphysis. Once the symphysis has been identified, the superior pubic rami can be exposed and followed laterally and deep into the pelvis to expose the endopelvic fascia (EPF) bilaterally. If the vas deferens draped by the peritoneum can be identified, the dissection is extended laterally to the medial borders of the vas. By using this systematic approach, the mesh or scarring from the previous surgery is often never encountered. If the mesh is seen, it is essential to keep the plane of dissection deep to the mesh at all times.

In patients with prior laparoscopic pre-peritoneal hernia repairs, tissue scarring can be more prominent. Again, the same principles are followed: a midline dissection into the retropubic space is developed, then extended laterally to the vas and deep along the EPF. A constant part of these complex dissections is early exposure of anatomical landmarks in the pelvis to help provide spatial orientation.

The Challenges of the Bladder Neck Dissection

Dealing with nuances of the bladder neck is probably the most challenging aspect of RALP. The unique variability of the anatomy at the bladder neck can pose quite a formidable task to even the most adept surgeon. The key is to recognize the anatomical landmarks and provide a precise dissection in a clear surgical field. The anterior bladder neck can be recognized in a variety of ways. One option is to observe the level of descent of the urethral catheter with a gentle tug. However, this maneuver can be compromised if there is a median lobe or a history of a prior TURP. The optimal method is to visualize the borders of the prostate laterally after the periprostatic fat has been cleared off. The cessation of the bladder fat as it approaches the prostate is usually the most reliable indicator of the boundary between the bladder and prostate. Once it is located, it should be dissected precisely to prevent inadvertent entry into the prostate. The authors recommend using the bipolar grasper and monopolar scissors to dissect on either side of the midline following the lateral contours of the prostate. If it is difficult to locate the planes of dissection, one should follow the bladder fibers down the midline as this will lead to entry into the anterior bladder at a safe location. An alternative method to identify the prostatovesical junction has been described by Tewari et al., where using blunt robotic instruments, the prostate is trapped on both sides and pulled proximally until there is a sudden feeling of "giving way" at its junction with the collapsed bladder.[6] Once the bladder has been entered, the urinary catheter can be identified and retracted superiorly with the fourth robotic arm to expose the posterior bladder neck.

The posterior bladder neck is best approached by incising the bladder neck full thickness and then dissecting directly downward. The bipolar grasper can be used to manipulate the posterior bladder neck and help identify the contour of the posterior plane. The dissection should be limited to the midline unless absolutely necessary, as lateral migration of the dissection will often lead to opening of the peripheral venous sinuses. If one sees vertically oriented white fibers during dissection, then these are of bladder origin. Incising these fibers horizontally will lead one into the correct plane to locate the seminal vesicles under the prostate (Fig. 16.4).

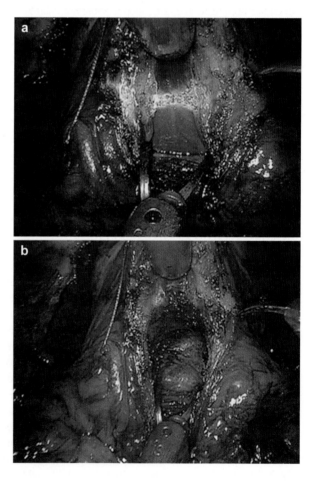

Fig. 16.4 (**a**) Posterior bladder neck dissection showing the white vertically oriented fibers and (**b**) completed posterior dissection exposing the seminal vesicles

Enlarged Prostate

Prostates that are larger than 100 g can also pose a surgical dilemma. These larger sizes pose many anatomical challenges as they often occupy a large portion of the pelvis, making exposure and rotation of the prostate difficult during dissection. In addition, larger prostates often have a generous blood supply and thick pedicles, further complicating the procedure. However, one advantage of large prostates is that they possess more obvious boundaries, which make the anatomical planes of dissection more distinct. It is important to carry out each stage of the procedure in a precise manner during RALP, as small mistakes have a tendency to produce an escalating "snowball" effect, leading ultimately to non-progression. However, if approached correctly, these cases can be performed safely with relative efficiency and low complication rates.

The authors recommend preoperative cystoscopy or transrectal ultrasound evaluation of all candidates during the first 20–25 cases of the learning curve and avoidance of such large prostates. The key to the dissection of an enlarged prostate is early identification and ligation of the dorsal venous complex (DVC). Opening the EPF, division of the puboprostatic ligaments, and early control of the dorsal vein will allow clear identification of the apical borders and reduces venous bleeding from large periprostatic veins throughout the remainder of the case.

The anterior bladder neck is once again potentially the most challenging aspect of the dissection, as the large volume of the prostate requires a technically precise dissection in the correct plane. It is important to provide adequate exposure to allow wide dissection without working in a tunnel with a deep hole. The key is to stay in the correct surgical plane between the vesicoprostatic junction; this is achieved by providing cranial retraction of the bladder with the fourth arm, producing an inverted-V shape of the detrusor musculature at the vesicoprostatic junction. Furthermore, traction can be applied on the Foley catheter by the assistant while visualizing the position of the Foley balloon on the bladder neck. Visual confirmation of where the perivesical fat stops at the vesicoprostatic junction is another technique in identifying the plane of dissection. The anterior bladder neck dissection should be approached in the midline following the vertical detrusor fibers, which are seen only if dissecting in the correct plane. Dissection should proceed strictly in the midline without deviating laterally, as this will minimize bleeding from large venous sinuses. Once the anterior bladder has been entered, the urinary catheter should be retracted anteriorly using the fourth arm to elevate the prostate superiorly, exposing the posterior bladder neck.

The posterior bladder neck dissection is difficult in that it requires dissecting deep in the posterior plane to reach the seminal vesicles. The key element in this dissection is maintaining a wide exposure by releasing the lateral bladder attachments to flatten out the posterior dissection, thus avoid working in a deep hole. Care must be taken to avoid extensive lateral dissection as bleeding from venous sinuses will increase, obscuring vision. Once the seminal vesicles are identified, the lateral bladder attachments are clipped with 10-mm Hem-o-lok® clips (Teleflex Medical, Research Triangle Park, NC) and divided. The keys to a successful bladder neck dissection are broad exposure, maintaining a relative bloodless operative field, and correct identification of surgical planes.

Prominent Median Lobe

The protrusion of a median lobe of prostatic tissue into the bladder neck can provide a surgical challenge, as it is often difficult to distinguish the true plane between the posterior bladder neck and the prostate. The first step in dealing with a median lobe is to diagnose its presence. This can be done preoperatively with cystoscopy or transrectal ultrasound. If the diagnosis is not made preoperatively, several clues during surgery can help with the diagnosis. Prior to the bladder neck dissection, a gentle tug on the urinary catheter will show contralateral deviation of the balloon away from the side of a unilateral median lobe enlargement. In patients with a circumferential or midline median lobe, the urinary catheter will not descend to the level of the true visualized bladder neck; this can be easily seen when inflating the Foley balloon with 40 cc of sterile water. The most definitive clue is the absence of the "drop-off" sign, which occurs when the Foley catheter is elevated while the bladder neck is opened with the forceps and the posterior bladder neck drops vertically downward into the body of the bladder in the absence of a median lobe. If the bladder base continues cranially, a median lobe is almost certainly present (Fig. 16.5). In this case, the lateral bladder attachments should be taken down to further expose the bladder base and trigonal area. With retraction on the anterior bladder neck, the median lobe can be delivered and elevated out of the bladder neck with the fourth arm. If the surgeon is unable to perform this, an alternative is to perform an anterior midline cystostomy to gain definitive visualization and assessment of the bladder neck anatomy. The median lobe can be lifted out of the bladder neck and retracted upward to locate the prostatic-posterior bladder neck junction.

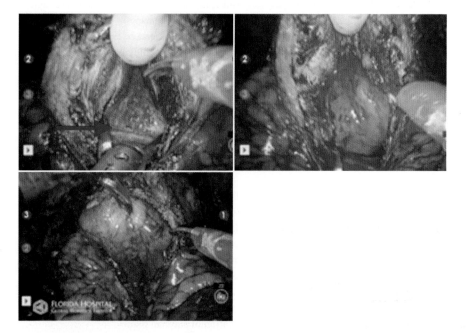

Fig. 16.5 Presence of median lobe with absence of "drop-off" sign as indicated by arrow

Prior to dissecting the posterior bladder neck, one must realize the presence of a voluminous median lobe will displace the bladder neck cranially, thus reducing its distance from the ureteral orifices. The location of the ureteral orifices must be identified prior to proceeding with the dissection of the posterior bladder neck. If there is any doubt as to the location of the orifices, intravenous administration of 1 ampule of indigo carmine (not methylene blue) about 15 min prior to beginning the bladder neck dissection followed by intravenous fluid bolus can often localize the orifices. It is essential to visualize a blue efflux of urine prior to commencing the dissection, as it will confirm both their location and integrity.

Once the median lobe has been retracted superiorly with the fourth arm, the first step in dissecting the posterior portion of the lobe is to score its border with the bladder circumferentially. The authors prefer to begin the dissection at the most lateral corners of the bladder, working their way medially below the median lobe. This allows optimal visualization of the corners and avoids working in a restricted hole. The bladder neck should then be divided full thickness. The posterior bladder dissection in these patients often varies from that of patients without a lobe, in that the lobe protrudes into the bladder. Therefore, the dissection should progress under the median lobe. Once the median lobe has been passed, the direction of dissection is downward along the contour of the bladder. If one continues to dissect along the horizontal plane of the adenoma, there may be inadvertent entry into the peripheral zone of the prostate. This step-like dissection is best performed by following the vertical detrusor fibers and keeping a wide plane of dissection.

Post-transurethral Resection of the Prostate

Many patients presenting with a diagnosis of prostate cancer have had a prior history of TURP or were diagnosed in such a manner. While the grade and stage of the cancer in these patients is variable, the optimal treatment is still often a radical prostatectomy. In patients diagnosed with prostate cancer via TURP, it is recommended to wait a minimum of 12 weeks to allow for healing and for inflammation to subside prior to RALP. The authors also advocate performing cystoscopy in these patients approximately 6 weeks post-TURP to make sure that the tissue has healed sufficiently. The most common challenge encountered in these patients is during the bladder neck dissection. The anatomy of the true bladder neck is distorted by the TURP, often making it difficult to locate and dissect the normal planes around the prostate.

When determining the plane of the vesicoprostatic dissection, the most optimal method to locate the bladder neck is by judging its location using visual clues. The 3D visualization provided by the *da Vinci*® system will often allow clean visualization of the contour and boundaries of the prostate. In addition, the perivesical fat ceases at the junction of the anterior bladder neck and prostate. It should be cautioned that using traction on the urinary catheter balloon to detect the location of the bladder neck in these patients can be misleading, as the balloon will often descend into the prostatic fossa. A generous TURP can lead to a large prostatic fossa into which the catheter balloon can lodge, distorting the perception of the bladder neck to a more distal location. To overcome this, the Foley catheter balloon can be inflated with 40–45 cc of sterile water in order to ascertain the line of prostatovesical dissection. After the anterior bladder neck and prostate junction is determined, the Foley catheter balloon should be deflated back to 10–15 cc for the remainder of the case, as a large balloon will hinder dissection. In these specific patients, it is often best to approach the bladder neck dissection in the midline to quickly enter the bladder, elevating the prostate using the urinary catheter, and surveying the anatomy from the inside.

Identifying the posterior bladder neck often provides the most ominous challenge due to the fact that the true anatomy is obscured either by regrowth of the adenoma or the reurothelialization of the vesicoprostatic junction, making it difficult to distinguish the boundary between the bladder and the prostate. The authors recommend that the ureteral orifices be identified prior to commencing dissection, as they are often close to the site of the posterior dissection. As described previously, indigo carmine can be used to visualize the ureteral orifices.

The posterior bladder neck should be approached with cautious optimism. The previous history of TURP (or in certain transurethral microwave thermotherapy [TUMT] or transurethral needle ablation [TUNA] cases) will often decimate the true surgical planes, especially at the level of the seminal vesicles, creating a challenging scenario. The key to the posterior bladder neck dissection in these patients is to incise full thickness and carrying the dissection inferiorly, making sure not to advance forward into the prostate tissue or to advance too cranially into the bladder toward the ureters. Usually the best practice is straight downward to locate the seminal vesicles, keeping in mind that a 30° camera is used during this dissection.

If, after a prolonged period (approximately 30 min), no efflux is visualized and the bladder neck dissection has been performed, then the integrity of the orifices should be tested. This is to ensure that no injury to the ureters has occurred during the isolation of the seminal vesicles and vas deferens. Urine output can be encouraged using small fluid boluses with diuretics if necessary; a 500-cc bolus of normal saline with 10 mg of lasix is often sufficient. If the aforementioned indigo carmine test is not successful, then a 5 French pediatric feeding tube can be placed intra-abdominally through the assistant trocar and advanced up the ureters bilaterally using the robotic instruments. If a ureteral injury is identified, the best method of treatment is usually reimplantation after excision of the injured and devascularized segment.

The Challenges of the Prostatic Apical Dissection

Handling of Accessory Pudendal Arteries

Several studies using Doppler flow ultrasound has shown that arterial insufficiency following radical prostatectomy is a contributing factor to port-operative erectile dysfunction.[7] Accessory pudendal arteries have been anatomically isolated during radical prostatectomy procedures with increased frequency, mainly due to improved intra-operative 3D magnification. The incidence of large accessory pudendal arteries in open radical prostatectomy series is reported to be 4%.[8] With the assistance of higher magnification, the incidence of accessory pudendal arteries during laparoscopic radical prostatectomy ranges from 25% to 30%.[9, 10]

Rogers et al. have shown that preservation of the accessory pudendal arteries directly correlates with improved recovery of sexual function and interval to recovery after radical prostatectomy by twofold.[8] With the assistance of higher magnification, Matin has shown that preservation of the accessory pudendal arteries was successful in 78.3% of the cases.[9]

Accessory pudendal vessels may be seen either coursing across the anterolateral aspect of the bladder and prostate beneath the EPF or emerging laterally through the levator ani musculature near the apex of the prostate gland. These vessels travel distally beneath the puboprostatic ligaments, alongside the deep dorsal vein complex to exit the pelvis through the genitourinary diaphragm to provide penile circulation.

Upon identification of an accessory pudendal vessel, the authors recommend completing the EPF dissection on the contralateral side first. When returning to the side of the accessory pudendal vessel, the EPF is opened sharply and the levator ani muscle is swept laterally from the prostate. The puboprostatic ligaments are divided and the lateral aspect of the dorsal vein complex with the adjacent accessory pudendal is exposed. The lateral pelvic fascia is then opened superficial to the pudendal and a combination of sharp and blunt dissection is used to free the vessel from the prostate and subsequently the dorsal vein complex (Fig. 16.6). As it courses adjacent to the apex of the prostate, occsionally the accessory pudendal gives off several small branches to the prostate, which need to be controlled with the bipolar graspers. Care must be taken to avoid excessive handling or traction on the vessel as this may lead to avulsion. The vessel must be released from the adjacent dorsal vein complex distally to allow suture ligation of the DVC; maintaining adequate pnemoperitoneum will assist with this dissection as it minimizes venous bleeding from the accessory pudendal.

Handling of the DVC

Incision of the EPF and identification of the DVC can lead to extensive bleeding that causes obscured vision, if not dissected in the proper planes. Using the 0° binocular lens, the following important landmarks need to be identified: bladder neck, base of the prostate, levator

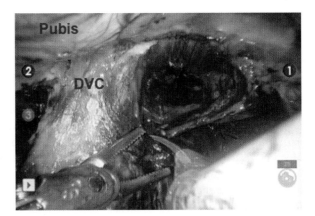

Fig. 16.6 Dissection and isolation of accessory pudendal artery as indicated by arrow

ani muscles, and apex of the prostate. Once adequate exposure has been obtained, the EPF is opened immediately lateral to the reflection of the puboprostatic ligaments bilaterally. The EPF is best opened at the base of the prostate using cold scissors. This is the area with the largest amount of prostate mobility and space between the prostate and the levator ani. Proceeding from the base to the apex, the levator fibers are pushed off of the prostate until the DVC and urethra are visualized. Dissect only that which is necessary to get in a good DVC stitch. Extensive dissection of the apex at this stage of the procedure can lead to unnecessary bleeding; the full apical dissection is best performed at the end of the procedure.

Many different sutures and types of needles are used for this purpose; however, the authors use a nonbraided absorbable suture (#1-Caprosyn™, Covidien, Dublin, Ireland) on a CT-1 needle. The needle is placed between the DVC and urethra in the visible notch, which is easily identified after incising the EPF and rotating the camera laterally. After suture placement, the authors prefer to ligate the DVC with a slip knot as it prevents the suture from loosening as it is tied.

If a slip knot is not feasible, an alternative method of ligating and dividing the DVC is described by Ahlering and associates, who use a 45-mm Endo-GIA stapling device (Ethicon, Somerville, NJ). According to their report, the one-step stapling and dividing method helps to protect the urethra.[11] Prior to employing the stapling device, a 22 French Foley catheter is placed to help protect the urethra, because it is difficult to staple through a 22 French catheter. They recommend clamping the DVC and waiting 30–60 s before firing the stapling device, as this compresses the edema from the tissue, creating a more secure staple line. Once the stapler is fired, the staple lines converge on top of the urethra in a V-configuration. In terms of oncologic control, Nguyen et al. showed no difference in the positive margin rate between sutured and stapled control of the DVC.[12]

After placement of the slip-knot on the DVC and before ligating the DVC, using the same Caprosyn™ suture, the authors place an anterior retropubic suspension stitch. This suture is used for suspending the urethra to the pubic bone to decrease post-operative urethral hypermobility to improve urinary incontinence (Fig. 16.7). The DVC is encircled and then stabilized against the pubic bone, thereby stabilizing the urethra anteriorly. Studies from open radical prostatectomy series have shown that the placement of the retropubic urethropexy suspension increases the likelihood of complete postoperative urinary continence by increasing the Valsalva leak-point pressure.[13]

Bladder Neck Reconstruction

After the removal of the prostate in patients with large glands, prominent median lobes or prior history of TURP, the bladder neck may be capacious. The authors recommend reconstructing the bladder neck prior to the performing the vesicourethral anastomosis in order to internalize the ureters away from the anastomotic sutures. The authors have found the most effective technique to be lateral closure of the bladder neck opening with 3–0 Monocryl™ suture (RB-1) (Ethicon, Inc., Somerville, NJ) in a figure of eight fashion at the 3 and 9 o'clock positions. The opening should be tailored to a 26 French caliber – this can be estimated against the diameter of the suction tip catheter that is 5 F. The authors have found that the traditional tennis racket closure on the anterior surface of the bladder leads

Fig. 16.7 Anterior suspension stitch. (**a**) After the EPF has been incised, the DVC is ligated with a Caprosyn™ suture; (**b**) using the same Caprosyn™ suture on a CT-1 needle held at a 90° angle, the needle is passed from right to left between the urethra and DVC; (**c**) the needle is placed through the periostium of the pubic tubercle; (**d, e**) a second pass between the urethra and DVC and through the periostium is performed; (**f**) the two ends of the suture are secured with a slip-knot to give the final configuration (Reprinted from Patel VR, Coelho RF, Palmer KJ, Rocco B, Periurethral suspension stitch during robot-assisted laparoscopic radical prostatectomy: description of the technique and continence outcomes. *Eur Urol.* 2009;56:472–478, with permission from Elsevier)

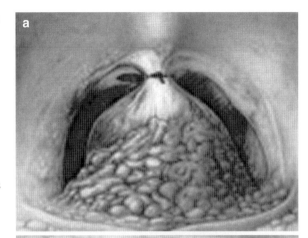

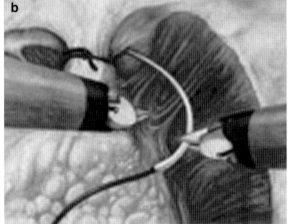

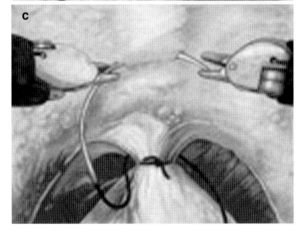

Fig. 16.7 (continued)

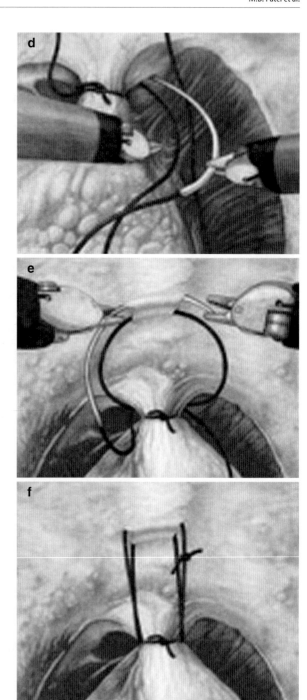

to medial migration of the ureteral orifices, causing a risk of injury to the ureters during the vesicourethral anastomosis.

The Vesicourethral Anastomosis

During the initial experience with robotic prostatectomy, it can be challenging to perform the vesicourethral anastomosis. One of the technical challenges can be to bring the posterior bladder neck down to the urethra. This difficulty can be obviated with a few simple steps. During the initial dissection, the peritoneum should have been mobilized lateral to the median umbilical ligaments and posteriolaterally to the intersection of the vasa bilaterally, providing adequate release of the bladder. The authors have incorporated a posterior reconstructive suture to re-approximate the proximal end of Denonvilliers fascia adjacent to the posterior bladder neck to the periurethral tissue near the rhabdosphincter on over 1,500 cases (Fig. 16.8). The authors use a double-armed (dyed and undyed) 3–0 Monocryl™ suture (RB-1), each 5 in. in length and connected at the terminal ends by a hand knot of eight throws. The undyed suture is used for re-approximating Denonvilliers fascia to the posterior periurethral tissue, while the dyed end of the suture is used for reapproximating the posterior lip of the bladder neck to the posterior lip of the urethral stump. Performing this reconstruction not only provides a tension-free vesicourethral anastomosis, but also provides improved urinary continence post-operatively.

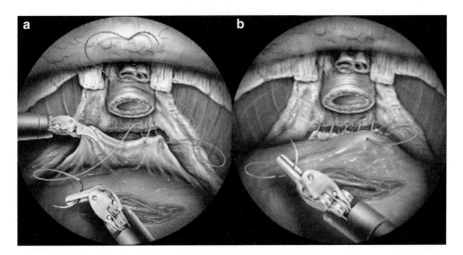

Fig. 16.8 Modified posterior reconstruction of the rhabdosphincter. The first layer (**a**) approximates the free edge of the remaining Denovilliers' fascia to the posterior aspect of the rhabdosphincter and the posterior median raphe using one arm of the continuous Monocryl™ suture. The second layer of the reconstruction (**b**) approximates the posterior bladder (2 cm posterosuperior to the bladder neck) to the initial reconstructed layer of posterior rhabdosphincter and Denovilliers' fascia, using the other arm of the Monocryl™ suture (From Coughlin G, Dangle PP, Nilesh NN, et al. Modified posterior reconstruction of the rhabdosphincter: application to robotic-assisted laparoscopic prostatectomy. *BJUI*. 2008;102(40):1482–1485. Reprinted with permission of Wiley)

The key to getting the bladder down to the urethra is the optimal placement of sutures and correct manipulation of the suture while sliding the bladder down to the urethra. The authors recommend taking generous bites (approximately 0.5–1 cm) of both the bladder neck and urethral tissue. The authors use the same double-armed suture as noted in the previous paragraph, but the length of each arm is 8 in. The anastomosis should be started on the outside-in of the bladder at the 5 o'clock position (if right-handed predominant suturing) and then inside-out at the same position on the urethra. The anastomosis is completed in a clockwise fashion using one arm of the suture, while the other end of the suture is used for completing the anastomosis in a counter-clockwise fashion. The two ends of the suture should be tied together on the same side of the anastomosis – never across the anastomotic line. Three passes through the bladder and two through the urethra are made before attempting to re-approximate the bladder neck to the urethral stump by placing tension on the suture. The mechanics of manipulating the stitch during the descent of the bladder are important to getting a close, tension-free approximation. The suture should be pulled directly vertically in a hand-over-fist manner using the two needle drivers. This provides the optimal angle and tension for the suture, allowing the bladder to slide down with the least difficulty. If there is still the presence of some tension or separation of the anastomosis, the authors recommend using the fourth robotic arm to hold the anastomosis together while placing reinforcing sutures to relieve the problem.

If a situation is encountered that the two will not reapproximate, one option is to move the location of the bladder neck anteriorly as the anterior portion of the bladder is likely to roll forward more easily. This can be performed by opening the bladder neck anteriorly in the midline, then suturing the area of the true bladder neck closed. This will move the bladder neck to a more maneuverable position.

If there is difficulty in performing an intracorporal knot during the anastomosis, an alternative method, as described by Shalhav et al., is to use a Lapra-Ty clip (Ethicon Endo Surgery, Cincinnati, OH) as a substitute for knot tying.[14] The vesicourethral anastomosis is performed using a double-armed suture composed of 3–0 Vicryl™ (Ethicon, Inc., Somerville, NJ) and 3–0 Monocryl™, each 6 in. in length and connected at the terminal ends by a hand knot and a Lapra-Ty clip. Their anastomosis is started at the posterior bladder neck (6 o'clock position), running the left arm of the suture toward the 11 o'clock position. Upon completion, the suture line was cinched with a Lapra-Ty clip at the level of the tissue. The same sequence was repeated on the right side with another clip applied at the 12 o'clock position. The clip has shown to maintain tensile strength for 14 days and is completely absorbed within 90 days.[15]

Conclusion

During the initial learning curve, the surgeon should be selective of patient population in order to decrease patient morbidity and mortality. Every attempt should be made to avoid patients with a BMI < 30; with prostate sizes less than 60–70 g as proven by transrectal ultrasound; with prior history of previous abdominal surgery (e.g., hernia repair); with previous TURP, TUNA, hormonal therapy, and/or radiation therapy; with identified large median lobes and/or history of chronic prostatitis; and with the clinical indications for a pelvic lymph node dissection. Also, patients should have a prostate-specific antigen (PSA) level of less than ten and a lower volume of Gleason Grade 6 cancer; this will decrease the likelihood of positive surgical margins in the initial cases. In addition, to diminish the impact of suboptimal nerve sparing, patients with low Sexual Health Inventory for Men (SHIM) scores or those in whom preservation of sexual function is not important should be in the initial group of patients.

With growing experience of the robotic team and confidence of the surgeon, preoperative screening will become unnecessary and the patient profile may be extended to obese patients, larger prostates, previous abdominal surgeries, RPLND, clinical T3 cancers, poor Gleason grades (8–10), or salvage prostatectomy.

References

1. Menon M, Shrivastava A, Tewari A, et al. Laparoscopic and robot assisted radical prostatectomy: establishment of a structured program and preliminary analysis of outcomes. *J Urol.* 2002;168(3):945-949.

2. Perer E, Lee D, Ahlering T, Clayman R. Robotic revelation: laparoscopic radical prostatectomy by a nonlaparoscopic surgeon. *J Am Coll Surg.* 2003;10:1738-1741.

3. Lavery H, Palmer KJ, Coughlin G, Patel VR. The advanced learning curve in robotic prostatectomy: a multi-institutional survey. *J Endourol.* 2007;21(Suppl 1):8-61.

4. Venkatesh V, Landman J, Sundaram CP, et al. Prevention, recognition, and management of laparoscopic complications in urologic surgery. *AUA Update Ser.* 2003;12(40):322-331.

5. Litwiller JP, Wells RE Jr, Halliwill JR, et al. Effect of lithotomy positions on strain of the obturator and lateral femoral cutaneous nerves. *Clin Anat.* 2004;17:45-49.

6. Tewari A, Rao SR. Anatomical foundations and surgical manoeuvres for precise identification of the prostatovesical junction during robotic radical prostatectomy. *BJU Int.* 2006;98:833-837.

7. Mulhall JP, Slovick R, Hotaling J, et al. Erectile dysfunction after radical prostatectomy: hemodynamic profiles and their correlation with the recovery of erectile function. *J Urol.* 2002;167(3):1371-1375.

8. Rogers CG, Trock BP, Walsh PC. Preservation of accessory pudendal arteries during radical retropubic prostatectomy: surgical technique and results. *Urology.* 2004;64(1):148-151.

9. Matin SF. Recognition and preservation of accessory pudendal arteries during laparoscopic radical prostatectomy. *Urology.* 2006;67(5):1012-1015.

10. Secin FP, Touijer K, Mulhall J, Guillonneau B. Anatomy and preservation of accessory pudendal arteries in laparoscopic radical prostatectomy. *Eur Urol.* 2007;51(5):1229-1235.

11. Ahlering TE, Eichel L, Edwards RA, Lee DI, Skarecky DW. Robotic radical prostatectomy: a technique to reduce pT2 positive margins. *Urology.* 2004;64(6):1224-1228.

12. Nguyen MM, Turna B, Santos BR, et al. The use of an endoscopic stapler vs suture ligature for dorsal vein control in laparoscopic prostatectomy: operative outcomes. *BJU Int.* 2008; 101(4):463-466.

13. Campenni MA, Harmon JD, Ginsberg PC, Harkaway RC. Improved continence after radical retropubic prostatectomy using two pubo-urethral suspension stitches. *Urol Int.* 2002;68(2): 109-112.

14. Shalhav AL, Orvieto MA, Chien GW, Mikhail AA, Zagaja GP, Zorn KC. Minimizing knot tying during reconstructive laparoscopic urology. *Urology.* 2006;68(3):508-513.

15. Anderson KR, Clayman RV. Laparoscopic lower urinary tract reconstruction. *World J Urol.* 2000;18:349-354.

Difficulties in Robotic-Assisted Nerve-Sparing Radical Prostatectomy

17

Gerald Y. Tan, Philip J. Dorsey Jr., and Ashutosh K. Tewari

Introduction

Serum prostate-specific antigen (PSA) screening, coupled with a rising incidence of needle biopsies in asymptomatic men, have all contributed to prostate cancer becoming the most common cancer in men in the United States[1,2] and other parts of the world.[3] With increasing evidence of improved long-term survival and progression-free outcomes,[4-7] radical prostatectomy has become increasingly popular as the treatment of first choice for organ-confined disease.

Since its inception in 2001, robotic-assisted radical prostatectomy has become immensely popular with both urologists and their patients, with over 55,000 radical prostatectomies being performed with *da Vinci*® robotic assistance (Intuitive Surgical, Inc. Sunnyvale, CA) in the United States in 2007.[8] The benefits of the *da Vinci*® robotic system over conventional laparoscopy are readily apparent: superior ergonomics, optical magnification of the operative field within direct control of the console surgeon, and enhanced dexterity, precision, and control of operative movements.

Nonetheless, robotic-assisted nerve-sparing radical prostatectomy (RARP) remains a difficult procedure to do well, although the learning curve is less steep than that for laparoscopic radical prostatectomy. Surgeon caseload and institutional volume have been shown in numerous studies to impact significantly on surgical outcomes.[9-11] Recent published meta-analyses comparing robotic-assisted radical prostatectomy with open and laparoscopic approaches have reported an overall complication rate of up to 33% for centers performing RARP.[12,13] Major complications associated with RARP include vascular injury and bleeding, lymphocele, injury to ureter or bladder, anastomotic leakage, bowel injury, obturator nerve injury, port site hernia, gas embolism, and robot malfunction.

In addressing the difficulties encountered by surgeons performing RARP, this chapter is organized as follows: (1) dealing with intraoperative complications; (2) avoiding

A.K. Tewari (✉)
Ronald P. Lynch Professor of Urologic Oncology and Director,
Lefrak Institute of Robotic Surgery Brady Foundation,
Department of Urology Weill Medical College of Cornell University,
New York Presbyterian Hospital,
New York, USA
e-mail: ashtewarimd@gmail.com

A.M. Al-Kandari and I.S. Gill (eds.), *Difficult Conditions in Laparoscopic Urologic Surgery*,   **229**
DOI: 10.1007/978-1-84882-105-7_17, © Springer-Verlag London Limited 2011

perioperative complications; and (3) optimizing pathologic and functional outcomes following surgery.

Dealing with Intraoperative Complications

Bleeding, Vascular Injury and Hematoma

Vascular injury and clinically significant bleeding requiring transfusion may result from injury to the inferior epigastric vessels, external iliac vein, Santorini's plexus, as well as bleeding from small vessels. Of these, inferior epigastric vessel injury during port placement remains the most common cause of vascular injury during RARP, usually occurring during insertion of the trocars at the pararectal line. Inferior epigastric vessel bleeding is usually discovered early in the operation, and may be controlled via bipolar coagulation, clips or, if persistent, suturing through the abdominal wall using a straight needle. Occasionally, the tamponading effect of the pneumoperitoneum may cause this injury to go unnoticed until the insufflations pressure is reduced, usually at the end of the procedure. If undetected and not redressed, persistent postoperative bleeding, and hematoma formation will ensue. This unpleasant scenario is best circumvented by carefully observing the shadow cast by the abdominal vessels during port placement with a 30° upward lens to avoid injury, and diligently inspecting the port sites during port removal with controlled desufflation of the pneumoperitoneum before final removal of the robotic lens.

Injury to the external iliac vein (EIV) may occur during lymph node dissection, or due to manipulation of robotic instruments without adequate visual control. In this situation, experienced surgeons often temporarily raise the pneumoperitoneum insufflation pressures to 20-cm water to slow down the bleeding, and proceed to repair the injury robotically with haemostatic Prolene™ 4/0 sutures (Ethicon, Inc., Somerville, NJ). Should robotic repair of the EIV injury proves unsuccessful, it may be necessary to convert to an open laparotomy.

Significant venous bleeding may also arise during dissection of Santorini's dorsal venous complex (DVC). Despite adequate ligation of the DVC, significant bleeding may reoccur during subsequent apical dissection. Encountering this, the insufflation pressure should be temporarily increased, the operative field irrigated and bleeding points accurately identified. If the prostatectomy is completed, firm caudal traction of the Foley catheter balloon inflated with 50-cc saline for 5–10 min is a helpful maneuver for tamponading bleeding from the DVC. Definitive control of these bleeding points may then be achieved robotically with Vicryl™ 0 running sutures (Ethicon, Inc., Somerville, NJ).

The small vessels at the lateral pedicle and lateral aspect of the prostate gland may also be a source of significant bleeding during RARP. If possible, use of cautery coagulation should be avoided for optimizing nerve preservation. Judicious placement of Hem-o-lok® clips (Teleflex Medical, Research Triangle Park, NC) are often sufficient for adequate vascular control. In rare situations, haemostatic sealants such as FloSeal™ (Baxter International Inc., Deerfield, IL) or TachoSil® (Nycomed, Zurich, Switzerland) may be further needed to control bleeding and ensure adequate homeostasis both during and after the procedure.[14]

Colon and Small Intestine Injury

Bowel injury is a severe potential complication during RARP which may be life threatening if not recognized early. With a reported incidence of 0.4–3.5% in various series of RARP,[14,15] it most commonly arises inadvertently during trocar insertion in patients with previous abdominal surgery and peritoneal adhesions, during passage of instruments and needles through the lateral ports, or due to cautery injury of viscera during surgical dissection or specimen extraction when the midline port incision is extended. Minor serosal abrasions may be repaired robotically with Vicryl™ 3/0 sutures.

Bowel perforation due to surgical dissection usually presents within 24–72 h postoperatively as fever, leucocytosis, vomiting, and persistent abdominal tenderness or guarding. If suspected, these patients should be placed on nil-by-mouth regimes, given broad-spectrum intravenous antibiotic coverage. Given its potential for fatality if not rectified promptly, surgeons should harbor a low threshold for bringing a suspected patient back to the operating theater for exploratory laparotomy and repair of bowel injury.

In the authors' practice, the following steps have been routinely adopted to minimize the possibility of colonic and bowel injury: (1) ensuring the patient is strapped and placed in full steep Trendelenburg position before commencement of port insertion; (2) making efforts to adequately mobilize the caecum and descending colon before insertion of the lateral trocars if these are adherent to the abdominal wall; (3) visually ensuring that the caecum and descending/sigmoid colon are adequately mobilized to ensure unobstructed passage of instruments and needles through the lateral ports; (4) use of an extended length (5–12 mm caliber) bariatric port (VersaPort™ Plus V2, Covidien, Dublin, Ireland) to deliver the right robotic instrument; and (5) minimizing intra-abdominal passage of laparoscopic Endo Shears™ scissors (Covidien, Dublin, Ireland) by employing the robotic needle drivers to snap off the sutures at the desired length instead. This ensures that retrieval of needles through the assistant port occurs under direct vision to avoid undetected intestinal serosal lacerations.

Rectal Injury

The incidence of rectal injury has been reported as 0.7–8.0% in various laparoscopic radical prostatectomy series, and less than 1% in contemporary robotic series.[16] It usually occurs during posterior dissection of the prostate gland, where desmoplastic reaction has caused the planes of Denonvilliers' fascia to become matted and fibrotic. Known risk factors include periprostatic fibrosis, previous prostate or rectal surgery, radiotherapy, previous hormonal therapy, and chronic prostatitis. Blunt posterior dissection should be avoided at all times. If suspected intraoperatively, rectal injury may be confirmed either by digital rectal examination, or by the presence of bubbles on rectal insufflation with air following copious irrigation of the operative field with water.

In both published laparoscopic and robotic series, most cases have recovered without consequence by: (1) intraoperative closure of the lesion with two-layer sutures; (2) interposition of healthy omentum between rectum and urethra to minimize the risk of rectourethral fistula formation; and (3) subsequent parenteral nutrition for 4 days and residual free enteral feeding for 6 days.[16-19] Diverting colostomy is generally only performed for patients with massive fecal spillage, previous radiotherapy, or a tense suture line.[20]

Obturator Nerve Injury

Injury to the obturator nerve (L2–L4) can occur during pelvic lymphadenectomy as a result of cautery injury, excessive traction, sharp transection, or entrapment with clips, and is often accompanied with a visible "obturator jerk." Clinical sequelae of obdurator nerve injury may be both sensory or motor, including pain or anesthesia over the medial aspect of the thigh, and weakness of thigh adduction. Neuropraxia from traction or thermal injury generally recovers within 6 weeks.[20,21] However, iatrogenic nerve transection should be repaired with an end-to-end tension-free coaptation, aligning the fascicles to give the best results. Spaliviero et al.[22] from the Cleveland Clinic reported their experience with a case of laparoscopic reapproximation of the transected ends of the obdurator nerve during laparoscopic radical prostatectomy. Using four 6-0 nylon epineural sutures under the direction of an on-site plastic surgeon to achieve a tension-free anastomosis of the cut ends (Fig. 17.1), the patient recovered with minimal neurological sequelae at 6 months' follow-up.

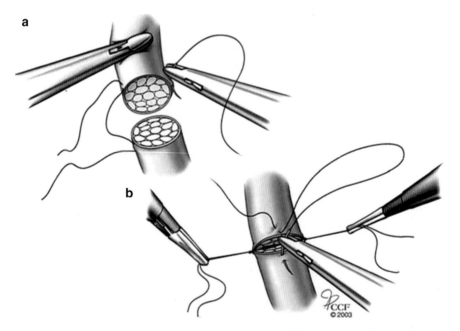

Fig. 17.1 Laparoscopic reapproximation of transected ends of obdurator nerve using 6-0 nylon. (Reprinted from Spaliviero et al.[22] With permission from Elsevier)

Large Median Lobes and Ureteric Orifice Injury

Inadvertent injury to the ureteric orifices may occur during the dissection of the posterior bladder neck or during vesicourethral anastmosis, particularly in patients with a large prostate or median lobe (Fig. 17.2) where bladder neck division has been extended close to orifices to ensure complete clearance of prostatic tissue.[23,24] Undetected, the injury may result in postoperative uraemia and flank pain from iatrogenic upper tract obstruction, requiring secondary procedures to redress this avoidable complication. To prevent ureteral orifice injury in cases where they are poorly visualized, double-pigtail ureteral stent insertion during robotic-assisted radical prostatectomy for accurate visualization and preservation of the ureteral orifices should be considered.[25 27]

In the authors' practice, they employ a 0-Vicryl™ suture on a GS-21 needle (Covidien, Dublin, Ireland) placed through the median lobe for improving anterior traction by the assistant. Intravenous furosemide and indigo carmine are then administered for accurate identification of both ureteral orifices, posterior bladder neck transection is completed under optical magnification, and radical prostatectomy proceeds in the standard fashion. Post-prostatectomy, an in situ ureteral intubation with 6-F double-pigtail ureteral stents (Sof-Flex® stent, Cook Medical Inc., Bloomington, IN) is performed at this point prior to vesicourethral anastmosis construction. The soft-tipped guidewire is introduced through the patent lumen of the suction trocar. The introducer tip is then grasped using both left and right robotic forceps and gently passed through the ureteral orifice along the axis of the distal ureter (Fig. 17.3a). Care is taken not to cause inadvertent ureteral perforation at this point by watching for signs of buckling of the guidewire. The radio-opaque 6-French double pigtail Sof-Flex® stent is then passed over the guidewire in a retrograde fashion using a modified Seldinger technique (Fig. 17.3b). The guidewire is then removed after correct positioning of the stent, and the procedure repeated on the contralateral side (Fig. 17.3c). The authors then complete the vesicourethral anastomosis with continuous running 2-0 Monocryl™ sutures (Ethicon, Inc., Somerville, NJ) (Fig. 17.3d). Postoperatively, upright abdominal roentograms are performed to confirm accurate stent position. The stents are removed cystoscopically 6 weeks after surgery to allow adequate time for resolution of edema and optimal healing at the anastomosis before instrumentation.

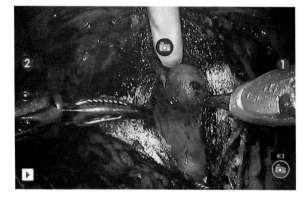

Fig. 17.2 Large median lobe visualized after anterior bladder neck dissection (From El Douaihy et al.[27] Reprinted with permission from Mary Ann Liebert, Inc.)

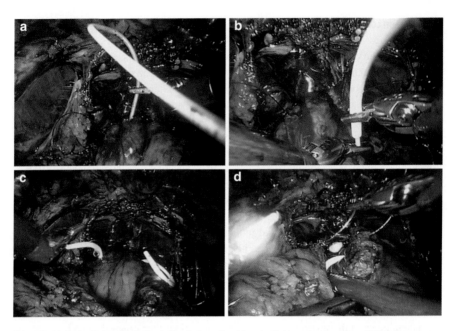

Fig. 17.3 (**a**) Robotic manipulation of soft-tipped guide wire into ureteral orifice. (**b**) Radio-opaque 6-F d*ouble pigtail stent* railroaded over the introducer. (**c**) Bilateral JJ stents in place just prior to the beginning of the anastomosis. (**d**) Construction of vesicourethral anastomosis with running continuous suture – the stents serve as visible landmarks for avoiding iatrogenic ureteral orifice injury (From El Douaihy et al.[27] Reprinted with permission from Mary Ann Liebert, Inc.)

Ureteral injury may also occur during dissection of the posterior bladder neck and extended pelvic lymph node dissection, particularly in patients with previous transurethral resection of prostate where the posterior anatomy may be distorted. In these cases, leakage of intravenous indigo carmine and furosemide from the cut ends of the distal ureter confirms the diagnosis and localizes the injury. Intra-operative repair may be performed by end-to-end ureterorrhaphy over a ureteral stent and/or placement of a double J-stent if not completely transected. Failing this, the distal ureter may be reimplanted robotically to the bladder dome at the end of the surgery over a similar ureteral stent.

Robot Malfunction

Perioperative failure of any of the many components involved in the robotic system can result in operative delays, cancelled surgery or conversion to an open or pure laparoscopic approach. While the manufacturers of the *da Vinci*® Surgical System do not release data on the reliability and failure rates of their systems, various authors have reported an incidence of technical malfunction at 0.5–2.6% in their series.[28,29] In their multi-institutional review of 8,240 cases in 11 institutions, Lavery et al. reported that critical malfunctions requiring the shut-down of the system occurred in 34 cases (0.4%), resulting in case cancellation or conversion to laparoscopic or open procedures.[30] Reported causes for robot malfunction included failures in power supply (15%), optics (34%), robotic arms (34%), failure of the masters (10%), and an unknown cause of malfunction (7%). Associated patient injury occurred in 4.8% of all robotic failures.

In the few instances of disabling robot malfunction encountered in the authors' institution with three *da Vinci*® systems, most malfunctions are correctable by simply undocking the robotic cart and instruments from the patient and rebooting the system again. On the rare occasion that the malfunction could not be rectified, the anesthetized patient was transferred from one operating suite to an adjacent suite with a functional *da Vinci*® system, and the surgery was completed using the new robotic system without complication.

Allograft Injury in the Renal Transplant Patient

Technical advances in renal transplantation, especially in living-related donor nephrectomies, coupled with improvements in immunosuppressive therapy regimes, have resulted in renal allograft recipients living longer and healthier lives of significantly better quality. The reported incidence of localized prostate cancer in these males varies from 1.8% to 3.1%, and is likely to increase with such men living longer lives with regular PSA surveillance.[31,32] To the extirpative urologist, preoperative strategies are required to overcome the unique challenges posed by such patients – how to avoid injury to the renal allograft, transplanted ureter and ureteroneocystotomy; technical modifications for pelvic lymph node sampling over the allograft; and possible delayed wound healing from chronic immunosuppression. Graft failure is devastating, with reported 5-year survival rates of 57–64% following this complication.[33]

In the authors' experience of performing RARP in the renal allograft patient[34] (Fig. 17.4), the following technical modifications were adopted to minimize risk of allograft injury: (1) use of an extended length (5–12-mm caliber) bariatric port (VersaPort™ plus V2) to bypass the allograft site and deliver the ipsilateral robotic arm directly into the pelvis; (2) development of the retropubic space from the contralateral side; (3) meticulous posterior dissection of the seminal vesicles to avoid possible injury along the course to the transplanted

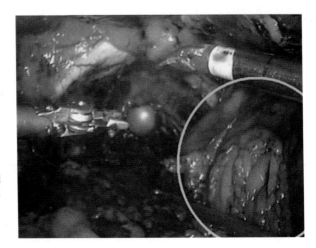

Fig. 17.4 Intraoperative view of heterotopically placed renal allograft in right iliac fossa during robotic-assisted radical prostatectomy (From Jhaveri et al.[34] Reprinted with permission from Mary Ann Liebert, Inc.)

ureter; and (4) limited pelvic lymph node dissection on the side ipsilateral to the allograft. The authors have not found it necessary to intubate the transplant ureter via cystoscopy at commencement of surgery for better appreciation of its course, as recommended in some reports.[35]

Avoiding Perioperative Complications

Anastomotic Leak and Bladder Neck Strictures

Several large series have highlighted anastomotic strictures as being the most significant predictor for postprostatectomy incontinence (PPI) following radical retropubic prostatectomy[36–38]; its incidence occurring up to 20% in some series. However, there remains to date little published data on the association of urinary leak documented on postoperative cystography with continence outcomes after radical prostatectomy. Menon and colleagues[39] recently published the largest series of 3,327 patients with routine cystography prior to Foley catheter removal 7 days after RARP. These investigators documented cystographic leakage in 8.6% of their cohort – of these patients, 70% regained continence within 3 months, and 94% at 12 months. Of those with urinary leakage, 2.8% required secondary intervention to redress bladder neck contracture, and these were all associated with moderate to severe leakage on postoperative cystography.

Significant predictors of postoperative cystographic leakage in the reported literature include technically difficult anastomosis creation, unsatisfactory intraoperative flush test and urinary tract infections, previous transurethral prostate surgery, ischemic heart disease, intraoperative blood loss, mucosal eversion, and preservation of the prostatic urethra.[40,41] Previous studies[42,43] failed to demonstrate an association between urinary leakage with a higher risk of bladder neck strictures. Omitting routine cystography after radical prostatectomy has also not been associated with increased risk of urinary retention, infection, renal failure, or bladder neck strictures.[44] Given the current evidence, it would appear that postoperative urinary leakage is not significant for delayed continence recovery, although if present, it usually necessitates prolonged catheterization.

The authors have found that a biomechanics-based approach of providing circumferential support to the newly fashioned vesicourehtral anastomosis, coupled with relieving pelvic descent of the bladder, significantly lowered the incidence of anastomotic leaks and bladder neck contractures, while also hastening early return of continence.[45] This approach is described in detail in a later section.

Lymphocele and Lymphedema

Lymphoceles arise from leakage from transected lymphatic vessels, and occur most commonly after pelvic lymph node dissection. Risk factors include an extraperitoneal approach and extended lymphadenectomy for high-risk cancer.[14] If significant, they may cause pelvic pain, voiding dysfunction, leg edema, and deep venous thrombosis, requiring definitive treatment with sclerotherapy, percutaneous drainage, or surgical intervention.

Meticulous use of Hem-o-lok® clips, use of bipolar cautery instead of sharp scissor dissection, and avoiding excessive traction on lymphatic tissue are helpful for minimizing subsequent lymphocele formation. Stoltzenburg and colleagues also reported lower rates of lymphocele formation in patients undergoing extended pelvic lymphadenectomy with peritoneal fenestrations.[46]

Port Site Hernias

Incisional hernias are a rare complication of RARP, occurring in between 0.6% and 1% of reported series.[14] Port site hernias most commonly occur at the periumbilical site, where the incision is extended to facilitate prostatectomy specimen retrieval. Various port site closure devices are currently available.[47] Regardless of port site closure device employed, sutures should be secured under direct vision while the pneumoperitoneum is fully insufflated, as there is a risk of small bowel loops getting caught in the sutures once the abdominal cavity is desufflated.

Optimizing Functional Outcomes Following Surgery

Hastening Early Return of Continence

Next to developing metastatic progression of cancer following surgery, urinary incontinence remains the most feared complication of men undergoing radical prostatectomy.[10] The incidence of PPI at 12-month follow-up after RARP has varied from 2% to 15% in various reported meta-analsyses.[12,13] Urinary incontinence has the most negative effect on patients' quality of life, causing psychological distress and social inhibition for fear of public embarrassment. The chronic requirement for pads in patients treated conservatively, and cost of secondary procedures such as slings and artificial sphincters also place an onerous burden on healthcare systems and individual finances.[48]

Increasing age, shorter pre- and postoperative membranous urethral length, anastomotic strictures, obesity, low surgeon volume, variations of surgical technique, and previous prostate surgery have been reported as negative risk factors for delayed continence recovery and/or permanent incontinence following radical prostatectomy. Recent advances in elucidating the functional anatomy and physiology of the male continence mechanism from cadaveric and videourodynamic studies have enabled surgeons to propose innovative surgical techniques during radical prostatectomy for augmenting continence preservation and early return. These have included optimizing preservation of urethral rhabdosphincter length[49,50]; avoiding rhabdosphincter injury[51,52]; posterior reconstruction of Denonvilliers' musculofascial plate[53–55]; preservation of the bladder neck and internal sphincter[56]; bladder neck intussusception[57,58]; bladder neck mucosal eversion[59]; and preservation of the puboprostatic ligaments and arcus tendineus.[60,61]

The authors postulate that during conventional anastomosis following radical prostatectomy, the vesicourethral anastomosis and bladder neck become biomechanically unstable at the following sites: (1) tension is exerted on the healing anastomosis from spontaneous urethral stump recession into the pelvic floor; (2) the posteriorly deficient Ω (omega)-shaped urethral rhabdosphincter lies unsupported posteriorly, impairing efficient contraction of the sphincter mechanism; (3) the posterior bladder neck lies unsupported in the retrotrigonal fossa created by excision of the seminal vesicles; and (4) the anterior and lateral bladder neck lie unsupported as well (Fig. 17.5). The overall effect appears to be pelvic descent of the bladder presses on the unsupported anastomosis. As a result, during micturition, the contractile forces generated by the detrusor musculature are directed inferiorly at the anastomosis, causing additional stress on the continence mechanism (Fig. 17.6).

As such, the authors have developed the following paradigm of seven key principles for optimizing early continence recovery following radical prostatectomy, which is described as the anatomic restoration technique (ART): (1) preservation of anterior fibrotendinous support structures, chiefly the arcus tendineus and the puboprostatic ligaments; (2) optimization of functional membranous urethral length; (3) reinforcement of unstable posterior bladder neck in the unsupported retrotrigonal fossa left by excised seminal vesicles; (4) reinforcement of the posteriorly deficient Ω (omega)-shaped urethral sphincter complex for suspensory support; (5) fashioning of a tension-free, stable vesico-urethral anastomosis; (6) prevention of urethral stump recession and optimizing mucosal coaptation; and (7) alleviation of pelvic descent and downward pressure of the bladder on the anastomosis during micturition (Fig. 17.7a and b).

The benefits of this approach appear to be threefold. Firstly, it provides circumferential dynamic suspensory support for the urethral sphincter complex, as documented by

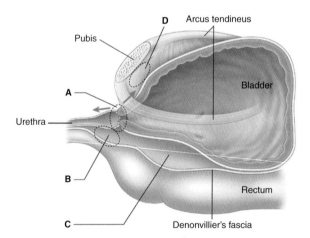

Fig. 17.5 Points of postulated biomechanical instability associated with the conventional vesicourethral anastomosis (sagittal view): (**a**) tension on the vesicourethral anastomosis from spontaneous urethral stump recession into the pelvic floor; (**b**) the posteriorly deficient Ω (omega)-shaped urethral rhabdosphincter lies unsupported posteriorly, impairing efficient contraction of the sphincter mechanism; (**c**) the posterior bladder neck lies unsupported in the retrotrigonal fossa created by excision of the seminal vesicles; (**d**) the anterior and lateral bladder neck lie unsupported as well (Reprinted from Tan et al.[45] With permission from Elsevier)

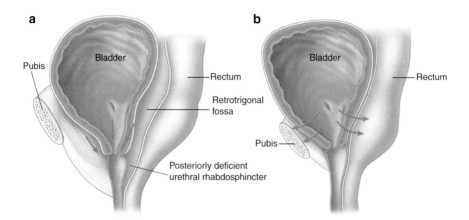

Fig. 17.6 Biomechanical forces acting on the vesicourethral anastomosis in the upright position. (**a**) In the conventional vesicourethral anastomosis, pelvic descent of the bladder presses on the unsupported anastomosis. During micturition, the contractile forces generated by the detrusor musculature are directed inferiorly at the anastomosis (*green arrows*), causing additional stress on the continence mechanism. (**b**) In the authors' technique, the bladder is hitched up anteriolaterally by the suspension sutures through the arcus tendineus, ameliorating downward tension on the healing anastomosis. During micturition, the same contractile forces (*green arrows*) are dissipated away from the anastomosis and urethral rhabdosphincter (Reprinted from Tan et al.[45] With permission from Elsevier)

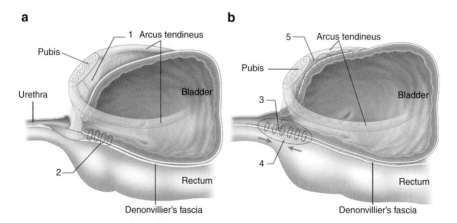

Fig. 17.7 (**a**) Anatomic restoration of vesicourethral junction: (1) Preservation of anterior support structures, i.e., puboprostatic ligaments and arcus tendineus; (2) posterior bladder neck reinforced with 0 Vicryl™ suture, obliterating retrotrigonal space. (**b**) Anatomic restoration of vesicourethral junction: (3) the posteriorly deficient urethral rhabdosphincter reinforced against Denonvilliers' musculofascial plate; (4) Denonvilliers' musculofascial plate reconstructed, preventing urethral stump recession, relieving tension on the anastomosis and improving mucosal coaptation at the anastomosis. The green arrows illustrate the improved apposition of the two ends of the anastomosis. (5) Anterior suspension sutures to the arcus tendineus and puboprostatic ligaments alleviate downward prolapse of the bladder on the anastomosis (Reprinted from Tan et al.[45] With permission from Elsevier)

postoperative cystographic studies (Fig. 17.8). Secondly, it avoids pelvic prolapse and downward pressure of the bladder on the healing anastomosis during micturition. Thirdly, tension at the anastomosis is relieved with improved mucosal apposition and coaptation. The authors recently reported their experience with ART in a cohort of 530 patients,[45] wherein continence was defined as zero pad usage. It was found that ART resulted in significantly earlier return of continence (38.6%, 82.6%, 90.5%, and 97.5% at 1, 6, 12, and 24 weeks follow-up, respectively), and significantly lower incidence of anstomotic strictures and clinically significant leaks compared to men receiving conventional anastomosis.

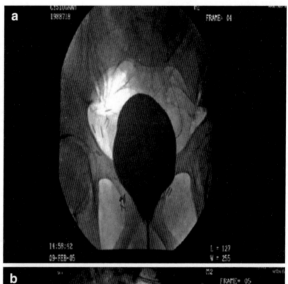

Fig. 17.8 (**a**) Postoperative cystogram in a patient with conventional anastomosis. Note the pelvic descent of the anastomosis. (**b**) Postoperative cystogram of a patient who underwent total anatomic restoration. Note the anastomosis and bladder neck being well suspended above the pubic ramus as a result of our technical modifications (Reprinted from Tan et al.[45] With permission from Elsevier)

Balancing Nerve Preservation with Oncologic Control

The prostate gland is enveloped by layers of the lateral pelvic fascia (LPF) carrying vessels and nerves (Fig. 17.9). The medial, well-defined component of the LPF is known as the prostatic fascia, and directly wraps around the prostate capsule. The laterally defined part of the LPF is the levator fascia, which lies on the levator ani (LA) muscles. Interposed between the prostatic fascia and the levator fascia, are the periprostatic venous plexus and the neurovascular tissue that travel distally to supply the sphincter, urethra, and cavernous tissue. These neural fibers can travel close to the vessels, or occasionally independently on the surface of prostate, or laterally on the rectum. Some of these vessels remain subcapsular for a short distance before dipping into the prostatic tissue. Excessive blunt dissection of these vessels can create an artificial transcapsular plane resulting in a capsular incision.

As such, the authors now adopt a risk-stratified approach toward nerve-sparing according to the patient's likelihood of ipsilateral extraprostatic extension of cancer (EPE) (Fig. 17.10). The patient's PSA, Gleason score, percentage of cancer in the biopsy, number of positive cores, presence of unilateral versus bilateral positive cores (used as a surrogate for high-volume cancer or multifocality), clinical stage, and findings of the endorectal magnetic resonance imaging in terms of cancer localization, volume, status of capsule, and periprostatic tissue are some parameters that the authors regularly use to select patients for a nerve-sparing prostatectomy. The authors' approach to nerve-sparing during robotic prostatectomy involves varying degrees of preservation of the nerve fibers in the various fascial planes. They are referred to as:

Grade 1 approach – Incision of the Denonvilliers' and LPF is taken just outside the prostatic capsule. This is only performed for patients with no to minimal risk of EPE.

Grade 2 approach – Incision through the Denonvilliers' (leaving deeper layers on the rectum) and LPF is taken just outside the layer of veins of the prostate capsule – this preserves most large neural trunks and ganglions, and is used for patients at low risk of EPE.

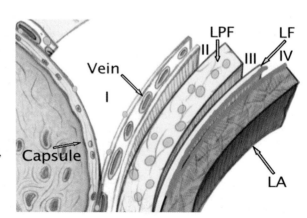

Fig. 17.9 Layers of fascia enveloping prostatic capsule, demonstrating the planes of dissection for differing grades (I–IV) of nerve-sparing

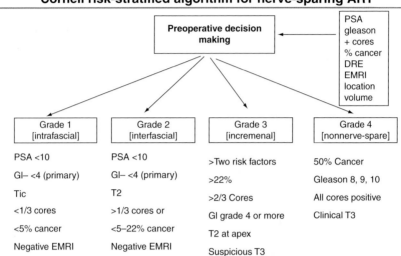

Fig. 17.10 Risk-stratified algorithm for athermal nerve-sparing robotic radical prostatectomy

Grade 3 (partial/incremental nerve-sparing) approach – Incision is taken through the outer compartment of LPF, excising all layers of Denonvilliers' fascia. This is performed for patients with moderate risk of EPE because some of the medial trunks are sacrificed while lateral trunks are preserved.

Grade 4 (nonnerve-sparing approach) – A wide excision of the LPF and Denonvilliers' fascia containing the majority of the periprostatic neurovascular tissue is performed. In some of these patients, nerve advancement of the identifiable ends of the neurovascular bundle may be attempted.

In addition, the authors have adopted the following modifications to their athermal robotic nerve-sparing technique: (1) minimal periprostatic dissection because this may break or avulse the nerves; (2) limiting the dissection to the midline during bladder neck transection, as this will protect the predominant neurovascular plate (PNP) from thermal or mechanical damage; (3) athermal dissection of the seminal vesicles, as this should cause the least damage to the PNP and hypogastric nerve; and (4) avoiding use of cautery during the posterior prostate dissection.

The authors have found in their cohort of potent men who meet selection criteria for aggressive bilateral Grade 1 nerve-sparing (PSA <10 ng/dL, clinical stage ≤ T2, primary Gleason grade <4, cancer volume <5% in all cores, and absence of cues suggestive of extraprostatic extension on endorectal MRI and during surgery), 95% of these hitherto potent men had partial erections with and without use of PDE5 inhibitors, and 86% had erection sufficient for penetrative intercourse at a mean follow-up of 26 weeks. The positive surgical margin rate in this cohort was 8.5%.

In conclusion, nerve preservation should no longer be considered a distinct step of radical prostatectomy, but rather an overarching surgical priority to be relentlessly pursued at all stages of this complex operation, since one or more components of the tri-zonal architecture are usually at risk during any given step. Preoperative risk stratification of likelihood of extracapsular extension of cancer helps the surgeon decide the level of aggressiveness to adopt for nerve-sparing. In the authors' experience, gentle athermal dissection of the robotic procedure will help optimize postoperative potency outcomes without compromise of cancer clearance outcomes.

Future Directions

Despite its relative infancy, there has been an unprecedented explosion in demand for robotic-assisted radical prostatectomy, both in the United States and increasingly in other parts of the world. Nonetheless, robotic-naïve surgeons with no prior experience at the robotic console still encounter significant obstacles in climbing the learning curve. The high costs of purchasing and housing a dedicated dry lab "training" *da Vinci*® system and the cost of surgical expendables used during training cases in wet labs usually mean that console experience obtained at various hands-on courses is often limited and fleetingly transient.

The dV-Trainer (Mimic Technologies Inc., Seattle, WA) has been developed in collaboration with Intuitive Surgical Inc., as a solution to some of these current obstacles in surgical training.[62,63] It consists of a master console with finger cuff telemanipulators connected to a binocular 3D visual output that aims to reproduce the look and feel of the *da Vinci*® console. The program encompasses exercises in *EndoWrist*® manipulation (Intuitive Surgical, Inc., Sunnyvale, CA), camera control, clutching, object transfer and placement, needle handling, needle driving, knot tying, and suturing. Researchers at the University of Nebraska are also working to produce a *da Vinci*® compatible virtual reality simulator, using kinematic data from the *da Vinci*® console through LabVIEW (National Instruments, Austin, TX) to drive simulation software (Cyberbotics Ltd., Lausanne, Switzerland).[64,65] Medical Education Technologies, Inc. (Sarasota, FL) has also made an attempt to produce a robotic surgery simulator (RSS) for its SurgicalSIM® package, although the reception to this has yet to be reported. With exciting technological advances in robotic-assisted urologic surgery taking place,[65] the authors look forward to the development of their craft in the next few years with great interest.

Authors' Disclosures of Potential Conflicts of Interest

- Gerald Y. Tan discloses that he receives financial support from the Ferdinand C. Valentine Fellowship in Urologic Research, New York Academy of Medicine; the John Steyn Travelling Fellowship in Urology, Royal College of Surgeons of Edinburgh; and the Medical Research Fellowship, National Medical Research Council, Singapore.
- Ashutosh K. Tewari discloses that he receives a research grant from Intuitive Surgical Inc., Sunnyvale, CA.

References

1. Penson DF, Rossignol M, Sartor AO, Scardino PT, Abenhaim LL. Prostate cancer: epidemiology and health-related quality of life. *Urology*. 2008;72(Suppl 6A):3-11.
2. Jemal A, Siegel R, Ward E, et al. Cancer statistics, 2008. *CA Cancer J Clin*. 2008;58:71-96.
3. Quinn M, Babb P. Patterns and trends in prostate cancer incidence, survival, prevalence and mortality. Part 1: International comparisons. *BJU Int*. 2002;90(2):162-173.
4. Lu-Yao GL, Yao S. Population based study of long-term survival in patients with clinically localized prostate cancer. *Lancet*. 1997;349:906-910.
5. D'Amico DV, Whittington R, Malkowicz SB, et al. Biochemical outcome after radical prostatectomy, external beam radiation therapy, or interstitial radiation therapy for clinically localized prostate cancer. *JAMA*. 1998;280(11):969-974.
6. Bill-Axelson A, Holmberg L, Ruutu M, et al. Radical prostatectomy versus watchful waiting in early prostate cancer. *N Engl J Med*. 2005;352(19):1977-1984.
7. Bill-Axelson A, Holmberg L, Filen F, et al. Radical prostatectomy versus watchful waiting in localized prostate cancer: the Scandinavian prostate cancer group-4 randomized trial. *J Natl Cancer Inst*. 2008;100(16):1144-1154.
8. Su L. Role of robotics in modern urologic practice. *Curr Opin Urol*. 2009;19:63-64.
9. Begg CB, Riedel ER, Bach PB, et al. Variations in morbidity after radical prostatectomy. *N Engl J Med*. 2002;346(15):1138-1144.
10. Bianco FJ Jr, Reidel ER, Begg CB, Kattan MW, Scardino PT. Variations among high volume surgeons in the rate of complications after radical prostatectomy: further evidence that technique matters. *J Urol*. 2005;173:2099-2113.
11. Wilt TJ, Shamliyan TA, Taylor BC, MacDonald R, Kane RL. Association between hospital and surgeon radical prostatectomy volume and patient outcomes: a systematic review. *J Urol*. 2008;180:820-829.
12. Berryhill R Jr, Jhaveri J, Yadav R, et al. Robotic prostatectomy: a review of outcomes compared with laparoscopic and open approaches. *Urology*. 2008;72:15-23.
13. Ficarra V, Novara G, Artibani W, et al. Retropubic, laparoscopic and robot-assisted radical prostatectomy: a systematic review and cumulative analysis of comparative studies. *Eur Urol*. 2009;55(5):1037-1063.
14. Fischer B, Engel N, Fehr J-L, John H. Complications of robotic-assisted radical prostatectomy. *World J Urol*. 2008;26:595-602.
15. Hu JC, Nelson RA, Wilson TG, et al. Perioperative complications of laparoscopic and robotic assisted radical prostatectomy. *J Urol*. 2006;175:541-546.
16. Yee DS, Ornstein DK. Repair of rectal injury during robotic-assisted laparoscopic prostatectomy. *Urology*. 2008;72:428-431.
17. Guillonneau B, Rozet F, Cathelineau X, et al. Perioperative complications of laparoscopic radical prostatectomy: the Montsouris 3-year experience. *J Urol*. 2002;167:51-56.
18. Bishoff JT, Allaf ME, Kirkels WIM, Moore RG, Kavoussi LR, Schroder F. Laparoscopic bowel injury: incidence and clinical presentation. *J Urol*. 1999;161:887-890.
19. Guillonneau B, Gupta R, El Fettouh H, Cathelineau X, Baumert H, Vallancien G. Laparoscopic management of rectal injury during laparoscopic radical prostatectomy. *J Urol*. 2003;169:1694-1696.
20. Shekarriz B, Upadhyay J, Wood DP. Intraoperative, perioperative and long term complications of radical prostatectomy. *Urol Clin North Am*. 2001;28:639-653.
21. Stolzenburg JU, Rabenault R, Do M, et al. Complications of endoscopic extraperitoneal radical prostatectomy (EERPE): prevention and management. *World J Urol*. 2006;24:668-675.
22. Spaliviero M, Stenberg AP, Kaouk JH, Desai MM, Hammert WC, Gill IS. Laparoscopic injury and repair of obdurator nerve during radical prostatectomy. *Urology*. 2004;64:1030.

23. Sarle R, Tewari A, Hemal AK, Menon M. Robotic–assisted anatomic radical prostatectomy: technical difficulties due to a large median lobe. *Urol Int.* 2005;74:92-94.

24. Meeks JJ, Zhao L, Greco KA, Macejko A, Nadler RB. Impact of prostate median lobe anatomy on robotic-assisted laparoscopic prostatectomy. *Urology.* 2009;73:323-327.

25. Rehman J, Chughtai B, Guru K, Shabsigh R, Samadi DB. Management of an enlarged median lobe with ureteral orifices at the margin of bladder neck during robotic-assisted laparoscopic prostatectomy. *Can J Urol.* 2009;16:4490-4494.

26. Katz MH, Eng MK, Deklaj T, Zorn KC. Technique for ureteral stent placement during robot-assisted radical prostatectomy: safety measure during vesicourethral anastomosis when ureteral orifices are too close for comfort. *J Endourol.* 2009;23:827-829.

27. El Douaihy Y, Tan GY, Dorsey PJ Jr, Patel ND, Jhaveri JK, Tewari AK. Double pig-tail stenting of the ureters: technique for securing the ureteral orifices during robotic-assisted radical prostatectomy for large median lobes. *J Endourol.* 2009;23(12):1975-1977.

28. Borden LS Jr, Kozlowski PM, Porter CR, Corman JM. Mechanical failure rate of da Vinci robotic system. *Can J Urol.* 2007;14:3499-3501.

29. Zorn KC, Gofrit ON, Orvieto MA, et al. Da Vinci robot error and failure rates: single institution experience on a single three-arm robot unit of more than 700 consecutive robotic-assisted laparoscopic radical prostatectomies. *J Endourol.* 2007;21:1341-1345.

30. Lavery HJ, Thaley R, Albala D, et al. Robotic equipment malfunction during robotic prostatectomy: a multi-institutional study. *J Endourol.* 2008;22:2165-2168.

31. Magee CC, Pascual M. Update in renal transplantation. *Arch Intern Med.* 2004;164: 1373-1388.

32. Campagnari J, Ribeiro L, Mangini M, et al. Localized prostate cancer in patients submitted to renal transplant. *Int Braz J Urol.* 2002;28:330-334.

33. Marcen R, Pascual J, Tato JL, et al. Renal transplant outcome after losing the first graft. *Transplant Proc.* 2003;35:1679-1681.

34. Jhaveri JK, Tan GY, Scherr DS, Tewari AK. Robotic-assisted laparoscopic radical prostatectomy in the renal allograft transplant recipient. *J Endourol.* 2008;22:2475-2479.

35. Thomas AA, Nguyen MM, Gill IS. Laparoscopic transperitoneal radical prostatectomy in renal transplant recipients: a review of three cases. *Urology.* 2008;71:205-208.

36. Eastham JA, Kattan MW, Rogers E, et al. Risk factors for urinary incontinence after radical prostatectomy. *J Urol.* 1996;156:1707-1713.

37. Sacco E, Prayer-Galetti T, Pinto F. Urinary incontinence after radical prostatectomy: incidence by definition, risk factors and temporal trend in a large series with a long-term follow-up. *BJU Int.* 2006;97(6):1234-1241.

38. Park R, Martin S, Goldberg JD, Lepor H. Anastomotic strictures following radical prostatectomy: insights into incidence, effectiveness of intervention, effect on continence, and factors predisposing to occurrence. *Urology.* 2001;57:742-746.

39. Patil N, Krane L, Javed K, Williams T, Bhandari M, Menon M. Evaluating and grading cystographic leakage: correlation with clinical outcomes in patients undergoing robotic prostatectomy. *BJU Int.* 2009;103:1108-1110.

40. Gnanapragasam VJ, Baker P, Naisby GP, Chadwick D. Identification and validation of risk factors for vesicourethral leaks following radical retropubic prostatectomy. *Int J Urol.* 2008;12:948-952.

41. Ramsden AR, Chodak GW. Can leakage at the vesico-urethral anastomosis be predicted after radical retropubic prostatectomy? *BJU Int.* 2004;93:504-506.

42. Leibovitch I, Rowland RG, Little JS Jr, et al. Cystography after radical retropubic prostatectomy: clinical implications of abnormal findings. *Urology.* 1995;46:78-80.

43. Berlin JW, Ramchandani P, Banner MP, et al. Voiding cystography after radical prostatectomy: normal findings and correlation between contrast extravasation and anastomotic strictures. *AJR Am J Roentgenol.* 1994;162:87-91.

44. Guru KA, Seereiter PJ, Sfakianos JP, Hutson AD, Mohler JL. Is a cystogram necessary after robotic-assisted radical prostatectomy? *Urol Oncol*. 2007;25:465-467.

45. Tan GY, Jhaveri JK, Tewari AK. Anatomic restoration technique (ART): a biomechanics based approach to early continence recovery following minimally invasive radical prostatectomy. *Urology*. 2009;74(3):492-496.

46. Stolzenburg J-U, Wasserschied J, Rabenault R, et al. Reduction in incidence of lymphocele following extraperitoneal radical prostatectomy and pelvic lymph node dissection by bilateral peritoneal fenestration. *World J Urol*. 2008;26(6):581-586.

47. Shaher Z. Port closure techniques. *Surg Endosc*. 2007;21:1264-1274.

48. Brown JA, Elliott DS, Barrett DM. Postprostatectomy urinary incontinence: a comparison of the cost of conservative versus surgical management. *Urology*. 1998;51(5):715-720.

49. van Randenborgh H, Paul R, Kubler H, Breul J, Hartung R. Improved urinary continence after radical retropubic prostatectomy with preparation of a long, partially intraprostatic portion of the membranous urethra: an analysis of 1013 consecutive cases. *Prostate Cancer Prostatic Dis*. 2004;7:253-257.

50. Nyugen L, Jhaveri J, Tewari A. Surgical technique to overcome anatomical shortcoming: balancing post-prostatectomy continence outcomes of urethral sphincter lengths on preoperative magnetic resonance imaging. *J Urol*. 2008;179:1907-1911.

51. Steiner MS. Continence-preserving anatomic radical retropubic prostatectomy. *Urology*. 2000;55:427-435.

52. Montorsi F, Salonia A, Suardi N, et al. Improving the preservation of the urethral sphincter and neurovascular bundles during open radical retropubic prostatectomy. *Eur Urol*. 2005;48:938-945.

53. Rocco F, Carmignani L, Aquati P, et al. Restoration of posterior aspect of rhabdosphincter shortens continence time after radical retropubic prostatectomy. *J Urol*. 2006;175: 2201-2206.

54. Rocco B, Gregori A, Stener S, et al. Posterior reconstruction of the rhabdosphincter allows a rapid recovery of continence after transperitoneal videolaparoscopic radical prostatectomy. *Eur Urol*. 2007;51:996-1003.

55. Nguyen MM, Kamoi K, Stein RJ, et al. Early continence outcomes of posterior musculofascial plate reconstruction during robotic and laparoscopic prostatectomy. *BJU Int*. 2008;101: 1135-1139.

56. Licht MR, Klein EA, Tuason L, Levin H. Impact of bladder neck preservation during radical prostatectomy on continence and cancer control. *Urology*. 1994;44:883-887.

57. Cambio AJ, Evans CP. Minimising postoperative incontinence following radical prostatectomy: considerations and evidence. *Eur Urol*. 2006;50:903-913.

58. Walsh PC, Marschke PL. Intussusception of the bladder neck leads to earlier continence after radical prostatectomy. *Urology*. 2002;59(6):934-938.

59. Srougi M, Paranhos M, Leite KM, Dall'Oglio M, Nesrallah L. The influence of bladder neck mucosal eversion and early urinary extravasation on patient outcome after radical retropubic prostatectomy: a prospective controlled trial. *BJU Int*. 2005;95(6):757-760.

60. Stolzenburg JU, Liatsikos EN, Rabenalt R, et al. Nerve sparing endoscopic extraperitoneal radical prostatectomy – effect of puboprostatic ligament preservation on early continence and positive margins. *Eur Urol*. 2006;49(1):103-111.

61. Tewari AK, Bigelow K, Rao S, et al. Anatomic restoration technique of continence mechanism and preservation of puboprostatic collar: a novel modification to achieve early urinary continence in men undergoing robotic prostatectomy. *Urology*. 2007;69:726-731.

62. Mimic Technologies. dv Trainer brochure. Available at: http://www.mimic.ws/products/MIMIC-dV-Trainer-Brochure.pdf. Accessed July 30, 2009.

63. Sweet RM, McDougall EM. Simulation and computer-animated devices: the new minimally invasive skills training paradigm. *Urol Clin North Am*. 2008;35:519-531.

64. Brown-Clerk B, Siu KC, Katsavelis D, Lee I, Oleynikov D, Stergiou N. Validating advanced robotic-assisted laparoscopic training task in virtual reality. *Stud Health Technol Inform.* 2008;132:45-49.
65. Tan GY, Goel RK, Kaouk JH, Tewari AK. Technological advances in robotic-assisted laparoscopic surgery. *Urol Clin North Am.* 2009;36:237-249.

Difficulties in Laparoscopic Urologic Surgery in Kidney Transplant Patients and Obese Patients

18

Mahesh R. Desai and Arvind P. Ganpule

Introduction

Laparoscopic surgery has become an established procedure for surgical management of most benign and malignant urologic conditions. Laparoscopic nephrectomy can be performed either by a transperitoneal or retroperitoneal approach. The complexity of the surgery directly relates to the chronic kidney disease (CKD) for which the surgery is to be performed. Laparoscopic interventions may be required in the following situations namely, pretransplant nephrectomy for stones in the native kidney, pyonephrosis, autosomal dominant polycystic kidney disease (ADPKD), pretransplant orchidectomy for an intra-abdominal testis, post-transplant lymphocoele marsupilisation and laparoscopic-assisted placement of a Tenckoff catheter. The approach to any given case is a matter of personal preference – it should be chosen depending on the comfort level of the surgeon.

Laparoscopy becomes challenging in conditions such as xanthogranulomatous pyelonephritis (XGPN) and pyonephrosis in obese and CKD patients due to the attendant comorbidities. This chapter deals with the anticipated problems in treating obese patients and laparoscopy in patients with CKD.

Preoperative Evaluation for Laparoscopy in Kidney Transplant Patients

There should be close coordination between the nephrologist, anesthetists, and the surgeon. Preoperative dialysis needs, postoperative dialysis timings and dosage requirements should be determined. Patients on hemodialysis usually require dialysis preoperatively within 24 h of the surgery to reduce the risk of overload and hyperkalemia. Patients on peritoneal dialysis should preferably switch over to hemodialysis prior to surgery. In post-transplant patients, the nephrologist should be consulted for immunosuppressive dosing, monitoring and adjustment.

M.R. Desai (✉)
Department of Urology, Muljibhai Patel Urological Hospital, Nadlad, Gujarat, India
e-mail: mrdesai@mpuh.org

A.M. Al-Kandari and I.S. Gill (eds.), *Difficult Conditions in Laparoscopic Urologic Surgery*,   **249**
DOI: 10.1007/978-1-84882-105-7_18, © Springer-Verlag London Limited 2011

Pre-transplant Nephrectomy for Adult Polycystic Kidney Disease

Bilateral simultaneous or staged nephrectomy is needed in patients with adult polycystic kidney disease. The indications being large size, recurrent urinary tract infections (UTI), abscesses, calculus, and hemorrhage in the cysts.[1] Few studies have observed a increased risk of urosepsis with an origin in the cyst in patients who were not nephrectomised.[2] The tradeoff in this aspect is reduced risk of infection in patients who underwent nephrectomy, but at the cost of increased perioperative risk, loss of diuresis, and managing an anephric state.[3]

The other issue is if unilateral nephrectomy is better than bilateral nephrectomy. In the authors' experience, a bilateral simultaneous nephrectomy is preferred, as the patient is subjected to anesthesia once and hence, less perioperative risk. Furthermore, the authors have observed that if staged nephrectomies are performed a few days apart, the peritoneal adhesions hinder the dissection and make the procedure more challenging. Lastly, performing a bilateral simultaneous nephrectomy decreases the time to transplantation. On comparing the open approach with the laparoscopic approach, the hospital stay, blood transfusion rate and analgesic requirements are significantly less. In the authors' opinion, a shorter convalescence leads to better preoperative preparation for transplantation.[1]

Operative Considerations in ADPKD

The authors perform the procedure by a transperitoneal approach. The patient is placed in a 45-degree oblique position. Prior to induction, the patient is catheterized and a nasogastric tube is inserted to help decompress the stomach and the bladder and to avoid injury during port insertion. During positioning, utmost care should be taken to avoid airway-related mishaps and nerve injury. Bony landmarks and pressure points should be padded and the patient adequately strapped in.

The major concerns in a laparoscopic approach for ADPKD is positioning and placement of ports. The proper position should be selected after reviewing the CT scan. A surface marking of the landmarks should be performed. The authors prefer creating the pneumoperitoneum with a closed technique using a Verres needle. The needle is inserted in the midclavicular line and a 12-mm working port is inserted at this point. A 5-mm port is inserted subcostally for the left-hand instrument. The camera port is inserted towards the midline (Fig. 18.1). In addition to the above-mentioned port configuration, a port is inserted on the right side for liver retraction. On either side, an extra 5-mm port is inserted for retraction, if required.

The dissection starts by reflecting the colon along the white line, identifying the ureterogonadal packet and then proceeding towards the hilum. The renal vessels should be secured as quickly as possible (Fig. 18.2). A key point is that the dissection should be outside Gerota's fascia as this prevents rupture of the cysts, which contain a noxious fluid that may lead to chemical peritonitis. If a cyst accidently ruptures, every attempt should be made

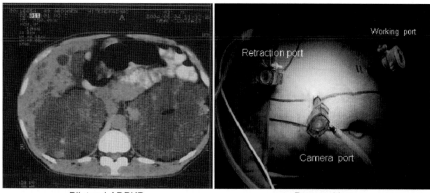

Bilateral ADPKD   Port position
CT scan helps in the assessment for port placement

Fig. 18.1 Port placement

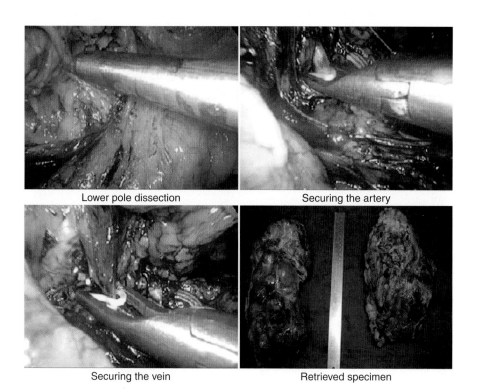

Lower pole dissection   Securing the artery

Securing the vein   Retrieved specimen

Fig. 18.2 Steps in pretransplant nephrectomy for bilateral ADPKD

to perform a thorough peritoneal lavage. Aspiration of these cysts may also be considered, as this maneuver reduces the amount of cystic fluid escaping into the peritoneal cavity, helps reduce kidney size, and ultimately aids retrieval. A potential problem in these patients is injury to adjacent organs which include intestines, colon, spleen, and liver.[1]

Some points of emphasis:

1. Proper preoperative assessment, which should include a CT scan
2. Adequate preoperative hemodialysis
3. Proper positioning and placement of ports for comfortable dissection
4. The dissection plane should be beyond cyst and Gerota's fascia to avoid cyst rupture. A thorough peritoneal lavage is necessary at the completion of the procedure.
5. Slow and meticulous dissection to prevent adjacent organ injury
6. The authors retrieve the specimen through a midline umbilical incision, as this helps to avoid incision in either iliac fossa. The specimen can be removed after morcellation, which appears to have the advantage of reducing the operative time and decreases the theoretical risk of hernias due to a shorter incision.[4] However, this does not offer an optimal histopathological evaluation.
7. In bilateral simultaneous procedures, prior to changing the position, ensure that there are no electrolyte disturbances before commencing the opposite side.
8. Bilateral simultaneous nephrectomy whenever possible.[1]

Pretransplant Nephrectomy in Infective Conditions and Previously Operated Cases

Laparoscopic nephrectomy is challenging in situations involving fibrosis and inflammation such as pyonephrosis, tuberculosis, and XPGN. Surgeons should embark on this surgical exercise only after gaining adequate surgical experience. Certain technical issues merit consideration while performing laparoscopic nephrectomy in this difficult patient group.

The Approach

The authors' preference is the transperitoneal approach since it offers a large working space and readily identifiable landmarks. This is especially important in situations such as nonfunctioning kidneys due to tuberculosis and XGPN where the course of the disease leads to abnormal orientation of hilar structures. An added advantage with the transperitoneal approach is that the bowel and the colon are adherent to the kidney. The approach also offers a unique opportunity to visualize the colon and adjacent structures and perform meticulous dissection, hence minimizing the chance of injury. It also facilitates the separation of colon and mesentery from the underlying gerotas.

However, one of the drawbacks of this approach is the potential exposure of the peritoneum to infective contents. In such situations involving pyonephrosis and/or XGPN, preplacing a percutaneous nephrostomy may also e helpful.

Securing the Hilum

Securing the hilum may be challenging in conditions involving renal tuberculosis and XGPN. With these two conditions, dense scarring of perihilar tissues may occur that make dissection of the hilum difficult. In contrast with calculus pyelonephritis, pyonephrosis, and ADPKD, the renal hilum is relatively spared and the main challenge lies in mobilizing the colon and other structures from the kidney. Although en bloc stapling of the renal hilum has been described in such situations, the authors prefer to individually ligate the artery and vein as much as possible. In situations where individual dissection of artery and vein is not possible laparoscopically, the authors prefer to transfix the pedicle through a small incision after the remainder mobilization of the kidney.

The authors retrospectively analyzed data from 84 patients with benign inflammatory diseases who underwent laparoscopic nephrectomy and compared their data with data from 94 matched patients undergoing open nephrectomy. The renal hilum was relatively unaffected in patients with pyonephrosis and calculus pyelonephritis. Pleural entry was more common ($P < 0.0001$) in the open group, and visceral injury was more common in the laparoscopic group ($P = 0.04$). Blood transfusion was necessary in 7% and 11% of patients in the laparoscopic and open groups, respectively. Open conversion was required in eight cases (ADPKD: three; pyonephrosis: two; XGPN and calculus pyelonephritis: three). Intestinal obstruction that required laparotomy and adhesinolysis developed in one patient in the laparoscopic group.[5] In many cases, previous peritoneal adhesions may have hampered the pneumoperitoneum with closed technique. In these situations, the use of open or Hasson's technique is prudent or alternatively, a subcostal access at the "palmars" point can be achieved. Later, a needloscope can be introduced through the Verres and the initial trocar introduced. This approach helps to avoid bowel injury. The debate continues as to whether a transperitoneal or retroperitoneal approach is advantageous in patients with XGPN.

Laparoscopic Marsupilisation of Post-transplant Lymphocoele

The incidence of post-transplant lymphocoele varies from 1% to 18%.[6,7] The treatment is indicated in expanding collections, causing obstruction and steady decline in function. The various treatment options available are needle aspiration and external drainage with or without sclerotherapy. Marsupilization of lymphocele can be done either with the open or laparoscopic technique. Laparoscopic marsupilization is a safe, effective method.

The Technique

After Foley catherization and nasogastric tube insertion, a Verres needle is placed at the umbilicus followed by insertion of a 10-mm port at the same site. The intra-abdominal pressure is kept at 15-mm Hg, and 5- and 10-mm trocars are then inserted under direct vision in the contralateral and ipsilateral iliac fossae, respectively. The key to success in this procedure is identification of vital structures, namely the ureter, the graft, and the bladder (Fig. 18.3).

The patient is placed in a head low position. Typically, the lymphocele is identified as a shining, bluish bulge separate from the allograft that typically transmits light. Upon identification, the lymphocele is further confirmed with needle aspiration. The fullest aspect of the bulge should be incised with a cautery or a scissors (Fig. 18.4). It is of utmost importance that all the bleeding edges be adequately secured. At times the omentum may be interposed in the lymphocele cavity, which improves results.

The head low position helps by allowing the bowel to fall away from the operative field. This, apart from identification of the lymphocele, also helps in preventing inadvertent injury to the intestines.

Before incising the lymphocele, it is of utmost importance to identify its limits. Gentle probing also helps in this regard and the lymphocele also readily transmits light. In

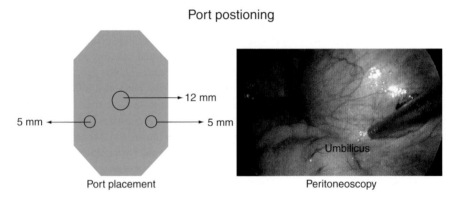

Fig. 18.3 Port placement for laparoscopic marsupilization of post-transplant lymphocele

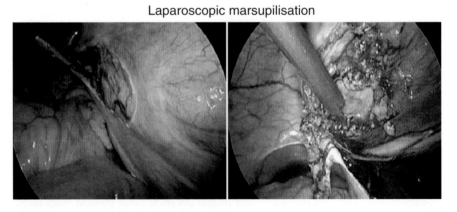

Fig. 18.4 Laparoscopic identification of a lymphocele

difficult situations, intraoperative laparoscopic sonography may be of benefit.[8] Filling and draining the bladder with an indwelling Foley catheter or alternatively probing the bladder with a laparoscopic grasper helps to prevent bladder injury. Matin and Gill[9] have described the use of an internalized peritoneal dialysis catheter for recurrent inaccessible lymphocele. In this technique, the lymphocele is localized with the help of a sonographically guided needle in the lymphocele cavity after port placement. The dissection proceeds meticulously around the needle until the collection. If an adequate omental tag cannot be brought down to the lymphocele, a cable catheter is placed. This technique cannot be used in infected lymphocele. The identification of lymphoceles will be difficult at times due to anatomic distortion or excessive fat. These problems can be overcome with the use of preplaced transperitoneal guidewires or angiography catheters.[10] This requires CT guidance and has a theoretical risk of peritoneal infection. Laparoscopic lymphocele marsupilization cannot be done in small symptomatic lymphocele, extremely lateral lymphocele, and those patients having extensive bowel adhesions or an interposing bowel.

Laparoscopic Assisted Insertion of a Continuous Ambulatory Peritoneal Dialysis (CAPD) Catheter

The perceived advantages of laparoscopic assisted insertion of a continuous ambulatory peritoneal dialysis (CAPD) catheter over open insertion is low incidence of visceral injury, improved ability to perform repair of hernia and omentectomy and the potential to perform the procedure as a day case. The laparoscopic approach can also be utilized as a rescue therapy for malfunctioning catheters.[11–13] The disadvantages are problems associated with pneumoperitoneum (such as decreased cardiac return), port site hernias, and occasional port-related visceral injuries.[14]

The Technique

The authors create an initial pneumoperitoneum and insert a 12-mm port at the umbilicus. Two 5-mm trocars are inserted in both the iliac fossa (Fig. 18.5). An 18-gauge diamond tip needle is inserted just beneath the umbilical port and a guide wire is passed, followed by a 14-F fascial dilator under vision. A Tenckoff catheter is passed under vision and sutured with the pelvic wall. Later, with the help of a dilator, the catheter is tunneled through the subcutaneous tissues, and then the catheter is flushed to prevent blockage. The authors feel that the advantage of using three ports is the ability to suture the catheter to the pelvic wall with intracorporeal sutures.

In a technique described by Hodgson et al., a novel method of two ports with a "add a cath" sheath is used.[14] Santarelli et al.[11] report on the use of laparoscopy for treating malfunctioning peritoneal dialysis catheters. According to their report, the major cause for malfunction was omental wrapping.

Laparoscopic assisted PD catheter insertion

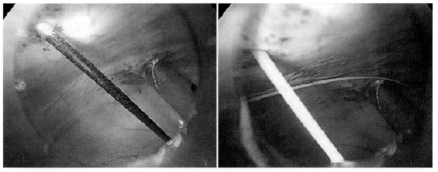

18 Gauge needle inserted under vision   Guide wire passed

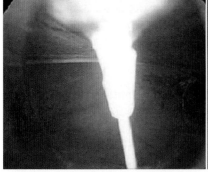 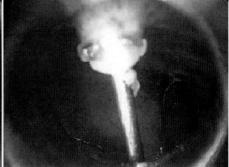

14 Fr Screw dilator   PD catheter passed over Alkens rod

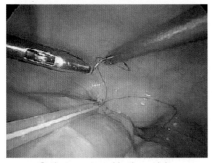

Catheter sutured in the pelvis

Fig. 18.5 Steps in the authors' technique of laparoscopic CAPD catheter placement

Laparoscopic Urology in Obese Individuals

Traditionally, obesity has been considered as a relative contraindication for laparoscopy.[15] Obese patients are considered to be at risk for a variety of reasons. They are at increased risk of developing heart disease, diabetes and hypertension. Obesity also poses a unique challenge to an anesthesia team as obesity is considered to be an independent risk factor for deep vein thrombosis.

Kurzer et al. describe a few modifications for laparoscopy in obese patients. The table should be customized to bear the additional weight of the patient. Pressure points should be adequately padded. Kurzer et al. describe the use of a bean bag for this purpose. The patients should also be placed on aggressive deep vein thrombosis prophylaxis.[15]

While achieving pneumoperitoneum, the ports should be placed more laterally than usual. Occasionally in these patients there may be a need to use extra long instruments and ports, particularly for the dissection of the upper pole. These strategically placed ports and instruments help reduce the distance to the kidney and prevent the bowel from obstructing the view. At the conclusion of the procedure, it is vital to close the ports (10 mm/12 mm) with a port closure device.

In their analysis of outcome in obese patients, Boorjian et al. concluded that body mass index (BMI) was not an independent predictor of positive surgical margins, complications, incontinence or erectile function in patients undergoing robot-assisted laparoscopic prostatectomy. They noted that these patients had longer operative room times which did not translate into greater risk of other complications.[16] The authors evaluated data from laparoscopic donor nephrectomies performed on donors that had a BMI of less than 30 and donors that had a BMI of more than 30. Patients with a higher BMI had significantly longer hospital stays and required more ports for dissection (Table 18.1). Jacobs et al. also compared markedly obese patients (BMI more than 35) and patients with BMIs less than 30 that were scheduled for laproscopic nephrectomy. They observed that the donor operation in the markedly obese patient was significantly longer by an average of 40 min. Obese patients were more also likely to have a conversion to open surgery.[17]

Table 18.1 Outcome in laparoscopic donors in relation to BMI

Parameter	Group 1 (BMI < 30) (n = 320)	Group 2 (BMI ≥ 30) (n = 41)	P-Value
Operative time (min)	156 ± 46.5	160 ± 54	NS
Number of ports	3.2 ± 0.5	4.0 ± 0.7	$P < 0.05$
Dose of analgesia (mg)	99 ± 64	110 ± 64	NS
Starting oral fluids (h)	19.7 ± 3	20 ± 3	NS
Drop in PCV (%)	4.8 ± 2.3	6.2 ± 3.2	NS
Duration of hospital stay (days)	3.0 ± 0.2	4.5 ± 0.6	$P < 0.05$
Warm ischemia (min)	5.8 ± 1.9	6.0 ± 2.0	NS
Total ischemia (min)	55 ± 8.7	58 ± 16	NS

Bivariate analysis of patients undergoing laparoscopic donor nephrectomy using Pearson's correlation coefficient (two-tailed). The only significant correlation found was the number of ports and the length of hospital stay

Conclusion

Risk reduction strategies in patients with chronic kidney disease and obesity involve proper preoperative evaluation, adherence to meticulous surgical principles, and adequate surgical expertise to deal with difficult situations and complications.

References

1. Desai MR, Nandkishore SK, Ganpule A, Thimmegowda M. Pretransplant laparoscopic nephrectomy in adult polycystic kidney disease: a single centre experience. *BJU Int*. 2008;101:94-97.
2. Rayner BL, Cassidy MJD, Jacobson JE, Pascoe MD, Pontin AR, van Zyl Smit R. Is preliminary bilateral nephrectomy necessary in patients with autosomal dominant polycystic kidney disease undergoing renal transplantation? *Clin Nephrol*. 1990;34:122-124.
3. Rozanski J, Kozlowska I, Myslak M, et al. Pretransplant nephrectomy in patients with autosomal dominant polycystic kidney disease. *Transplant Proc*. 2005;37:666-668.
4. Dunn MD, Portis AJ, Elbahnasy AM, et al. Laparoscopic nephrectomy in patients with end-stage renal disease and autosomal dominant polycystic kidney disease. *Am J Kidney Dis*. 2000;35(4):720-725.
5. Manohar T, Desai MM, Desai MR. Laparoscopic nephrectomy for benign and inflammatory conditions. *J Endourol*. 2007;21(11):1323-1328.
6. Howard RJ, Simmons RL, Najarian JS. Prevention of lymphoceles following transplantation. *Ann Surg*. 1976;184(2):166-168.
7. Braun WE, Banowsky LH, Straffon RA, et al. Lymphoceles associated with renal transplantation: report of 15 cases and review of the literature. *Am J Med*. 1974;57(5):714-729.
8. Abou-Elela A, Reyad I, Torky M, Meshref A, Morsi A. Laparoscopic marsupilization of post-renal transplantation lymphoceles. *J Endourol*. 2006;20(11):904-906.
9. Matin SF, Gill IS. Laparoscopic marsupilization of the difficult lymphocele using internalized peritoneal dialysis catheter. *J Urol*. 2000;163:1498-1500.
10. Tie MLH, Rao M, Russell C, Burapa K. Transperitoneal guide-wire or drainage catheter placement for guidance of laparoscopic marsupilization of lymphocoeles postrenal transplantation. *Nephrol Dial Transplant*. 2001;16:1038-1041.
11. Santarelli S, Zeiler M, Marinelli R, Monteburini T, Federico A, Ceruado E. Videolaparoscopy as rescue therapy and placement of peritoneal dialysis catherers: a thirty-two case single centre experience. *Nephrol Dial Transplant*. 2006;21:1348-1354.
12. Crabtree FH, Fishman A. A laparoscopic approach under local anesthesia for peritoneal dialysis access. *Perit Dial Int*. 2000;20:757-765.
13. Skipper K, Dickerman R, Dunn E. Laparoscopic placement and revision of peritoneal dialysis catheters. *JSLS*. 1999;3(1):63-65.
14. Hodgson D, Rowbothom C, Peters JL, Nathan S. A novel method for laparoscopic placement of Tenckhoff peritoneal dialysis catheters. *BJU Int*. 2003;91:885-886.
15. Kurzer E, Leveillee R, Bird V. Obesity as a risk factor for complications during laparoscopic surgery for renal cancer: multivariate analysis. *J Endourol*. 2006;20(10):794-799.
16. Boorjian SA, Crispen PL, Carlson RE, et al. Impact of obesity on clinicopathological outcomes after robot-assisted laparoscopic prostatectomy. *J Endourol*. 2008;22(7):1471-1476.
17. Jacobs SC, Cho E, Dunkin BJ, et al. Laproscopic nephrectomy in the markedly obese living renal donor. *Urology*. 2000;56:926-929.

Difficulties in Laparoscopic Retroperitoneal Lymph Node Dissection

19

Ahmed E. Ghazi and Günter Janetschek

Nonseminomatous Germ Cell Tumors

Malignant testicular cancers, both seminomas and nonseminomatous germ cell tumors (NSGCT), can be cured with a very high success rate when correctly managed. For seminomas, retroperitoneal lymph node dissection (RPLND) is rarely indicated. For NSGCTs, which differ substantially from seminomas, the mainstays of successful management are RPLND and chemotherapy, used either alone or in combination. However, RPLND and chemotherapy are both associated with specific morbidities, which increase significantly if the two therapies are combined. Because the therapeutic efficacy of RPLND cannot be further improved significantly, the goal in management of low-stage NSGCT and especially of clinical stage I NSGCT is reduction in morbidity without compromising the cure rate.

Indications and Therapeutic Concepts

Clinical Stage I

About 25–30% of patients with clinical stage I NSGCT have occult lymph node metastases in the retroperitoneum that cannot be diagnosed preoperatively, even with the most sensitive imaging techniques available.[1,2] However, in up to 20% of patients whose lymph nodes give suspicious computed tomography (CT) results, the pathologic analysis shows stage I disease.[3]

In general, RPLND is considered the only method that can immediately and reliably identify lymph nodes suspected of metastatic involvement without the potential for false-positive results. In replacing open RPLND with laparoscopic RPLND, the aim is to decrease surgical morbidity substantially while maintaining a comparable diagnostic accuracy. Short-term morbidity is comparable to that of major intra-abdominal surgery, but long-term

A.E. Ghazi (✉)
Department of Urology, Krankenhaus der Elisabethinen Linz, Linz, Austria
e-mail: ahmed_ghazimd@yahoo.com

A.M. Al-Kandari and I.S. Gill (eds.), *Difficult Conditions in Laparoscopic Urologic Surgery*, 259
DOI: 10.1007/978-1-84882-105-7_19, © Springer-Verlag London Limited 2011

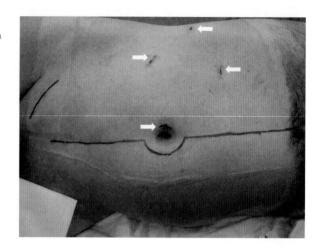

Fig. 19.1 Outline of the midline exploratory incision for open RPLND, contrary to the trocar site incisions for laparoscopic right RPLND (marked by the *arrows*)

morbidity is even more striking and includes loss of antegrade ejaculation and the formation of a long scar that impairs most young patients throughout their lives (Fig. 19.1).[4]

However, RPLND is considered in some countries as a second-line therapy with first-line therapy being either wait-and-see (low risk) or primary chemotherapy (high risk). There are, however, still several arguments in favor of RPLND. A relapse may be difficult to detect in a marker-negative patient. Therefore, wait-and-see is not a valid option in this situation. The same is true in a patient with poor compliance. Primary chemotherapy carries the risk of late recurrence with NSGCT containing chemoresistant tumor.[5] In summary, the indications for laparoscopic RPLND are the same as for open surgery. Previous surgery or obesity never were considered contraindications as neither resulted in conversion in the authors' series.

The concept presented here, although still debatable, is that RPLND should be performed for diagnostic purposes only, implying that treatment for patients with pathologic stage II will be combined with adjuvant chemotherapy.

Stage II After Chemotherapy

Stage IIa

This stage is treated similarly to clinical stage I with primary chemotherapy, and additional RPLND is usually not indicated.

Stage IIb

Due to high relapse rates after therapeutic RPLND for stage II NSGCT (between 34% and 55% for stage IIb),[4, 6, 7] relying on surgery alone in stage II disease without adjuvant chemotherapy would entail the same or even more problems as surveillance in clinical stage I disease. Therefore in tumors of 2–5 cm in size prior to chemotherapy, therapy is started with two cycles of PEB. Further chemotherapy, which is usually given to increase safety but has no more therapeutic impact once there is no more vital tumor, is replaced by laparoscopic RPLND. The benefit of this approach is twofold. The patient is spared unnecessary chemotherapy, and in a substantial proportion of patients, chemoresistant mature teratoma will be removed as well. Thereby, the effect of chemotherapy is well documented. Normalization of markers is a prerequisite to perform surgery. In the authors' experience, morbidity of laparoscopic RPLND is clearly less than morbidity of further chemotherapy. In this context, morbidity of chemotherapy increases exponentially cycle by cycle.

Stage IIc

Laparoscopic surgery is only indicated in selected smaller tumors where a unilateral surgical template is considered sufficient. The template has to include all visible tumors prior to chemotherapy. Three cycles of PEB are administered initially. The authors do not only remove a residual tumor, but always dissect the complete unilateral template.

Contraindications

Clinical Stage I

Persistently elevated tumor markers after orchiectomy, infection, and bleeding diathesis are the only contraindications. In this context, the half lives of alpha-fetoprotein and beta-human chorionic gonadotropin must be taken into consideration.

Stage IIb After Chemotherapy

Elevated tumor markers are a contraindication. Poor response to chemotherapy as assessed by the size of the residual tumor is not necessarily a contraindication if the tumor is believed to consist of mature teratoma. The anesthesiologist should be alert to the possibility that bleomycin may cause damage to the lungs.

Preoperative Measures

Preoperative staging includes chest radiography, ultrasonography of the abdomen and retroperitoneum, computed tomography of the chest and abdomen, and assessment of the tumor markers alpha-fetoprotein and beta-human chorionic gonadotropin. Bowel preparation, including a clear liquid diet and oral laxatives, is performed 1 day preoperatively. All patients receive low-dose antibiotic coverage. Typing and cross-matching are performed for two units of blood. As a preventive measure to avoid chylous ascites (which was observed in a few patients after postchemotherapeutic laparoscopic RPLND), patients are placed on a low-fat diet for 2 weeks postoperatively. The authors have not seen this complication since instituting this measure.

Template

Weissbach and Boedefeld (Fig. 19.2)[8] have described templates that include practically all primary landing sites of lymph node metastases. If all lymphatic tissue is resected within these templates, there is only a minimal risk for a metastasis to be overlooked. The templates for the left and the right side differ substantially; only the template for right-sided tumors includes the interaortocaval tissue. The authors have developed a laparoscopic, split-and-roll technique that enables transection of all lumbar vessels and enables the authors to perform the same radical dissection as with open surgery.[9] Furthermore, the primary landing sites with regard to their ventro-dorsal location (Fig 19.3) were investigated. All patients with solitary metastases, and most patients (22 of 25) with multiple metastases, were detected ventral to the lumbar vessels. Therefore, it can be concluded that the primary landing sites are invariably located ventrally, whereas dorsal metastases result

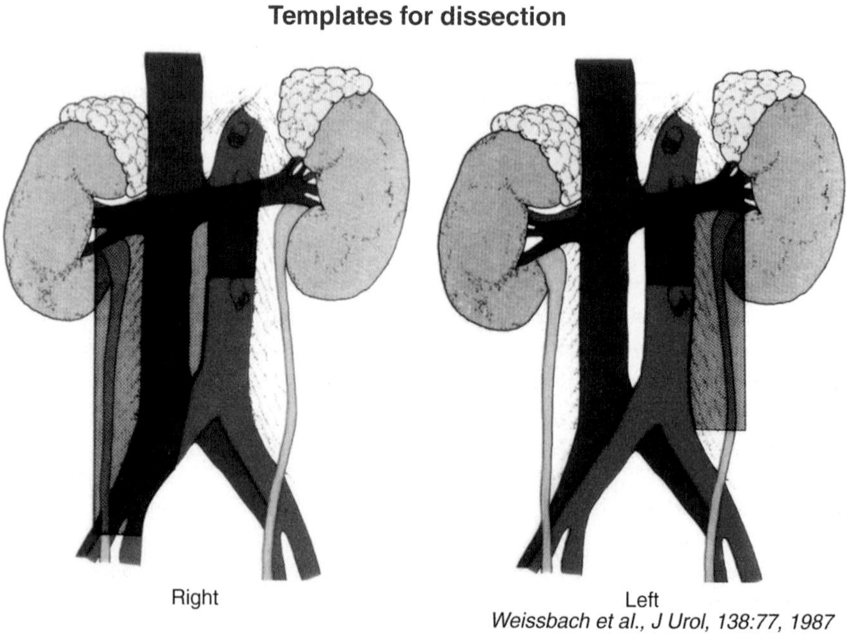

Templates for dissection

Right   Left
Weissbach et al., J Urol, 138:77, 1987

Fig. 19.2 Templates described by Weissbach and Boedefeld in 1987 for *right* and *left* laparoscopic RPLND (Adapted from Weissbach and Boedefeld[8])

Fig. 19.3 Ventral primary landing sites of metastasis from testicular cancer (*long arrow*), dorsal metastases result from further tumor spread (*short arrows*)

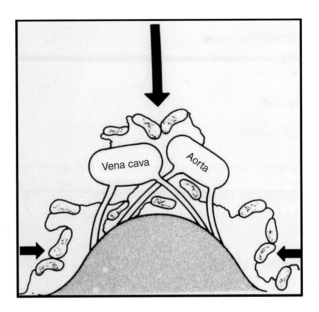

from further tumor spread.[2] Consequently, the authors no longer routinely transect all lumbar vessels to remove the tissue behind them; it is not required in diagnostic RPLND for clinical stage I tumors. This makes the laparoscopic procedure considerably easier, safer, and faster without affecting the diagnostic outcome or long-term survival.[10] Borders of the templates will be discussed in detail during description of the surgical technique.

The same procedure is performed in clinical stage IIB disease following chemotherapy. All tissue in which tumor was found before chemotherapy is removed and the ipsilateral template is dissected in the same fashion as in clinical stage I disease.

Equipment

The following tools have proved useful additions to the standard laparoscopic equipment. The authors exclusively use three-chip video cameras and 30°, 10-mm laparoscopes. The laparoscope is held and maneuvered by a robotic arm (AESOP, Computer Motion, Santa Barbara, CA). This robot is used to replace one assistant surgeon and has the advantage of providing stable video images even in lengthy procedures. An insufflator with a high flow rate (>12 L) has proved helpful because it prevents the pneumoperitoneum from collapsing during suction. A small surgical sponge that is held with a traumatic grasper is used for retraction, dissection, and hemostasis. A right-angle dissector (Snowden-Pencer® Brand Endo-Right Angle™ Dissector, Cardinal Health, Snowden Pencer® MIS Products, Tucker, GA) is applied for the dissection of vessels. The authors no longer use metallic clips, but have replaced them with Hem-o-lok® clips (Teleflex Medical, Research Triangle Park, NC).

Operative Technique

Clinical Stage I

Right Side

Patient Position

The patient is placed on the operating table with the right side elevated 45° upward so that by rotating the table he can be brought into a supine or lateral decubitus position without repositioning. In addition, the table is flexed at the level of the umbilicus. If necessary, the Trendelenburg or reverse Trendelenburg position is used (Fig. 19.4).

Initial Access and Trocars

A Veress needle is used for the initial stab incision to create the pneumoperitoneum whereas the Hasson cannula is reserved for patients who have previously undergone abdominal surgery. Only 10-mm trocars are used. The first trocar for the laparoscope is placed at the site of the umbilicus. Two secondary trocars for the surgeon are placed at the lateral edge of the rectus muscle, approximately 8 cm above and below the umbilicus. A retraction port is placed in the right flank a few centimeters medial to the tip of the 12th rib (Fig. 19.4).

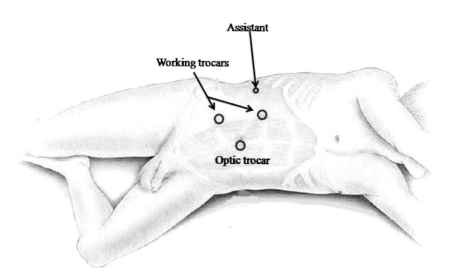

Fig. 19.4 Patient position and trocar arrangement for right laparoscopic RPLND

Exposure of the Template

Wide access to the retroperitoneum is a prerequisite for laparoscopic RPLND. Excellent access can be gained by wide dissection of the right colon and the duodenum in the plane of Toldt. As a first step, the peritoneum is incised along the line of Toldt from the cecum to the right colic flexure. This incision is carried cephalad parallel to the transverse colon and lateral to the duodenum along the vena cava, all the way up to the hepatoduodenal ligament. Caudally, the incision is carried along the spermatic vessels to the internal inguinal ring (Fig. 19.5). Next, the colon, the duodenum, and the head of the pancreas are reflected medially until the anterior surfaces of the vena cava, aorta, and left renal vein at its crossing with the aorta are completely exposed (Fig. 19.6).

Dissection of the Lymphatic Tissue Within the Template

At this point, the entire template described by Weissbach and Boedefeld[8] for right-sided tumors is accessible (Fig. 19.7). This template includes the interaortocaval nodes, the

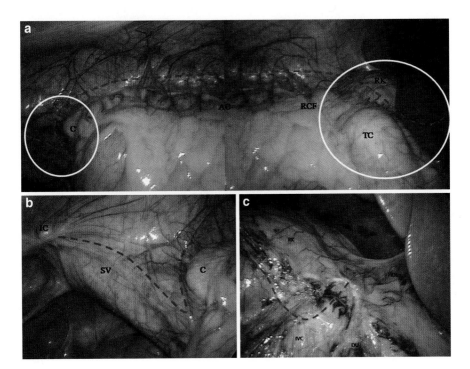

Fig. 19.5 Right-side laparoscopic RPLND. Peritoneal incision for right laparoscopic RPLND (**a**) Limits of peritoneal incision (*dotted line*). *C* cecum, *AC* ascending colon, *RCF* right colonic flexure, *TC* transverse colon, *RK* right kidney. (**b**) Caudal extension of the incision (*dotted line*) along the spermatic vessels to the internal inguinal ring. *IC* inguinal ring, *SV* spermatic vessels, *C* cecum. (**c**) Cranial extension of the incision (*dotted line*), with the transverse colon and liver retracted. *IVC* inferior vena cava, *DU* duodenum, *HDL* hepato-duodenal ligament, *RK* right kidney

Fig. 19.6 Right-side laparoscopic RPLND. Access to the retroperitoneum after dissection of the colon, duodenum, and head of pancreas (intraoperative site). *IVC* inferior vena cava, *AO* aorta, *LRV* left renal vein, *RRV* right renal vein, *RK* right kidney

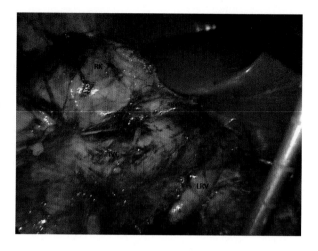

Template for right RPLND

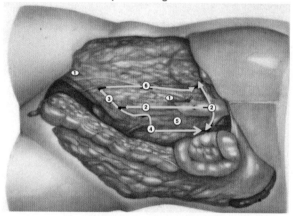

Fig. 19.7 Right-side laparoscopic RPLND. Template and incision lines. The numbers represent the various steps of dissection within the template. (1) Identification and dissection of the spermatic vessels, (2) dissection (splitting) of the lymphatic tissue overlying the IVC, (3) dissection of the lymphatic tissue at the lower border of the template, (4) dissection of the lymphatic tissue overlying the aorta, (5) dissection of the lymph node package within the interaortocaval space (medial to the IVC) and (6) dissection of lymph node package lateral to the vena cava and medial to the ureter (This image was published in *Atlas of the Urologic Clinics of North America*, Vol. 8, Janetschek G, Peschel R, Bartsch G, Laparoscopic retroperitoneal lymph node dissection, pp. 71–90, Copyright Elsevier, 2000)

preaortic tissue between the left renal vein and the inferior mesenteric artery, and all tissue ventral and lateral to the vena cava and right iliac artery and vein between the renal vessels and the crossing of the ureter with the iliac vessels. The template is bounded laterally by the ureter. As mentioned previously, the tissue behind the lumbar vessels and the vena cava

Fig. 19.8 Right-side
laparoscopic RPLND.
Excision of spermatic artery
and vein. Intraoperative site:
separate courses of
spermatic vein and artery.
IVC inferior vena cava, *AO*
aorta, *SA* spermatic artery,
SV spermatic vein

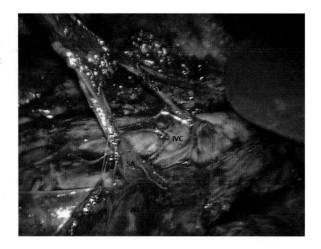

is not removed any longer during RPLND for diagnostic purposes. The spermatic vessels
are removed in their entire length.

Identification and Dissection of the Spermatic Vessels

The spermatic vein is dissected free along its entire course starting at the internal inguinal
ring. Provided radical orchiectomy has been adequately performed, the spermatic vessels
are ligated cephalad to the internal inguinal ring. One can be sure that the spermatic vessels
have been removed completely if this ligature can be identified. If not, the dissection within
the inguinal canal to remove remnants of the spermatic vein would be difficult and would
probably require an additional trocar in the ipsilateral lower abdomen, but the authors have
never confronted this problem. Special care must be taken when dissecting the opening of
the spermatic vein into the vena cava because the vein is liable to rupture at this point.
Cranially, the spermatic artery takes a separate course (Fig. 19.8); it is clipped and
transected at its crossing with the vena cava whereas its origin from the aorta is approached
later.

Dissection (Splitting) of the Lymphatic Tissue Overlying the Inferior Vena Cava (IVC)

The lymphatic tissue overlying the vena cava is split open from cranial (origin of renal
veins) to caudal (crossing of the right iliac artery), and its anterior and lateral surfaces are
dissected free. Both renal veins (upper border of template), as well as the anterior and
lateral surfaces of the IVC are dissected free (Fig. 19.9). This separates the template into
two distinct lymph node packages; the interaortocaval package and the package lateral to
the IVC. It is important to expose the lower edge of the left renal vein at this point of the
procedure as during dissection of the interaortocaval package from caudal in a cephalad
direction, the left renal vein can be injured easily if it is not clearly visible.

Dissection of the Lymphatic Tissue at the Lower Border of the Template

The lower border of the template is the point where the ureter crosses the right common iliac
artery. The lymph node package at this area is dissected, clipped, and transected (Fig. 19.10).

Fig. 19.9 Right-side
laparoscopic RPLND.
Following dissection of the
upper border of the template
(intraoperative site). *IVC*
inferior vena cava, *LRV* left
renal vein, *RRV* right renal
vein

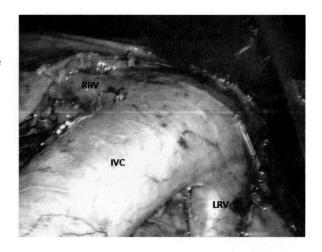

Fig. 19.10 Right-side
laparoscopic RPLND.
Clipping of the lymphatic
tissue at the lower border of
the template (intraoperative
site). *IVC* inferior vena cava,
U right ureter, *RCIA* right
common iliac artery, *LNP*
lymph node package

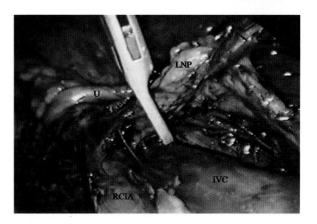

Dissection of the Lymphatic Tissue Overlying the Aorta

The lymphatic tissue overlying the right common iliac artery is incised up to the bifurcation and dissection is further continued to the origin of the inferior mesenteric artery. In
this area, the lymphatic tissue is usually dense, and care must be taken not to injure the
mesenteric artery. Cephalad to the artery, the lymphatic tissue is split along the left border
of the aorta so that the ventral surface of the aorta is completely freed up to the level of the
right renal artery, which is identified and dissected at this point. During this dissection, the
spermatic artery is clipped and transected, at its origin from the aorta.

Dissection of the Lymph Node Package Within the Interaortocaval Space (Medial to the IVC)

Now with exposure of both the IVC and aorta, the interaortocaval lymph node package is
dissected in a caudal to cranial direction. Starting with the caudal border of the dissection
(at the point where the ureter crosses the iliac vessels), where the lymphatic tissue was
clipped distally. The dissection is continued cephalic up to the right renal artery, which

Fig. 19.11 Right-side laparoscopic RPLND. Interaortocaval space after removal of lymphatic tissue (intraoperative site). *AO* aorta, *CSA* clipped spermatic artery, *LRV* left renal vein, *RRA* right renal artery, *IACS* interaortocaval space, *LV* spared lumbar vein, *IVC* inferior vena cava, *CSV* clipped spermatic vein

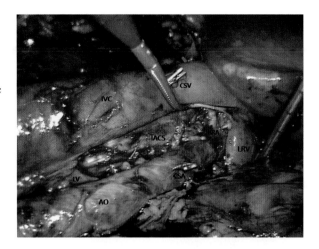

now can be identified as it courses across the interaortocaval space and, together with the previously exposed left renal vein, delineate the left cranial border of the dissection. The lumbar veins are exposed during dissection, but are only transected in exceptional cases to facilitate removal of the lymph nodes. The lymphatic package is then freed cranially (Fig. 19.11). When dissecting the cranial portions of the template, the liver must be retracted with a fan retractor.

Dissection of Lymph Node Package Lateral to the Vena Cava and Medial to the Ureter

The ureter, which defines the lateral border of the dissection, is usually identified during excision of the spermatic vessels. It is separated from the nodal package at its point of crossing with the iliac artery (Fig. 19.12a). Dissection is continued cranially along the ureter up to the renal hilum (Fig. 19.12b). At this point, the right renal artery is exposed and, together with the previously exposed right renal vein, delineates the right cranial border of the dissection. The package is then freed from any remaining attachments to the lateral surface of the IVC and down to the lumbar vessels (which are not transected) (Fig. 19.12c). Medial retraction of the IVC allows identification of the right sympathetic chain and lumbar arteries, lateral to the aorta. Finally, the lymph node package is freed from the right sympathetic chain. Although the postganglionic fibers are identified, they are not spared as maintaining dissection within a unilateral template preserves the contralateral sympathetic chain and subsequent ejaculation (Fig. 19.13).

Removal of the Nodal Package and Drainage

Now that the nodal packages are completely free, they are removed inside a specimen retrieval bag. A drain is not required. Finally, the colon and the duodenum are returned to their anatomic positions and secured with one suture, which is tied extracorporeally.

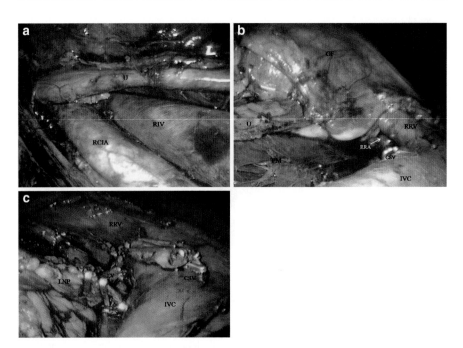

Fig. 19.12 Right-side laparoscopic RPLND. Dissection of lymph node package lateral to the vena cava and medial to the ureter (intraoperative site). (**a**) Distal border of dissection. Crossing of ureter with iliac artery. (**b**) Proximal ureter and Gerota's fascia separated from lymphatic tissue (This image was published in *Atlas of the Urologic Clinics of North America*, Vol. 8, Janetschek G, Peschel R, Bartsch G, Laparoscopic retroperitoneal lymph node dissection, pp. 71–90, Copyright Elsevier, 2000) (**c**) Dissection along the lateral surface of the vena cava. *U* ureter, *RCIA* right common iliac artery, *RIV* right iliac vein, *IVC* inferior vena cava, *RRV* right renal vein, *RRA* unexposed right renal artery, *CSV* clipped spermatic vein, *GF* Gerota's fascia (right kidney), *PM* psoas muscle, *LNP* lymph node package, *LV* spared lumbar vein

Fig. 19.13 Right-side laparoscopic RPLND. Intraoperative site after removal of lymph node package; the ureter is retracted ventrolaterally and the vena cava retracted medially. *IACS* interaorto-caval space, *IVC* inferior vena cava, *AO* aorta, *RRV* right renal vein, *RRA* right renal artery, *LA* lumbar artery, *LV* lumbar vein, *RSC* right sympathetic chain, *U* ureter, *RK* right kidney, *PM* psoas muscle

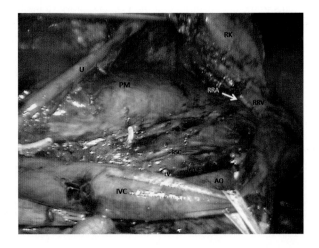

Left Side

Patient Position and Trocar Arrangement

The patient is in a right decubitus position. The trocars are placed as for right-sided tumors but in a mirror image array. Usually four 10-mm trocars will suffice because the bowel has to be retracted in rare cases only.

Exposure of the Template

The peritoneum is incised along the line of Toldt from the left colic flexure to the pelvic brim and distally along the spermatic vein to the internal inguinal ring (Fig. 19.14). It is essential also to incise the splenocolic ligament (Fig. 19.15). If the resulting exposure is not ideal, the peritoneal incision is continued cephalad lateral to the spleen up to the diaphragm. The spleen is then completely freed so that it can be rotated 180° medially. This maneuver allows the upper retroperitoneum to become freely accessible. However, this dissection of the spleen is required only in a minority of cases. The dissection of the colon must be continued until the anterior surface of the aorta is exposed completely in the plane of Toldt (Fig. 19.16). Normally the colon falls away from the operative site because of gravity and a retractor is required only in a few exceptional cases.

Dissection of the Lymphatic Tissue Within the Template

At this point, the entire template described by Weissbach and Boedefeld[8] for left-sided tumors is accessible. This does not include the interaorto-caval tissue, but the preoartic

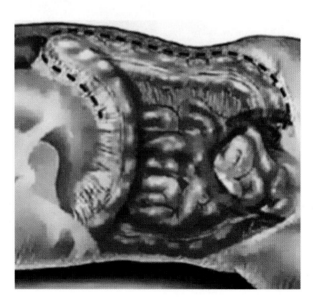

Fig. 19.14 Left-side laparoscopic RPLND. Peritoneal incision (*dotted line*)

Fig. 19.15 Left-side laparoscopic RPLND. Incision of the splenocolic ligament (intraoperative site). *SCL* splenocolic ligament, *LK* left kidney

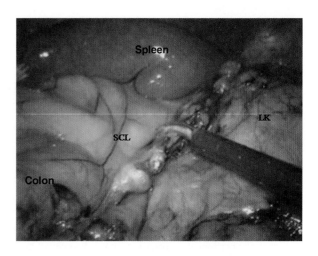

Fig. 19.16 Left-side laparoscopic RPLND. Exposure of the left retroperitoneum following medial displacement of the colon (intraoperative site). *LK* left kidney, *TL* tail of pancreas, *AO* aorta, *LRV* left renal vein

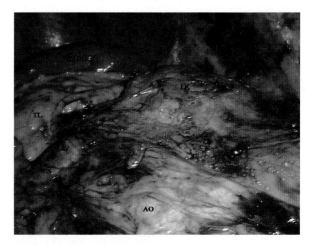

tissue between the left renal vein and the inferior mesenteric artery, all the tissue lateral to the aorta and the left common iliac artery. The lymphatic tissue ventral to the aorta below the inferior mesenteric artery is preserved. The lateral border of dissection is the ureter. The spermatic vessels are also removed in their entire length.

Identification and Dissection of the Spermatic Vessels

The spermatic vessels are dissected free along their entire course from the internal inguinal ring to its opening into the renal vein (spermatic vein) and origin from the aorta (spermatic artery) (Fig. 19.17), transected and removed. Before division of the opening of the spermatic vein into the left renal vein, it is wise to first completely dissect the left renal vein and its tributaries.

Fig. 19.17 Left-side laparoscopic RPLND. Dissection of spermatic artery and vein (intraoperative site). *Inset*: separate courses of spermatic vein and artery. *AO* aorta, *LRV* left renal vein, *LK* left kidney, *Sp. Vessels* spermatic vessels, *SA* spermatic artery, *SV* spermatic vein

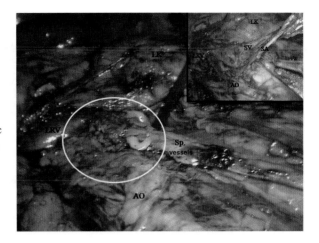

Dissection of the Upper Border of the Template

Following removal of the spermatic vein, the exposed left lumbar vein is transected between clips at its opening in the renal vein. The underlying left renal artery is then dissected free, delineating the upper border of the template (left renal hilum). The lymphatic tissue is then separated from the upper border of the template (Fig. 19.18), to avoid injury of the left renal hilum during further steps.

Lateral Border of the Template

The ureter, which defines the lateral border of the template, is then identified cranially and separated from the lymphatic tissue along its course caudally. Care must be taken to preserve the connective tissue that provides the blood supply of the ureter.

Lower Limit of the Template

The lymphatic tissue overlying the common iliac artery is split open starting at the crossing of the artery with the ureter, which delineates the distal border of the template. From there, the dissection is continued cephalad.

Dissection of the Lymphatic Tissue Ventral and Lateral to the Aorta

The previous dissection is continued along the ventral surface of the aorta until the level of the inferior mesenteric artery, which is circumvented and preserved. Directly above the mesenteric artery, the lymph package is separated as the lymphatic tissue ventral to the aorta below the inferior mesenteric artery is preserved. Dissection is then continued along the ventral and medial border of the aorta up to the level of the renal hilum, which was previously identified. Accessory arteries to the kidney may be encountered during the dissection between the aorta and the kidney; severing these arteries may result in troublesome bleeding and potential loss of renal function. The dissection is then continued along the lateral surface of the aorta, down to the origin of the lumbar arteries. As a last step, the lumbar vessels are separated from the lymphatic tissue to the point in which they disappear in the layer between the spine and the psoas muscle. Directly lateral to that point, the

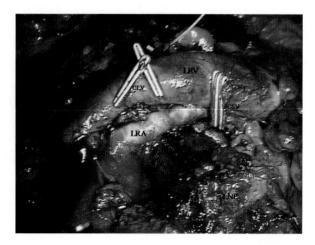

Fig. 19.18 Left-side laparoscopic RPLND. Lymphatic tissue is then separated from the upper border of the template (intraoperative site). *LRV* left renal vein, *LRA* left renal artery, *CLV* clipped lumbar vein, *CSV* clipped spermatic vein, *LNP* lymph node package (This image was published in *Atlas of the Urologic Clinics of North America*, Vol. 8, Janetschek G, Peschel R, Bartsch G, Laparoscopic retroperitoneal lymph node dissection, pp. 71–90, Copyright Elsevier, 2000)

sympathetic chain is encountered (Fig. 19.19). The postganglionic fibers, although readily identified in most cases, are not preserved.

Removal of the Nodal Package

The nodal package is completely free and can be retrieved (Fig. 19.20). Finally, the colon is returned to its normal anatomic position and secured in place with one extracorporeally tied suture.

Stage II After Chemotherapy

Unilateral RPLND is performed within the same template used for clinical stage I disease. Bilateral RPLND is not attempted – in the authors' series, the residual tumor was located within the unilateral template. The operative technique was same as for clinical stage I disease with the following to be taken into consideration; displacement of the bowel was feasible in all cases, although chemotherapy rendered identification of the tissue layers more difficult. Small venous branches draining the tumor must be meticulously dissected before they are clipped and transected. This is particularly true in cases of tumor-free residuals after embryonal carcinoma, which may be tightly adherent to the surrounding veins, especially the vena cava. Mature teratomas are usually well delineated (Fig. 19.21a and b).

Fig. 19.19 Left-side laparoscopic RPLND. Dissection of the lymphatic tissue ventral and lateral to the aorta (intraoperative site). *IMA* inferior mesenteric artery, *LNP* spared lymph node package below the level of the inferior mesenteric artery, *AO* aorta, *LA* lumbar artery, *LSC* left sympathetic chain, *LRV* left renal vein, *LRA* left renal artery

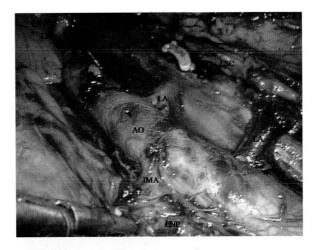

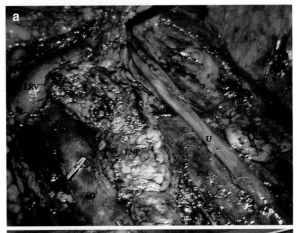

Fig. 19.20 Left-side laparoscopic RPLND. (**a**) Intraoperative site following complete dissection of the lymph node package. (**b**) Operative site after removal of all lymph nodes within the template. *LNP* lymph node package, *AO* aorta, *LRV* left renal vein, *LRA* left renal artery, *CLV* clipped lumbar vein, *CSV* clipped spermatic vein, *LA* lumbar artery, *U* ureter, *PM* psoas muscle

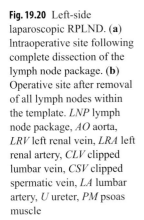

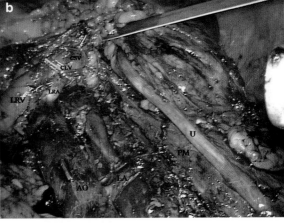

Fig. 19.21 Laparoscopic RPLND for clinical stage II tumor after chemotherapy (*left side*). (**a**) 4-cm residual tumor (mature teratoma) delineated by the aorta, left renal vein, and a lower pole renal artery. (**b**) Intraoperative site after removal of the tumor. *AO* aorta; *LRV* left renal vein, *LPA* lower pole artery, *T* tumor, *GF* Gerota's fascia of left kidney, *PM* psoas muscle (This image was published in *Atlas of the Urologic Clinics of North America*, Vol. 8, Janetschek G, Peschel R, Bartsch G, Laparoscopic retroperitoneal lymph node dissection, pp. 71–90, Copyright Elsevier, 2000)

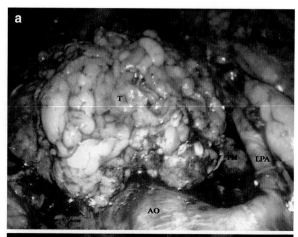

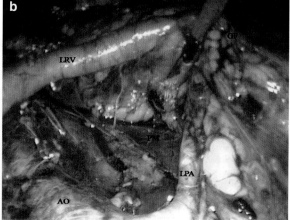

Methods to Overcome Difficulties During Laparoscopic RPLND

Split and Roll Technique

To avoid iatrogenic organ injury, the surgeon should maintain clear dissection borderlines by remaining on the vessels at all times during dissection.

Exposure

As with any surgical procedure, gaining exposure is of utmost importance. Insufficient exposure because of protruding segments of small or large bowel may render the operation difficult, dangerous, or even impossible. The authors have never converted to laparotomy because of insufficient exposure, but in a few cases exposure was a major problem. The fan retractor for the liver may be used to retract the duodenum as well. Additional retraction of the bowel can be achieved by surgical sponges held with traumatic graspers. Only in exceptional cases is it necessary to insert an additional trocar in the midline just caudal to the costal margin for the introduction of a second fan retractor. With the latter measure, sufficient exposure was achieved in all instances.

Technique of Dissection and Hemostasis

The most useful tools for achieving bloodless dissection and adequate hemostasis are bipolar coagulation and the harmonic scalpel (Ultracision Harmonic scalpel, Ethicon Endo-Surgery, Cincinnati, OH). The authors have found using these tools makes dissection easier, safer, and faster. A small clamp for bipolar coagulation allows for meticulous dissection of delicate structures, whereas broader bipolar forceps provide highly efficient hemostasis. In the authors' hands, these tools have proved so efficient that they have even supplanted the argon beam coagulator.

In open surgery, acute bleeding can be stopped instantaneously with the index finger of the surgeon. In laparoscopy, a small surgical sponge held with a traumatic grasper can be used to substitute for the surgeon's finger (Fig. 19.22). Once the bleeding has been stopped temporarily with this technique, the surgeon need not rush since there is plenty of time to undertake the necessary steps.

The authors' animal studies and clinical experience have shown that most venous bleedings, including those resulting from small leaks in the vena cava, can be stopped with the help of fibrin glue (Tisseel, Baxter, Deerfield, IL). A special laparoscopic applicator is available from the manufacturer with two separate channels for the two components of fibrin glue (Duplojet syringe apparatus, Baxter, Deerfield, IL) (Fig. 19.23). The edges of larger defects are approximated with a grasper or clips and then sealed with fibrin glue. In addition, a strip of oxidized regenerated cellulose or other hemostatic agents can be used

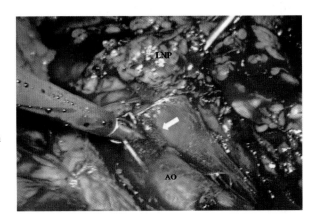

Fig. 19.22 Acute bleeding can easily be stopped by pressure applied with a surgical sponge held with a traumatic grasper. *AO* aorta, *LNP* lymph node package

Fig. 19.23 Small defect in the vena cava sealed with fibrin glue. *VC* vena cava (This image was published in *Atlas of the Urologic Clinics of North America*, Vol. 8, Janetschek G, Peschel R, Bartsch G, Laparoscopic retroperitoneal lymph node dissection, pp. 71–90, Copyright Elsevier, 2000)

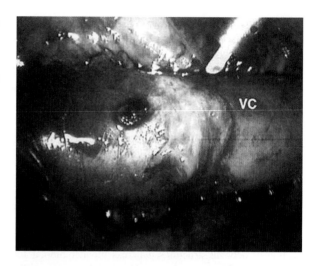

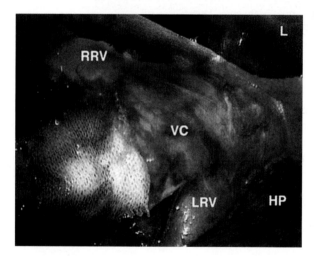

Fig. 19.24 Large defect in the wall of the vena cava that could be approximated but not completely closed with clips. It was then sealed with fibrin glue, and the tightness of the repair was enhanced using a strip of oxidized regenerated cellulose. *VC* vena cava, *RRV* right renal vein, *LRV* left renal vein, *L* liver, *HP* head of pancreas (This image was published in *Atlas of the Urologic Clinics of North America*, Vol. 8, Janetschek G, Peschel R, Bartsch G, Laparoscopic retroperitoneal lymph node dissection, pp. 71–90, Copyright Elsevier, 2000)

to enhance the tightness of the repair (Fig. 19.24). However, these are inappropriate for active arterial bleeding.

In cases of arterial bleeding, clips can be extremely useful, or, alternatively, a suture bolstered with clips may allow the quick closure of significant defects. This can be easily accomplished by tying a knot at the free end of a short stitch and a PDS locking clip (Lapra-Ty, Ethicon Endo-Surgery, Inc., Cincinnati, OH) applied between the knot and the needle to close the free end. The locking clip acts as a bolster allowing fast hemorrhage

Fig. 19.25 Closure of a defect in the aorta using a suture bolstered with clips (*arrow*). *AO* aorta, *LNP* lymph node package

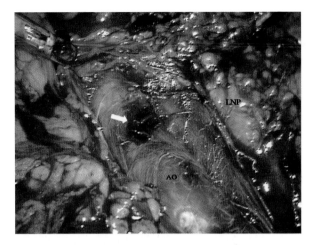

control by passing the needle through the free edges of the defect and applying gentle traction on the stitch. A second clip may be applied at the exit site of the stitch to secure it in place under gentle tension, thus obviating the need to waste time on intracorporeal knot-tying during ongoing bleeding (Fig. 19.25). Finally, the surgeon should not hesitate to add an extra 5-mm trocar to manage the situation, as this may make the difference between a laparoscopic procedure and a conversion.

Lymphocele Formation

Lymphocele formation can be another troublesome postoperative complication. The best treatment in this situation is prevention; the use of clips on the resected margins of tissue should help minimize lymphocele formation. In addition, the authors usually never leave a suction drain and never retroperitonealize the great vessels at the end of the procedure. In the authors' opinion, these measures contribute to reduced lymphocele formation.

Preservation of Antegrade Ejaculation

Loss of antegrade ejaculation is the most common long-term functional complication of bilateral RPLND. This problem can be overcome by performing either a template dissection[10] or nerve-sparing RPLND.[11] The postganglionic fibers of the right sympathetic nerve travel through the interaortocaval space. The corresponding fibers of the left side are found within the left para-aortic nodes. In a right template dissection, the right postganglionic fibers are resected while all fibers of the left side remain intact. With a left template dissection, all left postganglionic fibers are resected while the right fibers remain intact as long as the interaortocaval space is not approached. Complete unilateral destruction of the sympathetic nerve does not result in loss of antegrade ejaculation as long as the contralateral nerve remains intact. It has been known since 1964 that destruction of the sympathetic chain on one side does not result in aspermia as long as the contralateral side is intact.[12]

The authors have followed this strategy in their work and in 100 of their stage I patients, the antegrade ejaculation rate was 100% (three patients were lost during follow-up). In stage II patients, antegrade ejaculation was preserved in 57 out of 59 patients.

With the introduction of nerve-sparing RPLND, Donohue was able to improve the ejaculation rate from 70% to almost 100%. However, Donohue simultaneously introduced nerve-sparing dissection along with unilateral template dissection, sparing the contralateral sympathetic chain[13] and as mentioned above, preservation of a unilateral sympathetic chain is alone enough to prevent aspermia. Therefore, additional preservation of the ipsilateral nerve by a nerve-sparing technique is not required. Dissection of the postganglionic fibers is required in bilateral RPLND only, and such a dissection via laparoscopic techniques is feasible.

Quality of Life

Because excellent results are achieved by RPLND, surveillance, and risk-adapted chemotherapy, treatment-dependent quality of life has become a major issue. To exclude the bias of the surgeon, a quality-of-life study has been performed in cooperation with psychiatrists at the authors' center.[14] A questionnaire including 39 questions was distributed to 119 patients and completed in personal interviews by 118 for a compliance rate of 99.2%. The questionnaire included questions about the patients' satisfaction, their treatment experience, and its side effects. Patients were asked about the period of time needed before they were able to perform gentle physical exercise, return to normal activities, and were free of symptoms. Other questions addressed interest in sexual activity, whether the patient felt "lovable," experienced any problems in his partnership, psyche, or social life, and whether he was anxious about losing his job or had emotional problems associated with the loss of a testicle or the RPLND procedure. The open RPLND group included 53 patients (47.3%). The laparoscopic RPLND group comprised 59 patients (52.7%).

Surprisingly, both laparoscopic and open RPLND were better tolerated than chemotherapy. Open RPLND impairs the quality of life much more than laparoscopic RPLND. There was not a single item on the questionnaire in which open RPLND was superior to laparoscopy. The patients who participated in the study preferred laparoscopic RPLND to all other treatment modalities.

Results

Clinical Stage I/Pathologic Stage I

The quality of RPLND can be best judged by analysis of the relapse rate within the retroperitoneum, because any tumor left behind will become obvious within a short period of time. The relapse rate outside the retroperitoneum, however, does not rely on surgery. Among 115 clinical stage I patients operated between August 1992 and April 2006, 79 were pathologic stage I. The mean follow-up was 63 (6–113) months. There were five relapses (5.8%), three in the lung, one marker only, and one (1.15%) in the retroperitoneum.

Closer analysis of this retroperitoneal relapse revealed that it was not due to insufficient histology, but false-negative histology. This patient was cured with two cycles of PEB and laparoscopic RPLND on the contralateral side.

Antegrade ejaculation was preserved in 104/105 patients (99%).

Clinical Stage I/Pathologic Stage II

Twenty-six out of 105 patients were pathologic stage II. They all received two cycles of adjuvant chemotherapy (PEB). There was not a single relapse after a mean follow-up of 47 (4–97) months.

Pathologic Stage II After Chemotherapy

Between February 1995 and April 2006, laparoscopic RPLND was performed in 47 consecutive stage IIb patients and 18 selected stage IIc patients. There was not a single conversion among the 65 patients, in contrast to the 2.7% conversion rate in clinical stage I. A single major complication occurred – a delayed bleeding that was managed laparoscopically. In seven patients, a chylous ascites occurred that was always managed conservatively (low-fat diet, middle-chain triglycerides). The authors now start this diet postoperatively in every patient over a period of 3 weeks and have not seen this complication since. Histology revealed mature teratoma in 24 patients, necrosis in 39 patients, active NSGCT in 1/64 patients, and active seminoma in 1/1 patients. With a mean follow-up of 38 (3–73) months, there was a single relapse (1.5%) (mature teratoma at the inner inguinal ring outside the surgical template). That patient was cured by another RPLND.

Cost Effectiveness

Although costs are not a not a primary issue yet, they have been taken into consideration. In the authors' series, the surgery per se was found to be less expensive if performed by open surgery rather than laparoscopy. However, if the cost of hospital stay were included, both totals are almost equal. Another factor that has not been considered in most studies is the time to convalescence, especially considering the fact that most of our patients are young, productive individuals. If this factor was added, laparoscopic RPLND was definitely found to be on the winning side.[15]

Discussion

Surgical efficiency of laparoscopic RPLND at least equals that of open surgery. Direct comparison of our data with contemporary large open series shows; that blood loss and operative time are equal, but hospital stay is clearly shorter.[16] More importantly, the rate of major complications observed with open surgery is significantly higher (5.4%), including severe complications such as nephrectomy due to a lesion of the renal artery, bowel necrosis requiring colostomy following a lesion of the superior mesenteric artery, and an ileus followed by relaparotomy. The rate of minor complications was 14.2% in the open group. The major long-term morbidity consists in loss of antegrade ejaculation. Dissection within the unilateral diagnostic templates results in injury of the ipsilateral sympathetic chain only, whereas the contralateral side remains intact.[12] The quality of diagnostic RPLND is best judged by the rate of retroperitoneal relapse in pathologic stage I. This rate was 1.15% in the authors' series compared to 1.8% after open RPLND.[16] The value of laparoscopic RPLND after chemotherapy is well documented by the low complication and relapse rate.

References

1. Freedman LS, Jones WG, Peckham MJ, et al. Histopathology in the prediction of relapse of patients with stage I testicular teratoma treated by orchidectomy alone. *Lancet.* 1987;330: 294-298.
2. Holtl L, Peschel R, Knapp R, et al. Primary lymphatic metastatic spread in testicular cancer occurs ventral to the lumbar vessels. *Urology.* 2002;59:114-118.
3. Bussar-Maatz R, Weissbach L. Retroperitoneal lymph node staging of testicular tumours TNM study group. *Br J Urol.* 1993;72(2):234-240.
4. Javadpour N. Predictors of recurrence in stage II nonseminomatous testicular cancer after lymphadenectomy: implications for adjuvant chemotherapy. *J Urol.* 1985;134:629.
5. Ronnen EA, Kondagunta GV, Bacik J, et al. Incidence of late-relapse germ cell tumor and outcome to salvage chemotherapy. *J Clin Oncol.* 2005;23:6999-7004.
6. Donohue JP, Thornhill JA, Foster RS, et al. The role of retroperitoneal lymphadenectomy in clinical stage B testis cancer: the Indiana University experience (1965 to 1989). *J Urol.* 1995;153:85-89.
7. Williams SD, Stablein DM, Einhorn LH, et al. Immediate adjuvant chemotherapy versus observation with treatment at relapse in pathological stage II testicular cancer. *N Engl J Med.* 1987;317:1433-1438.
8. Weissbach L, Boedefeld EA. Localization of solitary and multiple metastases in stage II nonseminomatous testis tumor as basis for a modified staging lymph node dissection in stage I. *J Urol.* 1987;138:77-82.
9. Janetschek G, Hobisch A, Holtl L, Bartsch G. Retroperitoneal lymphadenectomy for clinical stage I nonseminomatous testicular tumor: laparoscopy versus open surgery and impact of learning curve. *J Urol.* 1996;156:89-94.
10. Colleselli K, Poisel S, Schachtner W, Bartsch G. Nerve preserving bilateral retroperitoneal lymphadenectomy: anatomical study and operative approach. *J Urol.* 1990;144:293-298.
11. Donohue JP, Foster RS, Rowland RG, Bihrle R, Jones J, Geier G. Nerve-sparing retroperitoneal lymphadenectomy with preservation of ejaculation. *J Urol.* 1990;144:287-292.
12. Whitelaw GP, Smithwick RH. Some secondary effects of sympathectomy; with particular reference to disturbance of sexual function. *N Engl J Med.* 1951;245(4):121-130.
13. Donohue JP, Thornhill JA, Foster RS, Roland RG, Bihrle R. Retroperitoneal lymphadenectomy for clinical stage A testis cancer (1965 to 1989): modifications of technique and impact on ejaculation. *J Urol.* 1993;149:237-243.

14. Hobisch A, Tönnemann J, Janetschek G, et al. Morbidity and quality of life after open versus laparoscopic retroperitoneal lymphadenectomy for testicular tumour – the patient's view. In: Jones WG, Appleyard I, Harnden P, Joffe JK, eds. *Germ Cell Tumours VI*. London, UK: John Libbey; 1998:277.

15. Janetschek G. Laparoscopic retroperitoneal lymph node dissection. *Urol Clin North Am*. 2001;28:107-114.

16. Heidenreich A, Albers P, Hartmann M, et al. Complications of primary nerve sparing retroperitoneal lymph node dissection for clinical stage I nonseminomatous germ cell tumors of the testis: experience of the German Testicular Cancer Study Group. *J Urol*. 2003;169: 1710-1714.

Difficulties in Laparoscopic Radical Cystectomy

20

Amr M. Abdel-Hakim, Ahmed S. El-Feel, and Mahmoud A. Abdel-Hakim

Bladder cancer is a common malignancy of the urinary tract. It accounts for 63,000 new cases and 13,000 deaths annually in the USA.[1] Radical cystectomy remains the primary line of treatment for muscle invasive disease. Laparoscopy has been successfully used in urological surgery, mainly for the kidney and the prostate. Laparoscopic radical cystectomy was the natural development for successful urological laparoscopy.

Laparoscopic cystectomy was first reported in 1992, followed in 1995 by the first report of laparoscopic radical cystectomy (LRC).[2,3] Soon after, reports on small series of LRC appeared in the literature followed by larger series with reproducible results.[4–14]

Open radical cystectomy (ORC) remains the gold standard treatment for muscle invasive bladder cancer despite its substantial morbidity, even in centers with large volume and experience. Major complications occur in 10–12% with an overall complication rate of 30–60%; wound complications accounted for 10% and perioperative mortality were reported in 2–5% of ORC.[15]

More than 700 LRC from 14 countries have been documented in the ongoing international registry of LRC initiated by Inderbir Gill in 2005.[16] LRC provides excellent visualization and decreased blood loss allowing highly precise technical operation. Smaller skin/fascial incisions decrease pain and shorten convalescence, with the potential for decreasing perioperative complications. By minimizing bowel manipulation and its exposure to the atmosphere, postoperative ileus may be reduced. LRC must deliver loco-regional oncologic clearance comparable to ORC, thereby guaranteeing equivalent oncologic outcomes. Therefore, data requires careful scrutiny to ensure that soft tissue margins, nodal yields, local recurrences, and cancer-specific survival meet the standards established by ORC.[16]

Difficulties in LRC

Difficulties in LRC will be discussed as difficulties in access, difficulties in cystectomy, and difficulties of urinary diversion.

A.M. Abdel-Hakim (✉)
Department of Urology, Cairo University, Cairo, Egypt
e-mail: aahakim@gmail.com

A.M. Al-Kandari and I.S. Gill (eds.), *Difficult Conditions in Laparoscopic Urologic Surgery*,
DOI: 10.1007/978-1-84882-105-7_20, © Springer-Verlag London Limited 2011

Difficulties of Access

Difficulties in access mean either difficulty to initiate pneumoperitonium and/or proper port placement. These difficulties may be related to the patients' body mass index (BMI), stature, and/or previous surgeries. In obese patients there is higher liability to induce extra peritoneal insufflation.

Initiation of pneumoperitonium through the umbilicus may be difficult. In this case, one can use an alternative site in the midclavicular line three to four fingers below the costal margin (Fig. 20.1). The latter site has many advantages, namely the needle passes through two points of obvious resistance: the external oblique aponeurosis and the peritoneum. Secondly, it is away from major vessels, namely the aorta and the inferior vena cava. Lastly, it can be used in cases with previous midline incisions.

After induction of pneumoperitonium, the first or camera port is introduced, usually at the umbilicus. In cases of patients of short stature, it is advisable to introduce the camera port 1 in. above the umbilicus for better ergonomic port placement.

Previous surgery in general can pose difficulties of access, due to possible visceral adhesions to the anterior abdominal wall. The most common incisions encountered are McBurney, inguinal, and midline subumbilical incisions. To obtain safe access, the Veress subcostal insufflation site can be used to initiate pneumoperitonium. The camera ports can be applied cephalad to the midline incision (Fig. 20.2). A visual port can be used to apply the first port under direct vision. This reduces the difficulty of access and reduces the possibility of organ injury. The Hasson technique can be a safe alternative.[17]

Secondary ports are introduced under vision. Sometimes it is wiser to delay application of one or more ports until the adhesions from previous surgery are dissected using the rest of the ports. This is most common at the site of the right 10-mm port that can be masked by omental or bowel adhesions following appendectomy (Fig. 20.3).

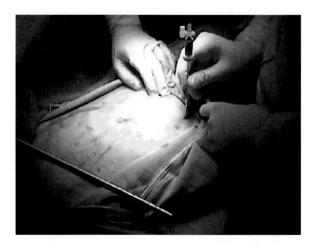

Fig. 20.1 Right subcostal access for insufflations

Fig. 20.2 Camera port 1 in. above the umbilicus (to avoid a midline scar incision)

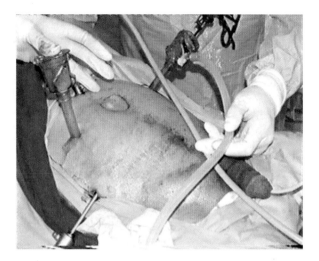

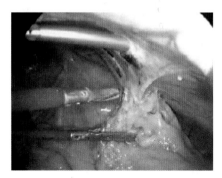

Fig. 20.3 Intraperitoneal adhesions following appendectomy

Vascular Injuries During Access

Injuries can be inflected either by the Veress needle or by the ports. The aortic bifurcation and common iliac vessels are at the level of the umbilicus and can be punctured by the Veress needle. If the needle aspirates blood, it should be slightly withdrawn until no blood is aspirated and pneumoperitonium initialized.

After rapid port application, the site of injury is inspected. If the injury is small, compression by mounted gauze or laparoscopic suture can be applied. Major vascular injury may require immediate laparotomy and formal repair. Inferior epigastic artery injury can occur during port placement and is diagnosed by blood trickling from the port. If the bleeding is not controlled by compression using the port, a full thickness suture under laparoscopic guidance using a fascial closure needle usually controls the injury (Fig. 20.4).

Fig. 20.4 Control of bleeding
from inferior epigastric
artery using the fascial
closure device

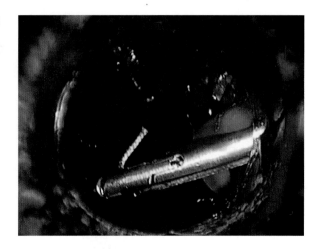

Visceral Injuries During Access

Injury to colon or small intestine can be suspected when colored or malodorous fluid is aspirated through the Veress needle. These organs must be carefully examined once the camera is introduced. Usually no further treatment is required. Less commonly, laparoscopic suturing is indicated. Visceral injury can occur during their release from adhesions to the anterior abdominal wall to allow proper secondary port placement. Injury is suspected by visualization of bowel contents or the mucosa.

The injured bowel loop should be completely mobilized to allow proper closure in layers. If mobilization cannot be safely accomplished or closure is not satisfactorily performed, immediate conversion and formal repair must be established.

Difficulties During Cystectomy

After establishing pneumoperitoneum and ergonomic port placement, difficulties can arise either from the large size of the mass limiting the working space around the bladder or from severe adhesions. Adhesions are usually secondary to previous urologic surgery to the bladder and/or the ureter(s). Less commonly adhesions and obliteration of the planes can result from the tumor itself or from previous aggressive resection and biopsies of the bladder tumor.

Difficulty caused by tumor size can be avoided by proper case selection. The problem of tumor size can be circumvented by prosperous assistance, application of an extra (sixth) port and by working through the side with more working space first. Sometimes, retrograde cystectomy can be attempted. After controlling the bladder pedicle on the side with reasonable working space, the cave of Ritzus is opened. The bladder is freed anteriorly. The lateral endopelvic fascia is incised. The sides of the prostate are freed, the deep dorsal complex is controlled and the urethra is divided. Then the prostate is reverted cephalad by pulling on the divided urethral catheter in order to dissect the prostate in retrograde manner. This allows the bladder mass to migrate upwards increasing the working space. Then one should proceed from the side with wider working space that is usual the contralateral side of the tumor.

However, large bladder masses are better managed by ORC, since they require a big abdominal incision to extract.

Previous bladder surgery does not usually cause severe technical difficulty. The bladder can be sharply mobilized from the rectus abdominus muscle. Care must be taken to avoid injury to the bladder (and hence tumor spillage) by working always close to the anterior abdominal wall (Fig. 20.2). The real challenge is caused by previous open ureteral surgeries as the ureter becomes adherent to the external iliac artery, and more dangerously to internal iliac vessels.

In the authors' cystectomy series, this difficulty was encountered in six cases. The affected ureter is usually dilated with thick wall (Fig. 20.5). The ureter should be exposed from a fresh area more proximal to the site of surgery and mobilized as distal as possible. Then the iliac artery is also exposed until the adhesion site. This is usually accomplished during the lymphadenectomy. The ureter is then approached from the medical side that is exposed during posterior bladder dissection and exposure of the ipsilateral seminal vesicles. By careful blunt and sharp dissection, working towards the ureter and always visualizing the external iliac artery, the ureter was freed in five of the six cases. In the last case, the ureter was mobilized proximal and distal to external iliac artery. The ureter was then divided at the site of arterial adhesion distally in the pelvis and its end sent for frozen section; the ureter was pathologically free. Then the ureter was divided proximal to the adhesions to the artery, leaving the part adherent to the artery in place. The anterior and lateral walls of the adherent short ureteral segment were excised and submitted to pathological examination that confirmed absence of malignant involvement.

Adhesions to the rectum with replacement of the perirectal fat by fibrofatty tissue, increases the risk of rectal injury. Rectal injury can occur 0.5–9% of cases during laparoscopic prostatectomy.[18–21] In cases with adhesions, electrocautary should be avoided in this area. Combined blunt and sharp dissection should be used.

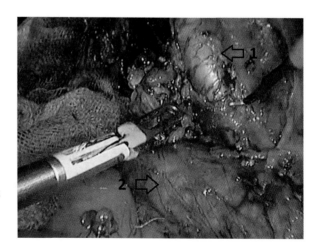

Fig. 20.5 Adhesions resulting from a previous ureteral surgery (1 – External iliac artery; 2 – Dilated ureter)

Fig. 20.6 Gross lymph-adenectomy (1 – External iliac artery; 2 – External iliac lymph nodes adherent to the external iliac vessels; 3 – Left ureter)

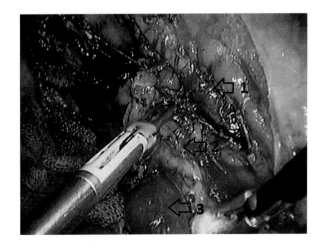

After complete separation of specimen, the rectum should be tested for possible injuries. This best accomplished by filling the pelvis with saline and air is injected in a rectal tube. If small injury is detected, it can be repaired either laparoscopically or formally repaired during open diversion. If the injury is severe and cannot be securely closed, one should consider a terminal colostomy and a rectal bladder diversion.

Laparoscopic lymphadenectomy, particularly in the presence of gross lymphadenopapathy carries the risk of vascular injury (Fig. 20.6)

External iliac vein injury was encountered in one case in the authors' ongoing series of more than 110 LRC. The injury was detected immediately and repaired by Prolene™ (Ethicon, Inc., Somerville, NJ) 5/0 laparoscopic suturing.

Obturator nerve injury during pelvic lymphadenectomy is rare. When tension-free primary repair is not feasible, nerve grafting can be used. However, even without a nerve repair, conservative management with physiotherapy can compensate for the defect.[22]

Difficulties of Diversion

All types of urinary diversion have been used in association with LRC. Diversion was done laparoscopically in some early reports.[4, 6] Others have performed the diversion through a mini laparotomy to exteriorize the selected bowel loop. Small midline incisions, extended port site (Fig. 20.7) or small Pfannenstiel incisions have been used.[23] After preparation of the pouch extracorporeally, uretero-intestinal and the urethro-intestinal anastomoses can be done conventionally or laparoscopically.

Currently the authors exteriorize the ileum through a 7-cm Pfannenstiel incision, prepare a Y-pouch, and perform the stented uretero-ileal anastomosis conventionally. The pouch is repositioned intraobdominally and the wound is closed. The urethroileal anastomosis is performed by continuous freehand laparoscopic suture.

Difficulties of diversion can occur due to either short ureters, urethroileal anastomosis, and/or ureteric stenting.

Fig. 20.7 Extended right
10-mm port site for the
neobladder preparation in a
patient with a previous
midline incision

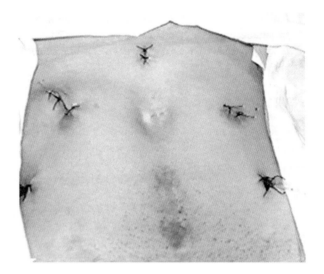

Short Ureters

The problem of short ureters can be overcome by selecting the proper type of ileal neo-bladder. The Studer technique with a long "chimney" can overcome this hurdle.[24] The Y-bladder has the advantage of "taking the ileum to the ureters" and not the reverse. Therefore, the ureters are kept in place; the extra few centimeters needed to carry the ureter to the ileum medially are not required.[23,25]

Urethroileal Anastomosis

To avoid a loop with short mesentery, the selected loop should be tested laparoscopically if a high minilaparotomy or port site incisions are selected for pouch reconstruction. The midpoint of the selected loop is pushed down to the urethra to confirm a tension-free urethro-ileal anastomosis. A small Pfannenstiel incision avoids this problem, since the selected loop can be drawn to the urethra.

During urethroileal anastomosis, twisting of the pouch mesentery should be avoided. This is even more important if the anastomosis is performed laparoscopically. To facilitate the urethro-ileal anastomosis the authors have adopted two maneuvers. First, a very long silk suture that is attached to the urethral catheter marks the lowest part of ileal opening. The catheter is removed, allowing the silk suture to hang out of the urethra. Pulling of the silk suture drives the ileal opening to the urethra. Second, the Denonvillier fascia posterior to the urethral stump is sutured to the remnants of the peritoneal reflection of the rectovesi-cal pouch anterior to the rectum. The same principle was used by Rocco after laparoscopic radical prostatectomy.[26] This maneuver helps stabilize the urethral stump intra-abdominally, facilitating the urethroileal anastomosis.

Preservation of the puboprostatic ligaments anteriorly may also help. After performing these sutures, the ileourethral anastomosis is started. The silk suture is pulled out of the urethra and the anastomosis completed over a 22 F silicon Foley catheter.

Stenting

Stenting of the uretero-ileal anastomosis is usually performed by extracorporeal stents. This tends to prolong the hospital stay, increase the chance of urinary leakage after stent removal from the pouch wall, and may increase the chance of wound infection. In the last 29 cystectomies of the authors' ongoing series, the combination of the 7-cm Pfannenstiel incision and the use of 28-cm, 7 F double-J stents has shortened the hospital stay from a mean of 11 days to only 5 days (A. M. Abdel-Hakim, unpublished data, February 2010).

Difficulty in removal of the double J stents was encountered in two cases. The stents migrated up the pouch and were hidden by the folded neobladder. The patients were put in Trendlenburg position, the neobladder distended by saline and under fluoroscopic guidance the stents were removed. To avoid this problem, the double J stents are marked by a long silk suture that ties the two double Js and fixes them to the pouch's mucosa near the urethral opening. The silk suture can be easily found during cystoscopy even if the double Js are hidden.

References

1. Herr HW, Faulkner JR, Grossman HB, et al. Surgical factors influence bladder cancer outcomes: a cooperative group report. *J Clin Oncol.* 2004;22(14):2781-2789.
2. Parra RO, Andrus CH, Jones JP, Boullier JA. Laparoscopic cystectomy: initial report on a new treatment for the retained bladder. *J Urol.* 1992;148(4):1140-1144.
3. Puppo P, Perachino M, Ricciotti G, Bozzo W, Gallucci M, Carmignani G. Laparoscopically assisted transvaginal radical cystectomy. *Eur Urol.* 1995;27(1):80-84.
4. Gill IS, Fergany A, Klein EA, et al. Laparoscopic radical cystoprostatectomy with ileal conduit performed completely intracorporeally: the initial 2 cases. *Urology.* 2000;56(1):26-29.
5. Denewer A, Kotb S, Hussein O, El-Maadawy M. Laparoscopic assisted cystectomy and lymphadenectomy for bladder cancer: initial experience. *World J Surg.* 1999;23(6):608-611.
6. Türk I, Deger S, Winkelmann B, Schönberger B, Loening SA. Laparoscopic radical cystectomy with continent urinary diversion (rectal sigmoid pouch) performed completely intracorporeally: the initial 5 cases. *J Urol.* 2001;165:1863-1866.
7. Abdel-Hakim AM, Bassiouny F, Abdel Azim MS, et al. Laparoscopic radical cystectomy with orthotopic neobladder. *J Endourol.* 2002;16(6):377-381.
8. Moinzadeh A, Gill IS, Desai M, Finelli A, Falcone T, Kaouk J. Laparoscopic radical cystectomy in the female. *J Urol.* 2005;173(6):1912-1917.
9. Finelli A, Gill IS, Desai MM, Moinzadeh A, Magi-Galuzzi C, Kaouk JH. Laparoscopic extended pelvic lymphadenectomy for bladder cancer: technique and initial outcomes. *J Urol.* 2004;172:1809-1812.
10. Lane BR, Finelli A, Moinzadeh A, et al. Nerve- sparing laparoscopic radical cystectomy: technique and initial outcomes. *Urology.* 2006;68(4):778-783.

11. Arroyo C, Andrews H, Rozet F, Cathelineau X, Vallancien G. Laparoscopic prostate-sparing radical cystectomy: the Montsouris technique and preliminary results. *J Endourol.* 2005;19(3):424-428.

12. Gill IS, Kaouk JH, Meraney AM, et al. Laparoscopic radical cystectomy and continent orthotopic ileal neobladder performed completely intracorporeally: the initial experience. *J Urol.* 2002;168(1):13-18.

13. Beecken WD, Wolfram M, Engl T, et al. Robotic-assisted laparoscopic radical cystectomy and intra-abdominal formation of an orthotopic ileal neobladder. *Eur Urol.* 2003;44(3):337-379.

14. Balaji KC, Yohannes P, McBride CL, Oleynikov D, Hemstreet GP. Feasibility of robot-assisted totally intracorporeal laparoscopic ileal conduit urinary diversion: initial results of a single institutional pilot study. *Urology.* 2004;63(1):51-55.

15. Skinner DG, Crawford ED, Kaufman JJ. Complications of radical cystectomy for carcinoma of the bladder. *J Urol.* 1980;123(5):640-643.

16. Gill IS, Fergany AF. Laparoscopic radical cystectomy. *Urol Clin North Am.* 2008;35: 455-466.

17. Gill IS, Kerbl K, Meraney AM, Clayman RV. Basics of laparoscopic urologic surgery. In: Walsh PC, Retik AB, Vaughan ED, Wein AJ, Kavoussi LR, Novick AC, Partin AW, Peters CA, eds. *Campbell's Urology.* 8th ed. Philadelphia, PA: W.B. Saunders; 2002:3456.

18. Blumberg JM, Lesser T, Tran VQ, Aboseif SR, Bellman GC, Abbas MA. Management of rectal injuries sustained during laparoscopic radical prostatectomy. *Urology.* 2009;73(1): 163-166.

19. Guillonneau B, El-Fettouh H, Baumert H, et al. Laparoscopic radical prostatectomy: oncological evaluation after 1, 000 cases at Montsouris Institute. *J Urol.* 2003;169:1261-1266.

20. Rassweiler J, Sentker L, Seemann O, Hatzinger M, Rumpelt HJ. Laparoscopic radical prostatectomy with the Heilbronn technique: an analysis of the first 180 cases. *J Urol.* 2001;166:2101-2108.

21. Castillo OA, Bodden E, Vitagliano G. Management of rectal injury during laparoscopic radical prostatectomy. *Int Braz J Urol.* 2006;32:428-433.

22. Kirdi N, Yakut E, Meric A, Ayhan A. Physical therapy in a patient with bilateral obturator nerve paralysis after surgery. A case report. *Clin Exp Obstet Gynecol.* 2000;27:59-60.

23. Abdel Hakim AM. Urinary diversion during laparoscopic radical cystectomy. In: Montague D, Gill I, Angermeier K, Ross JH, eds. *Textbook of Reconstructive Urologic Surgery.* London, United Kingdom: Informa; 2008:305-310.

24. Studer UE, Danuser H, Thalmann GN, et al. Antireflux nipples or afferent tubular segments in 70 patients with ileal low pressure bladder substitutes: long-term results of a prospective randomized trial. *J Urol.* 1996;156(6):1913-1917.

25. Fontana D, Bellina M, Scoffone C, Poggio M, Guercio S. "Y" neobladder: preliminary results. *Eur Urol.* 2001;8(1): video J.

26. Rocco B, Gregori A, Stener S, et al. Posterior reconstruction of the rhabdosphincter allows a rapid recovery of continence after transperitoneal videolaparoscopic radical prostatectomy. *Eur Urol.* 2007;51:996-1003.

Arvind P. Ganpule, Shashikant Mishra, and Mahesh R. Desai

Introduction

Laparoscopic pyeloplasty was first described as a minimally invasive treatment option by Schuessler and colleagues in 1993,[1] and there are now several large published series with extended follow-up confirming long-term patency rates of 96–100%.[2–4] These results parallel the outcomes of the open pyeloplasty. As demonstrated with other minimally invasive operations, patients undergoing laparoscopic pyeloplasty have reduced analgesic requirements, hospital stays, and time until return of full activities compared with their open surgery counterparts. Although technically challenging, the low incidence of failure combined with reduced postoperative morbidity has made this an increasingly popular treatment option at various centers across the globe. This chapter discusses the possible difficulties a surgeon may encounter and also details the possible solutions to these problems.

Patient Selection and Indication

The authors feel that inexperience of the surgeon is a contraindication for laparoscopic pyeloplasty. As with any other procedure, the surgeon should be astute enough to select the proper case. An ideal case to start doing a laparoscopic pyeloplasty is an adult patient with a short segment ureteropelvic junction (UPJ) obstruction and a dilated extrarenal pelvis. As the surgeon gains experience, the surgeon should graduate to doing adult patients with intrarenal pelvis where a flap procedure may be required (Fig. 21.1).

As the surgeon ascends the learning curve, pediatric patients can be done. These small patients require miniature equipment and imaging equipment and good intracorporeal

M.R. Desai (✉)
Department of Urology, Muljibhai Patel Urological Hospital, Nadlad, Gujarat, India
e-mail: mrdesai@mpuh.org

A.M. Al-Kandari and I.S. Gill (eds.), *Difficult Conditions in Laparoscopic Urologic Surgery*,
DOI: 10.1007/978-1-84882-105-7_21, © Springer-Verlag London Limited 2011

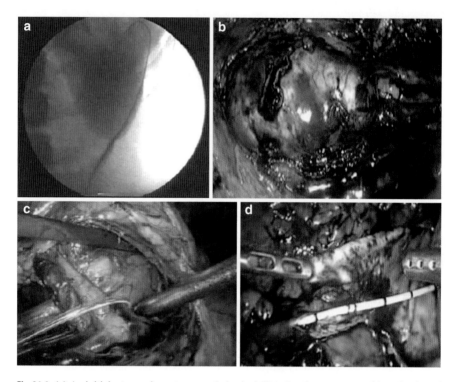

Fig. 21.1 (**a**) An initial retrograde ureterogram helps in delineating the anatomy and introduction of an open-end ureteral catheter. (**b**) An extrarenal pelvis with a short segment stricture is an ideal case when beginning to perform laparoscopic pyeloplasty. (**c**) Crossing vessels should be meticulously slinged and preserved. (**d**) Construction of a flap prior to pyeloplasty

suturing skills. Apart from this, a competent anesthetist trained in pediatric anesthesia should be available.

At the authors' center, residents are trained in the skills of intracorporeal suturing on dry and wet laboratory trainers. Such training is necessary before one starts doing cases. A variety of models have been described that include the use of chicken skin.[5] An indigenous model using a chicken carcass also is helpful in developing the art of intracorporeal suturing.

Muljibhai Patel Urological Hospital Model for Training in Laparoscopy

The chicken crop and esophagus were used to simulate the renal pelvis and ureter, respectively. These were exposed by reflecting the skin overlying the neck and thorax. The crop was thoroughly cleaned and filled with water via the esophageal end to simulate the dilated renal pelvis. Laparoscopic pyeloplasty was performed using the dismembered Anderson Hynes technique. The model was used over a period of 1 month by three urology trainees in their final year of training. They were assessed with respect to time needed to complete anastomosis and quality of anastomosis. At the end of four attempts of suturing, all trainees were able to satisfactorily complete a good quality ureteropelvic anastomosis in a mean time of 67.7 min (range 62–76 min). The conclusion of this study was that laparoscopic suturing skills require effective training and constant practice to perfect the technique. Adequate practice on this chicken model shortens the learning curve, makes the trainee more confident of his or her skills, and improves his operative performance.[4]

Operating Room Setup

The patient is placed in a flank position with the area to be operated up. The operating surgeon and first assistant stand on the contralateral side and the second assistant and operating room (OR) technician stand on the opposite side of the table. The monitor should be positioned angled at the feet with screens at a comfortable eye level to the surgeons. The tower containing the insufflators, light source, and camera plug-in should be on one side of the primary surgeon to facilitate visual monitoring of the pressure recordings. The electrocautery generator units are located near the patient's head end. The nurse places the working table at the foot end of the patient.

Retrograde Ureterogram and Stenting

A retrograde pyelogram can be performed at the time of stent placement if a prior contrast study has not adequately defined the anatomy of the UPJ and distal ureter. This information is particularly important in defining the length of the scarred segment following previous failed procedures. Unlike the era where the debate continued whether retrograde ureterogram is required or not, this is a necessity if one is planning the laparoscopic approach.

Stenting

The stent serves the purpose of identifying the ureter and spatulation intraoperatively, postoperatively it also acts like a splint in facilitating healing of the anastomosis. The various options available for stenting in laparoscopic pyeloplasty are:

1. Preoperative placement of stent
2. Intraoperative placement of open end ureteric catheter and converting it into a double J stent at the conclusion of the procedure
3. Placing a stent intraoperatively under laparoscopic vision
4. Antegrade stenting in pediatric patients
5. No stents at all

Preoperative Placement of Stent

Stenting the patient's obstructed ureter at least 1 week prior to laparoscopic pyeloplasty allows for passive dilation of the UPJ and ureter, which will aid in performing the reconstruction.

An extra-long stent reduces the risk of pulling the stent into the distal ureter during its laparoscopic manipulation. In the authors' opinion, however, the presence of a stent for a prolonged period of days or weeks prior to the pyeloplasty can result in inflammation, infection, and edema of the ureter, making suturing difficult. The authors do not place a stent preoperatively, and if it is already placed elsewhere, the authors recommend removal of any previously placed ureteral stent several days before the surgery, unless there are overriding reasons not to do so.

Use of Ureteral Catheter as a Splint and a Stent

This is a practice the authors follow at their institute. Prior to the pyeloplasty, the patient undergoes cystoscopy and retrograde dye study (Fig. 21.1). An open-ended pigtail ureteric catheter is then passed over the guidewire after removal of the cystoscope, and the catheter is positioned with its tip a few centimeters above the UPJ. It is helpful to have a distended renal pelvis for easier dissection. A urethral Foley catheter is placed, and the ureteric catheter is secured to the Foley catheter. The patient is then repositioned for the laparoscopic pyeloplasty. The ureteric catheter is included in the sterile preparation of the abdomen and kept in the field for access during surgery. During dissection of the retroperitoneum, the ureteric catheter may be manipulated to help identify the ureter and distend the pelvis. After the pyeloplasty is complete, double J stent can be easily placed under C arm.

Intraoperative Placement of Stent

Many surgeons place a stent through 3-mm port intraoperatively. The position of the stent in the bladder is confirmed by free efflux of urine or methylene blue instilled in the bladder. Alternatively, during the operation, a guidewire, passed through the ureteral catheter in a retrograde fashion, is brought out through one of the ports, the ureteral catheter is removed, and the ureteral stent is then passed antegradely and positioned in the pelvis prior to completion of the anastomosis.

Antegrade Placement of Stent

This is of particular utility in pediatric patients, as retrograde ureterogram and subsequent placement of stent is cumbersome, tedious, and at times may cause injury to the urethra and the ureter in these patients. In these cases, the authors gain antegrade access to the concerned renal unit and with the help of a double-lumen catheter place, and an open-end ureteral catheter is placed in the pelvis along with a nephrostomy. Intraoperatively the

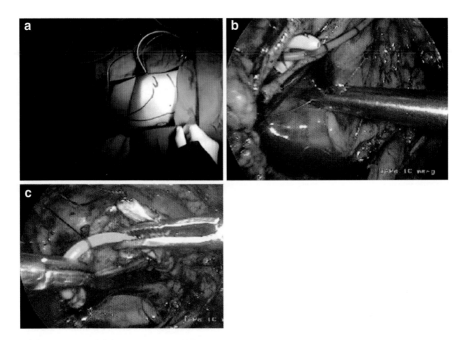

Fig. 21.2 (**a**) An open-end ureteric catheter and a nephrostomy are in place. (**b**) On opening the pelvis, the nephrostomy and the open-end catheter is in place. (**c**) Once the ureteric spatulation is completed, the ureteric catheter is advanced into the ureter

open-end ureteral catheter is advanced into the ureter and anastomosis performed over the stent; this avoids urethral instrumentation (Fig. 21.2).

It does not really matter whether one places a double-J stent in the ureter retrogradely preoperatively using cystoscopy, or intraoperatively in an antegrade manner, or postoperatively under C arm cover. It is the preference of the surgeon to utilize any of these techniques.

Approach

At the beginning of the procedure, an oro- or nasogastric tube is placed to decompress the stomach and a Foley catheter is inserted to drain the bladder. A bolster is placed on the table beneath the patient to secure the patient. Although the reteroperitoneal approach is performed with equivalent results to the transperitoneal approach, the choice of approach is a matter of surgeon preference. The transperitoneal approach offers space and latitude for movement of instruments and makes the dissection and suturing less challenging. The retroperitoneal approach offers fast access to the UPJ, since the collecting system is the most lateral structure. Compared with the transperitoneal approach, dissection of the crossing vessels is easier, but the anastomosis may be challenging.

The authors prefer the transperitoneal approach. Preparation of the bowel is important because it facilitates visualization by decompressing the colon and reduces the risk of fecal soiling in the event of bowel injury.

Positioning

The down leg is flexed, with padding positioned between the legs at right-angles to the upper leg. Intravenous lines or monitoring devices (e.g., blood pressure cuff) to which the anesthesiologist wishes to have quick access should be placed on the upper arm. The entire abdomen and back is shaved from the midline to the posterior axillary line and from xiphoid to pubis.

Port Placement

Port placement is mirrored for right- and left-sided cases. An initial 1-cm incision for introduction of the Veress needle and 10-mm camera port is placed midway between the umbilicus and the superior iliac crest just lateral to the rectus muscle. A clamp is used to spread the subcutaneous tissues down to the level of the fascia and the Veress needle is introduced. Typically, the first popping sensation indicates fascial entry and the second indicates entry into the peritoneal cavity. Saline injected into the hub of the Veress needle should flow easily into the peritoneal cavity and aspiration should not yield any gas, blood, or bowel contents. The abdomen is insufflated to 15 mmHg. While introducing the trocar, the tip of the trocar should be perpendicular to the skin and directed at the kidney. The port entry should not be oblique, to avoid surgical emphysema. A second 10-mm port is placed at the subcostal line in the perpendicular line starting from the first port and intersecting the coastal cartilage. The second and third trocar can be either a 5- or 10-mm depending on the side and the dominant hand of the operating surgeon. The camera port 10 mm is inserted at the junction of upper one third and lower two third at the lateral border of rectus belly. The camera port thus inserted lies opposite the level of pelvis. A 5-mm liver retraction port is also required for the right side. Adequate retraction of the liver is necessary at times. At the authors' center, liver is retracted with the help of a 5-mm locking Allis clamp that is introduced through the 5-mm port. This is inserted in the midline, just below the xiphoid cartilage. Care must be taken to prevent injury of the falciform ligament and prevent entrapment of the instruments by this structure. The authors prefer to fix the ports to prevent dislodgement.

Exposure of the Retroperitoneum

The extent of the dissection and medial colonic mobilization can be tailored somewhat depending on the position and ease of exposure of the UPJ. It is advisable to dissect only the pelvis and expose the UPJ and avoid dissecting the kidney.

After mobilization of the colon, the next step is to identify the ureter. Owing to the presence of the stent or a pigtail catheter, identification of ureter becomes easy. The gonadal vein can also help identification. When a tubular structure is identified and there is a question of whether or not it represents ureter, contact with an instrument will show peristalsis. Once identified, the ureter is then elevated and traced to the area of the UPJ. If identified, the crossing vessels should be meticulously preserved. The authors prefer to dissect these vessels with minimal use of energy with the help of a right-angled dissector. Once these are identified, they are slinged either with the help of a red rubber catheter or with the help of a feeding tube. Unlike the ureter, the pelvis can be gently grasped during the dissection; care should be taken to avoid use of crushing clamps. Another alternative could be the use of a straight needle directed directly down the anterior abdominal wall, and hitch the most anterior part of the pelvis (Fig. 21.3).

Incision of the Ureteropelvic Junction

The principle of any pyeloplasty is to produce a ureteropelvic junction that is funnel shaped, dependent, and without tension. The incision on the pelvis is done with the help of cutting scissors or roticulator scissors. The incision on the pelvis is scored to avoid disorientation. A stay suture is taken at the superior most aspect of the pelvis. Care is to be exercised while incising the pelvis is to avoid cutting too little or too much (excess), to avoid cutting into

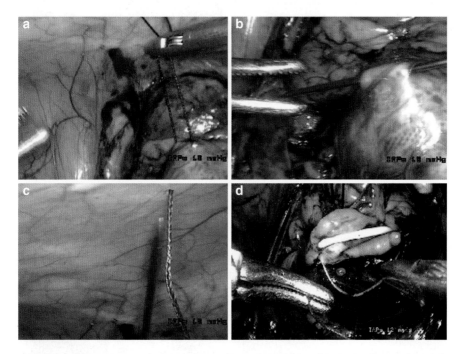

Fig. 21.3 (**a–c**) A straight needle inserted through the abdominal wall helps in slinging the pelvis which, apart from orientation, also helps in traction. (**d**) The long threads of the anterior layer help in suturing of the posterior layer. The bent needle helps in suturing

the calyces, maintain the orientation of the flap of the incised pelvis (this will be always oriented medially), and lateral spatulation of the ureter. From a ergonomic point of view, an important tip while spatulating the ureter is to incise the ureter with the right hand in a right-sided pyeloplasty, while one may use the left hand in a left-sided case (Fig. 21.4). A roticulator scissor helps in orienting the tip of the scissors in the lie of the ureter. The spatulation is made easier if a stent is in place. In this context, in the authors' opinion, if a pigtail catheter or an open end is in place, the catheter can be withdrawn and the spatulation can be made easier over the preplaced guide wire. The magnification offered by laparoscopy helps in meticulous spatulation incising the whole stenosed segment. The redundant flap of the pelvis helps in lateral spatulation of the ureter. In cases of crossing vessels, once the vessels are dissected and slinged, they may be transposed or relocated (Fig. 21.5).

Ureteric spatulation

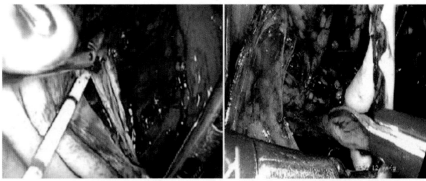

Ureter spatulation on the left side   Ureter spatulation on the right side

Fig. 21.4 From an ergonomic point of view, the right-sided ureteric spatulation is done with the right hand, while the left-sided one is done with the left hand

Tackling crossing vessel

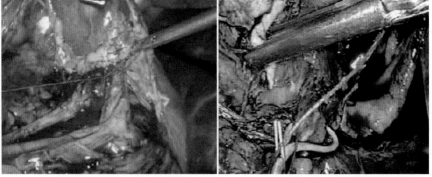

Hellstrom's relocation   Trasposition of Vessels

Fig. 21.5 The crossing vessels can be tackled either with Hellström's relocation or transposition.

In summary, the salient features and points to be meticulously followed in this step are:

1. Maintain orientation of the pelvis and ureter
2. Avoid use of excessive traction and crushing instruments on the parts to be reconstructed
3. Always keep the stent in view to avoid inadvertently cutting them
4. Use the pelvic flap prior to reduction to maintain orientation and traction
5. In case of calyces too close to the pelvis, incise the pelvis keeping the calyces in view to avoid cutting them.

Performing the Anastomosis

Before starting the anastomosis, the surgeon should personally prepare the suture material to be used for the anastomosis. The length of the suture material should be approximately 8 in. from the needle to the tail in adult patients and 6 in. in pediatric patients. It is a useful trick to make the needle "fish hook" shaped (Fig. 21.3) for ease in insertion of the needle in the edges and secondly to facilitate the easy passage of the needle through the port. If the needle is bent in such a way, it can be easily inserted or removed through 5-mm ports. The needle entry through the port should be always under vision, and if the needle is not straight, it should be straightened prior to removal. The "V" stitch is the most important stitch; an assistant can help in taking this stitch in by holding one edge of the spatulated ureter with a grasper introduced through an extra 5-mm port. The spatulated ureter should be sutured to the most dependent part of the pelvis. The authors prefer to suture the anterior layer first, the posterior layer is sutured last, excess threads at one end of the anterior suture line helps in suturing of the posterior layer (Fig. 21.3).

Exiting the Abdomen

The area of dissection is inspected under reduced insufflation pressures of 8 mmHg. In all cases a drain is kept. In ports that exceed 10 mm in size, the port closure is done with the help of Carter-Thomasen CloseSure System® (CooperSurgical, Inc., Trumbull, CT). If a pigtail catheter is used as a stent, it is replaced with a double J stent under fluoroscopy control at the conclusion of the procedure.

The patient is sent home on low-dose antibiotic prophylaxis until the stent is removed in the outpatient department 4 weeks following the operation. A diuretic renal scan is performed 6 months after the operation.

Conclusion

Laparoscopic pyeloplasty is a technically demanding procedure. It has a steep learning curve that can be overcome with skills learned in laboratory training. In the initial part of the learning curve, the surgeon should select cases judiciously. The key points in successfully accomplishing the procedure are proper port placement, meticulous dissection, adequate spatulation, and meticulous suturing. Proper instrumentation plays a pivotal role in success of the procedure.

References

1. Schuessler WW, Grune MT, Tecuanhuey LV, Preminger GM. Laparoscopic dismembered pyeloplasty. *J Urol*. 1993;150(6):1795-1799.
2. Chen RN, Moore RG, Kavoussi LR. Laparoscopic pyeloplasty. Indications, technique, and long-term outcome. *Urol Clin North Am*. 1998;25(2):323-330.
3. Bauer JJ, Bishoff JT, Moore RG, Chen RN, Iverson AJ, Kavoussi LR. Laparoscopic versus open pyeloplasty: assessment of objective and subjective outcome. *J Urol*. 1999;162:692-695.
4. Singh H, Ganpule A, Malhotra V, Manohar T, Muthu V, Desai M. Transperitoneal laparoscopic pyeloplasty in children. *J Endourol*. 2007;21(12):1461-1466.
5. Ooi J, Lawrentschuk N, Murphy DL. Training model for open or laparoscopic pyeloplasty. *J Endourol*. 2006;20(2):149-152.

Nasser Simforoosh, Alireza Aminsharifi, and Akbar Nouralizadeh

Introduction

For centuries, stone disease has been a common health problem – in fact, one of the first surgeries performed on humans was for stones – and traditional open surgery was utilized to manage the problems it caused.[1] Stone disease is still common today, but the pattern of practice in stone management has undergone a revolution in the last few decades. Nowadays, open surgery for stone disease is considered obsolete and has been almost totally abandoned.[2] The biggest blow to open stone surgery (OSS) occurred when extracorporeal shock wave lithotripsy (SWL) was applied successfully by Chaussy in Berlin.[3] Percutaneous nephrolithotomy (PCNL) and ureteroscopic lithotripsy (URL) were also great steps forward, and these procedures have major roles in managing large renal and ureteral stone disease in most parts of the world today. Pneumolithotripsy and laser lithotripsy technologies were another important achievement in dealing with stone disease during PCNL and URL. It is used commonly in many countries due to its efficacy, and especially because of its cost effectiveness. The introduction of flexible instruments also has facilitated navigation through the collecting system. Disposable flexible endoscopes seem to be promising alternative to the costly fiberoptic ones, and solve problems related to their cost and maintenance. All of the above measures, which are today referred to as "endourology," have resulted in putting the knife aside in almost all cases of stone disease.

In the era of minimally invasive endoscopic procedures and SWL, laparoscopy has a limited role in the urologist's armamentarium for surgical stone management.[4] However, in cases of large stones, single or combined endourologic procedures may not be more cost effective than a single, one-session approach for complete stone removal.[5] Therefore, OSS, including open ureterolithotomy, pyelolithotomy, and nephrolithotomy, still has a role in many centers. Laparoscopic stone removal is a valuable option in these situations, and offers a less morbid modality for removing large stones in the urinary tract. This chapter

N. Simforoosh (✉)

Department of Urology, Shahid Labbafinejad Hospital, Urology and Nephrology Research Center, Shahid Beheshti University of Medical Sciences, Tehran, Iran

e-mail: simforoosh@iurtc.org.ir

A.M. Al-Kandari and I.S. Gill (eds.), *Difficult Conditions in Laparoscopic Urologic Surgery*,   **305**
DOI: 10.1007/978-1-84882-105-7_22, © Springer-Verlag London Limited 2011

focuses on the potential difficulties and complications that may occur during laparoscopic stone surgery. Various approaches to deal with these difficulties will be discussed.

Laparoscopic Ureterolithotomy (LU): Difficulties and Their Management

Laparoscopic ureterolithotomy (LU) is an alternative option for removal of impacted ureteric stones larger than 15 mm,[6,7] or may be used as a salvage procedure in failures of SWL and/or ureteroscopic lithotripsy.[8] This technique usually results in complete stone removal through a single minimally invasive surgery with a reasonable operative time and short hospital stay.[9] Thus, the indications for laparoscopic ureterolithotomy in the era of modern endourology include stones that cannot be accessed ureteroscopically or cannot be fragmented (Fig. 22.1).

LU can be accomplished through a transperitoneal (TP) or retroperitoneal (RP) route. Although the preferred approach is mainly defined by a surgeons preference and experience, the authors prefer a TP approach, especially for the beginner or average laparoscopic surgeons. In comparison to the RP route, the TP approach provides a larger working space with familiar anatomic landmarks. Moreover, difficulties and complications may be handled better in a TP approach.[10] In the absence of dense retroperitoneal fibrosis, laparoscopic ureterolithotomy is almost an easy procedure, especially for beginners (Video Clip 22.1). However, laparoscopic ureterolithotomy for distal ureteral stones, especially those lodged behind the bladder and very close to ureterovesical junction, is more difficult and requires more expertise.

Stone Migration During LU

The ideal case for LU is a large, impacted ureteral stone. However, as in open ureterolithotomy, there is always a potential risk of upward stone migration during the procedure. To decrease the chance of stone migration to the kidney, ureteric dissection should be accomplished as gently as possible in a proximal to distal direction. Once the dilated ureter above the site of the impacted stone is identified, placement of a laparoscopic Babcock prevents stone migration during further ureter dissection. Placing the patient in a head up position, keeping the patient well hydrated, and intravenous infusion of 0.5mg/kg furosemide may also help prevent stone migration.

In cases of stone migration, the surgeon should open the ureter at the site of stone impaction. By passing a rigid or flexible ureteroscope through the lower abdominal 5-mm laparoscopic port, ureteroscopy can be easily performed up to the renal calices. Then, the migrated stone can be pushed back to the site of the ureteric incision by basketing or "milking" the ureter with the laparoscopic Babcock.

Difficulties in Stone Localization During LU

Sometimes, after the dissection of the ureter, it is difficult to localize the site of the stone. This may occur especially in obese patients and patients with dense, fibrotic adhesions around the ureter due to chronic inflammation or multiple sessions of SWL. Intermittent

Fig. 22.1 Preoperative (**a**) and postoperative (**b**) intravenous urography (IVU) following laparoscopic ureterolithotomy (**c**). Significant relief of obstruction is noted. (*Arrow* on **a** indicates the proximal ureteral stone, *U* ureter)

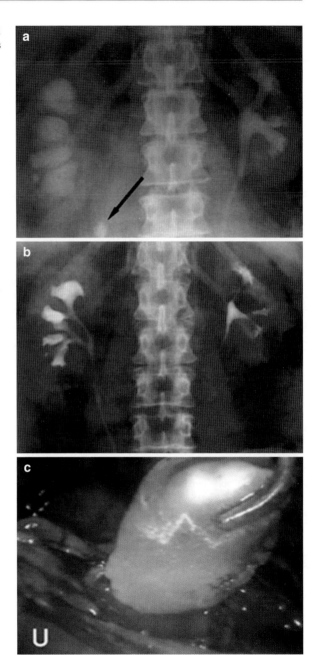

pressing of the dilated proximal ureter in a proximal to distal direction with the laparoscopic Babcock may help in locating the site of the impacted stone. Difficulty in localizing the stone due to severe periureteric fibrosis can be overcome by the use of fluoroscopy or intraoperative laparoscopic ultrasonography. If the stone still cannot be localized, the problem can be fixed by employing proximal and distal ureteroscopy after the ureter is opened at the site of its maximal dilation and a rigid or flexible ureteroscope is passed to the ureterotomy via the lower or upper abdominal trocars. After finding the stone, it can be removed through the ureteral incision by milking or basketing, or it can be fragmented in situ with pneumatic or laser lithotripsy.

Stone Adhering to the Mucosa

After the ureteral incision, sometimes the stone cannot be easily delivered because of its adherence to the ureteral mucosa. This is especially true in long-standing, large, impacted stones and those with multiple sessions of SWL. After proximal extension of the ureteral incision over the dilated proximal ureter, one can separate the "head" of the stone from the ureter with the aid of a laparoscopic hook. Then the rest of stone can be easily released from the ureteral mucosa using the laparoscopic Babcock. Levering the stone out of the ureter prevents its breakage and subsequent problems from small pieces. It has been recommended that direct stone grasping with the laparoscopic grasper should be avoided, especially when the stone is somewhat soft. Grasping the stone can break it with the possibility of migration.[11]

Lost Stone

Sometimes, after stone extraction, the stone may be lost before it is removed from the abdomen. To avoid this possibility, it is recommended that the surgeon place an endobag or its alternate in the abdomen before incising the ureter. The stone can then be placed into the bag just after it is removed. Sometimes, the stone is already fragmented (perhaps due to the effects of previous SWL), or it may be fragmented by the force of the graspers at the time of extraction. Having the bag near the field allows the surgeon to collect the fragments and prevent loss. However, in cases where the stone is lost, the stone usually stays medial to the ureter over the reflected colon. Changing the camera port may help in locating the lost stone.

Stenting and Suturing

Classically, both ureteral stenting and suturing have been recommended. Laparoscopic antegrade ureteral stenting is feasible by placing the double J or feeding tube into the laparoscopic suction and guiding it to the ureteral incision. However, there is evidence that ureteral stenting during LU could be obviated safely. Demirci and colleagues have demonstrated the safety of leaving the sutured ureterotomy without stenting.[12] Similar findings have been demonstrated by others as well.[8,9] Goel and Hemal recommend stenting only in cases of renal dysfunction and/or stone impaction.[13]

Suturing of the ureterotomy incision is usually a simple task. Laparoscopic magnification allows clear visualization of the mucosal apposition. Sometimes suturing is not possible due to severe inflammation and fragility of the tissue. Fixing a stent in the ureter and leaving the unsutured ureteral incision with an external draining catheter can be safely implemented in these circumstances.[5,8,9]

Ureteral Stricture

The incidence of ureteral stricture following LU has been reported between 2.5% and 20%.[14,15] Various contributing factors may have a role in the development of ureteral stenosis. Nouira and colleagues have recommended that adhering to the principles of ureterotomy closure during open surgery (i.e., loose sutures in order to just approximate the ureteral edges) may reduce the chance of ureteral stricture following LU.[14] They also believe that using a laparoscopic cold knife is more suitable than an electrical hook. However, in the authors' opinion, the use of a cutting-mode electrical hook is much easier and more popular.[5,9] To decrease the rate of stricture, the authors suggest that the cutting-electrical hook be applied only on the dilated ureter proximal to the stone. The extension of the hook-incision should be done with laparoscopic scissors.

Laparoscopic Pyelolithotomy (LP): Difficulties and Their Management

Compared with PCNL, the laparoscopic removal of renal pelvic stones has a limited role. Its indications also have not been clearly defined. There are a few comparative studies between PCNL and laparoscopic pyelolithotomy (LP) in the literature.[16,17] However, in situations of failed percutaneous access due to technical reasons, a laparoscopic approach in selected cases may provide similar success rates as open surgery. In the authors' option, LP can be reserved as an alternative approach in selected cases of large renal pelvis stones, stones resistant to fragmentation, and in patients with abnormal kidney anatomy. This technique allows en bloc stone extraction in a minimally invasive milieu. The procedure is easier in patients with an extrarenal pelvis. Partial staghorn stones are also appropriate for laparoscopic pyelolithotomy (Video Clip 22.2).

Dissecting the Renal Pelvis

Identification and dissection of the proximal ureter is the initial step during LP. Dissection over the proximal ureter usually guides the surgeon to the renal pelvis. Aggressive dissection over the ureteropelvic junction (UPJ), especially in the presence of inflammation, may lead to UPJ avulsion. In cases of avulsion, meticulous dissection and mobilization of the renal pelvis may allow laparoscopic reanastomosis following stone removal via the pyelotomy incision.

The renal pelvis should be released and dissected completely before pyelotomy. In patients with prior retroperitoneal surgery, a transperitoneal approach is recommended (Fig. 22.2). During LP, dissection should be done over the renal pelvis to prevent inadvertent

Fig. 22.2 Preoperative KUB (**a**) and IVU (**b**) of a patient with a large renal pelvis stone. Laparoscopic pelvic dissection and stone extraction have been carried out (**c**, **d**). (*U* ureter, *P* renal pelvis)

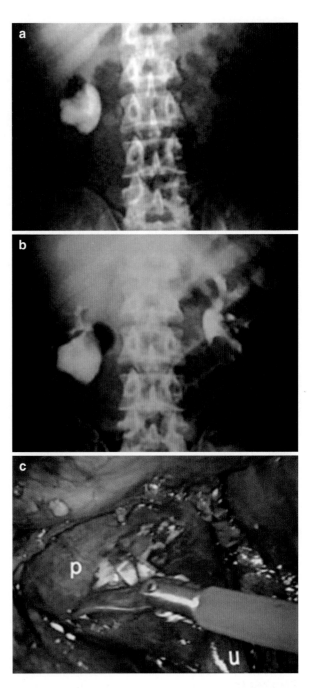

Fig. 22.2 (continued)

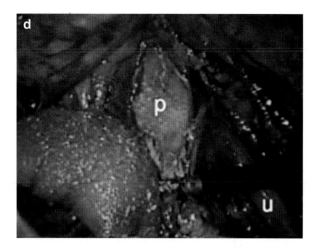

injury to the branches of the renal artery, renal vein, and aberrant vessels. Peripelvic inflammation, as well as a number of aberrant vessels, may be found while dissecting the pelvis, requiring expertise in laparoscopic dissection. Conversion to open surgery may be required due to significant perinephric adhesions and resultant difficulty in dissection.

Pyelotomy and Stone Removal

The pyelotomy incision can be made using a laparoscopic knife, or more popularly, a cutting-mode electrical hook. The incision may be longitudinal or transverse. Sometimes, especially in cases with a large, impacted stone, it is better to place two stay sutures at both ends of the pyelotomy incision to prevent incision extension during stone removal. These sutures also make pyelotomy closure easier. The pyelotomy may be well extended to the superior and inferior calyces or their infundibula. Gentle delivery of the "tail" of the stone from the UPJ, together with rotating and twisting maneuvers, help in the extraction of large stones. This invariably leads to delivering one end of the partial staghorn stone first, allowing manipulation of the other end.

One of the major limitations of the laparoscopic approach is the difficulty in retrieving the caliceal calculi.

In situations where the stone is too large for the port site, the stone can be placed in a laparoscopic sac and removed via the umbilical laparoscopic port site by extending the incision after pyelotomy closure. Alternatively, the stone can be fragmented within the endobag and removed via a lesser incision.

Stone Migration

Stone migration during LP usually occurs in the presence of a small renal pelvis stone that causes severe hydronephrosis. If the stone has migrated to the kidney, guiding a flexible or rigid ureteroscope to the pyelotomy incision via the lower abdominal laparoscopic port allows direct exploration of the calyces and stone removal under direct vision with a nitinol stone basket. Since the patient is in a lateral decubitus position, the migrated stone often falls into the upper pole calyces. Micali et al. have described removal of pelvic and caliceal calculi using a flexible cystoscope through the 10-/12-mm laparoscopic port.[18]

Pyelotomy Closure

Reconstructing the pyelotomy requires advanced laparoscopic skills in intracorporeal suturing. Sometimes the edges of the incised renal pelvis are inflamed and fragile, which makes suturing not possible. Antegrade placement of a ureteral stent and applying two sutures at both ends of the pyelotomy incision and tying them to each other usually fix the problem.[19] However, excessive manipulation in such situations may result in renal pelvis disruption.

Laparoscopic Nephrolithotomy

Staghorn renal stones are a challenging issue in urology. Even with the introduction of endourological methods, the management of staghorn renal stones remains difficult. Several series have considered open anatrophic nephrolithotomy for the management of staghorn renal stones, even in the era of endourology. Due to the high incidence of recurrence of staghorn stones, particularly those associated with an infective process, the complete removal of the stone is the ultimate goal in their management, a result that might not be attained even after several sessions of PCNL and/or SWL and/or retrograde intrarenal surgery.[6,20,21]

Laparoscopic anatrophic nephrolithotomy (LAN) may be considered as an alternative to open surgery of staghorn renal stones. Currently, there are only two reports on six cases of LAN in humans in the literature.[22,23] LAN is a complex laparoscopic procedure that requires full laparoscopic experience. Large burden, "en-bloc" (complete or partial) staghorn stones are appropriate candidates for LAN. Small burden stones, or stones with many particles in different calyces are very difficult for LAN. Renal vascular anatomy, stone size, and burden should be assessed preoperatively by computerized tomographic angiography.

After complete dissection of both renal artery and vein, Gerota's fascia is incised and the kidney fully mobilized within this fascia. Unless the renal parenchyma is atrophic, the renal artery should be clamped temporarily with a bulldog clamp. Through an incision of sufficient length on the Brodel line, the collecting system is sharply incised and the staghorn stone is mobilized intrarenally, rotated, and removed as completely as possible (Fig. 22.3).

In order to decrease warm ischemia time, both the collecting system and renal cortex can be closed with a single row of polyglactin 2–0 running sutures. The sutures are buttressed by applying Hem-o-lok® clips (Teleflex Medical, Research Triangle Park, NC)

Fig. 22.3 Preoperative KUB (**a**) and IVU (**b**) of an obese patient with a large complete staghorn renal stone (**c**) extracted by laparoscopic anatrophic nephrolithotomy (**d**). Sites of trocars are shown (**e**) (From Simforoosh et al.[23] Reprinted with permission from Wiley-Blackwell)

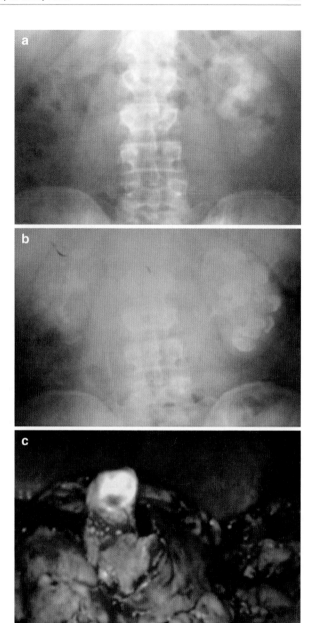

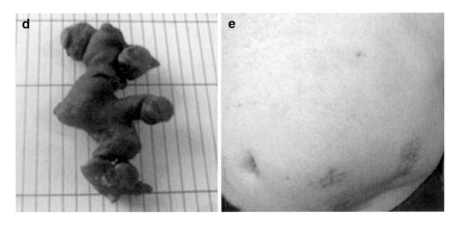

Fig. 22.3 (continued)

instead of tying knots. Intraoperative laparoscopic ultrasonography may be used to identify the site of the thinnest parenchyma and to detect possible residual stones (Video Clip 22.3).

Laparoscopic Management of Stone Disease in Anomalous Kidneys

Relative urinary stasis imposed by anomalies in the collecting system predisposes the kidney to urolithiasis and increases the risk of stone recurrence.

Ureteropelvic Junction Obstruction (UPJO) and Stones

There is a 70-fold increased risk of renal stone formation in patients with ureteropelvic junction obstruction (UPJO).[24] Since laparoscopy is becoming the standard of care in managing UPJO, a concomitant stone can be removed laparoscopically during a pyeloplasty procedure.[25,26] The stone can be removed by laparoscopic instruments if it is located in the renal pelvis or at visible areas of the kidney. Furthermore, navigation within the collecting system is possible using flexible or rigid endoscopes. After localizing the hidden stone, it can be managed with basketing and/or pneumatic or laser lithotripsy under direct vision.

The authors have used a rigid ureteroscope and pneumatic lithotriptor successfully during laparoscopy for management of stones in kidneys with UPJO. In case of failure, intraoperative ultrasound can also be used to find stones in the kidney. Sometimes after stone localization with intraoperative ultrasonography, nephrotomy over the stone is necessary for en-bloc stone extraction. This is especially true when the stone is located in inaccessible calices in the hydronephrotic system. Nephrotomy can be done without hilar clamping since the renal cortex is usually thin when it is associated with UPJO.

Horseshoe Kidney

Relative urinary stasis and abnormal anatomy of the collecting system in patients with a horseshoe kidney put them at risk of urolithiasis, with an incidence rate of 21–60%. Various single or combined endourologic procedures, such as SWL and PCNL, can provide up to 90% of stone-free rate in these patients.[27–29] Laparosopic pyelolithotomy is an alternative option in patients with a horseshoe kidney that have a large burden stone in the renal pelvis or isthmus. There are several advantages to a laparoscopic approach in removing stones from a horseshoe kidney. The whole procedure can be done under direct vision without any need of radiation exposure. There is no glomerular damage and there is a reduced chance of hemorrhage. The stone can be removed in one piece, especially if it is located in the renal pelvis (Fig. 22.4). When UPJO is associated with horseshoe kidney, pyeloplasty can be performed simultaneously. During laparoscopy, care should be taken not to injure the anomalous vascular supply to the horseshoe kidney (Video Clip 22.4).

Cross-Fused Kidney

The authors have successfully removed a stone from a cross-fused ectopic kidney. It was very difficult to find a bare area of pelvis for pelviotomy due to abnormal vascular anatomy, but with great care and patience, a large stone was extracted en-bloc from the kidney.

Pelvic Kidney

While laparoscopic assisted PCNL is standard of care for minimally invasive management of stones in a pelvic kidney,[30] large stones, especially in the renal pelvis, can be removed by laparoscopy. Since the kidney is located in a lower anatomic position in the abdomen, transperitoneal laparoscopy is the best alternative to open surgery in these circumstances (Fig. 22.5).

The authors successfully removed a kidney stone from the renal pelvis of a pelvic kidney, but unfortunately, the stone was dropped and lost during surgery. The procedure was not converted to open surgery, and postoperative imaging revealed that the lost stone was behind the spleen. The stone did not cause any clinical problems during follow-up and was left intact.

Retrocaval Ureter

If a stone is present in a kidney with a retrocaval ureter, laparoscopic stone removal can be performed directly, or by using another endourologic means, such as flexible or rigid ureteroscopy or a percutanous approach. The authors have reported six cases of retrocaval ureter, with one case associated with a 12mm renal pelvis stone. The stone was removed with laparoscopic grasping forceps in one piece.[31]

Fig. 22.4 Preoperative KUB (**a**) and IVU (**b**) of a patient with a large renal pelvis in his horseshoe kidney. The stone was removed by laparoscopic pyelolithotomy (**c**). The renal pelvis was easily accessed during laparoscopy due to its anterior position

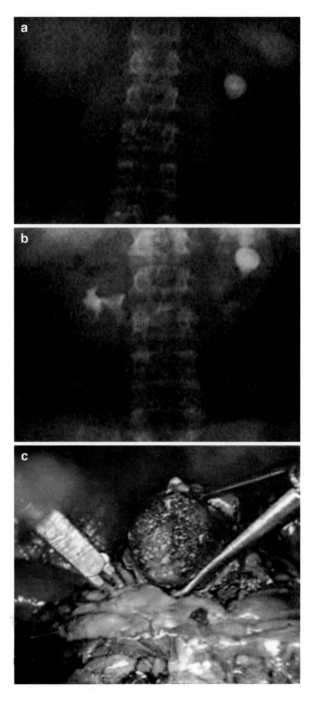

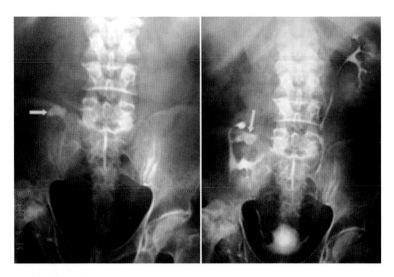

Fig. 22.5 Preoperative KUB (*left*) and IVU (*right*) of a patient with an upper calyx stone in his ectopic kidney (indicated by *arrows*). The patient was successfully managed by laparoscopic-assisted PCNL

Conclusion

Although laparoscopic stone surgery has a limited role in management of urolithiasis, it can be offered as a proper alternative to open stone surgery. Proper case selection for laparoscopic ureterolithotomy, pyelolithotomy, and especially laparoscopic anatrophic nephrolithotomy is key in preventing complications during the procedure. However, most of the difficulties during these procedures can be managed without the need for an open conversion.

References

1. Herr HW. 'Cutting for the stone': the ancient art of lithotomy. *BJU Int.* 2008;101(10): 1214-1216.
2. Segura JW, Preminger GM, Assimos DG, et al. Ureteral Stones Clinical Guidelines Panel summary report on the management of ureteral calculi. *J Urol.* 1997;158(5):1915-1921.
3. Chaussy C, Eisenberger F, Forssmann B. Extracorporeal shockwave lithotripsy (ESWL): a chronology. *J Endourol.* 2007;21(11):1249-1254.
4. Desai RA, Assimos DG. Role of laparoscopic stone surgery. *Urology.* 2008;71(4):578-580.
5. Gaur DD, Trivedi S, Prabhudesai MR, Madhusudhana HR, Gopichand M. Laparoscopic ureterolithotomy: technical considerations and long-term follow-up. *BJU Int.* 2002;89(4): 339-343.
6. Lingeman JE, Matlaga BR, Evan AP. Surgical management of upper urinary tract calculi. In: Wein AJ, Kavoussi LR, Novick AC, Partin AW, eds. *Campbell-Walsh Urology.* 9th ed. Philadelphia, PA: Saunders; 2007:1431-1507.

7. Basiri A, Simforoosh N, Ziaee AM, Shayaminasab H, Moghaddam SMM, Zare S. Retrograde, antegrade and laparoscopic approaches for the management of large, proximal ureteral stones: a randomized clinical trial. *J Endourol.* 2008;22(12):1-4.

8. Kijvikai K, Patcharatrakul S. Laparoscopic ureterolithotomy: its role and some controversial technical considerations. *Int J Urol.* 2006;13(3):206-210.

9. Simforoosh N, Basiri A, Danesh AK, et al. Laparoscopic management of ureteral calculi: a report of 123 cases. *Urol J.* 2007;4(3):138-141.

10. Harewood LM, Webb DR, Pope AJ. Laparoscopic ureterolithotomy: the results of an initial series, and an evaluation of its role in the management of ureteric calculi. *Br J Urol.* 1994;74(2):170-176.

11. Yadav R, Kumar R, Hemal AK. Laparoscopy in the management of stone disease of urinary tract. *J Minim Access Surg.* 2005;1:173-180.

12. Demirci D, Gülmez I, Ekmekçioğlu O, Karacagil M. Retroperitoneoscopic ureterolithotomy for the treatment of ureteral calculi. *Urol Int.* 2004;73(3):234-237.

13. Goel A, Hemal AK. Upper and mid-ureteric stones: a prospective unrandomized comparison of retroperitoneoscopic and open ureterolithotomy. *BJU Int.* 2001;88(7):679-682.

14. Nouira Y, Kallel Y, Binous MY, Dahmoul H, Horchani A. Laparoscopic retroperitoneal ureterolithotomy: initial experience and review of literature. *J Endourol.* 2004;18(6):557-561.

15. Lee WC, Hsieh HH. Retroperitoneoscopic ureterolithotomy for impacted ureteral stones. *Chang Gung Med J.* 2000;23(1):28-32.

16. Goel A, Hemal AK. Evaluation of role of retroperitoneoscopic pyelolithotomy and its comparison with percutaneous nephrolithotripsy. *Int Urol Nephrol.* 2003;35:73-76.

17. Meria P, Milcent S, Desgrandchamps F, Mongiat-Artus P, Duclos JM, Teillac P. Management of pelvic stones larger than 20 mm: laparoscopic transperitoneal pyelolithotomy or percutaneous nephrolithotomy? *Urol Int.* 2005;75(4):322-326.

18. Micali S, Moore RG, Averch TD, Adams JB, Kavoussi LR. The role of laparoscopy in the treatment of renal and ureteral calculi. *J Urol.* 1997;137:463-466.

19. Shah SR. Modified method for closure of transverse pyelotomy incision in Gil-Vernet pyelolithotomy operation. *Tech Urol.* 1999;5(2):106-107.

20. Matlaga BR, Assimos DG. Changing indications of open stone surgery. *Urology.* 2002;59:490-493.

21. Esen AA, Kirkali Z, Guler C. Open stone surgery: is it still a preferable procedure in the management of staghorn calculi? *Int Urol Nephrol.* 1994;26:247-253.

22. Deger S, Tuellmann M, Schoenberger B, Winkelmann B, Peters R, Loening SA. Laparoscopic anatrophic nephrolithotomy. *Scand J Urol Nephrol.* 2004;38:263-265.

23. Simforoosh N, Aminsharifi A, Tabibi A, et al. Laparoscopic anatrophic nephrolithotomy for managing large staghorn calculi. *BJU Int.* 2008;101(10):1293-1296.

24. Husmann DA, Milliner DS, Segura JW. Ureteropelvic junction obstruction with concurrent renal pelvic calculi in the pediatric patient: a long term follow up. *J Urol.* 1996;156:741-743.

25. Srivastava A, Singh P, Guptam M, et al. Laparoscopic pyeloplasty with concomitant pyelolithotomy – is it an effective mode of treatment? *Urol Int.* 2008;80(3):306-309.

26. Eden CG, Moon DA, Gianduzzo T. Concomitant management of renal calculi and pelvi-ureteric junction obstruction with robotic laparoscopic surgery. *BJU Int.* 2006;97(3):653-654.

27. Mosavi-Bahar SH, Amirzargar MA, Rahnavardi M, Moghaddam SM, Babbolhavaeji H, Amirhasani S. Percutaneous nephrolithotomy in patients with kidney malformations. *J Endourol.* 2007;21(5):520-524.

28. Symons SJ, Ramachandran A, Kurien A, Baiysha R, Desai MR. Urolithiasis in the horseshoe kidney: a single-centre experience. *BJU Int.* 2008;102:1676-1680.

29. Irani D, Eshratkhah R, Amin-Sharifi A. Efficacy of extracorporeal shock wave lithotripsy monotherapy in complex urolithiasis in the era of advanced endourologic procedures. *Urol J.* 2005;2(1):13-19.

30. Mousavi-Bahar SH, Amir-Zargar MA, Gholamrezaie HR. Laparoscopic assisted percutaneous nephrolithotomy in ectopic pelvic kidneys. *Int J Urol.* 2008;15(3):276-278.
31. Simforoosh N, Nouri-Mahdavi K, Tabibi A. Laparoscopic pyelopyelostomy for retrocaval ureter without excision of the retrocaval segment: first report of 6 cases. *J Urol.* 2006;175(6):2166-2169.

Difficulties in Laparoscopic Ureteral and Bladder Reconstruction

23

Rakesh V. Khanna, Ricardo Brandina, Andre Berger, Robert J. Stein, and Inderbir S. Gill

Ureteral reconstruction may be required in the setting of iatrogenic injury to the ureter, infectious strictures from tuberculosis, or schistosomiasis, endometriosis, trauma, or malignancy.

Injury to the ureter is most commonly iatrogenic in nature. These occur most commonly in gynecological, colorectal, or urological procedures. Mechanism of injury may include transection, ligation, cautery injury, or devascularization. If not recognized and repaired intraoperatively, patients may present postoperatively with a urine leak or fistula.

A number of techniques exist for ureteral reconstruction. These include ureteroureterostomy, ureteroneocystostomy, psoas hitch, Boari flap, ileal ureter, and transureteroureterostomy (TUU). The choice of technique is dependent on the length and location of injury. These should be assessed by either intravenous urogram, computed tomography (CT) urogram, retrograde pyelography, ureteroscopy, or a combination of these techniques. In patients with a nephrostomy tube preoperatively, antegrade nephrostogram is often used in evaluating the proximal extent of injury. Additional preoperative investigations include a measurement of both total and ipsilateral renal function, especially when nephrectomy, ileal substitution or TUU is considered, and in cases of ureteroneocystostomy, an estimate of bladder capacity can be obtained. Augmentation cystoplasty remains the most widely accepted technique for patients requiring surgical augmentation of bladder capacity for protection of the upper urinary tract and provides urinary continence in patients with bladder dysfunction secondary to reduced functional capacity or poor compliance.[1,2]

With increasing experience in minimally invasive urology, a laparoscopic approach for each of these reconstructive techniques has been described. In general, the laparoscopic approach aims to duplicate the principles of open surgery. In the appropriate patient, laparoscopy offers the advantages of decreased pain and shorter convalescence.

R.V. Khanna (✉)
Glickman Urological and Kidney Institute; Cleveland Clinic, Cleveland, OH, USA
e-mail: khannar@ccf.org

A.M. Al-Kandari and I.S. Gill (eds.), *Difficult Conditions in Laparoscopic Urologic Surgery*,
DOI: 10.1007/978-1-84882-105-7_23, © Springer-Verlag London Limited 2011

Boari Flap

The Boari flap is commonly used for ureteroneocystostomy when ureteral pathology is located mid ureter. In order to minimize the risk of flap ischemia, the ratio of flap length to base width should not exceed 3:1 (Fig. 23.1a, b). The length and location of the stricture is defined by preoperative imaging. If a large bladder flap is to be created, preoperative assessment of bladder capacity and compliance is performed. Reconstruction is facilitated by large bladder capacity with good compliance and minimal scarring from previous radiation therapy, abscess, urinoma, or benign prostatic hyperplasia. If collecting system decompression is required preoperatively, consideration should be given to nephrostomy tube placement as edema and inflammation from the ureteral stent can increase difficulty with mobilization and make visualization of the strictured segment of ureter more difficult.

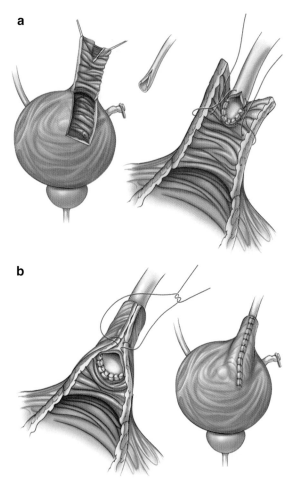

Fig. 23.1 Laparoscopic Boari flap. (**a**) Bladder flap is created. The ureter is spatulated and the dorsal aspect anastomosed to the flap. (**b**) Flap is tubularized and the remainder of the bladder defect is closed (Reprinted with permission, Cleveland Clinic Center for Medical Art & Photography © 2010. All Rights Reserved)

Technique

Positioning and Port Placement

The patient is given a dose of antibiotic preoperatively to cover urinary pathogens. The patient is secured in a low lithotomy position with 30° Trendelenburg (Fig. 23.2). After being prepped and draped, a Foley catheter is placed in the bladder. For a left-sided stricture, the surgeon stands on the left side of the patient whereas the assistant is on the right side. A 12-mm camera port is placed at the umbilicus. A 5-mm and 12-mm port is placed at the right and left lateral border of the rectus muscle two fingerbreadths below the umbilicus. A fourth 5 mm port is placed two fingerbreadths superior to the anterior superior iliac spine to serve as an assistant port. For a right-sided stricture, the surgeon stands on the right side and the port positions are reversed.

Procedure

The line of Toldt is incised and the colon is reflected medially. The ureter is identified at the level of the iliac vessels and mobilized as distally as possible (Fig. 23.3a–f). In the absence of a ureteral stent, a normal ureter will often be dilated proximal to the level of obstruction. To aid with the dissection, a vascular loop can be passed around the ureter and brought out through one of the trocars to place the ureter on traction.[3] As the ureter is mobilized, care is taken to preserve the adventitial tissue in order to maintain the blood supply of the ureter. The diseased segment of ureter is then excised and sent for pathology. In cases where stricture etiology is unclear, frozen section analysis should be obtained. The ureter is then mobilized at least 4–5 cm proximally and spatulated on its ventral aspect.

Attention is then turned to the bladder. The peritoneum overlying the bladder is incised and the urachus is divided. The bladder is freed anteriorly by dissecting the space of

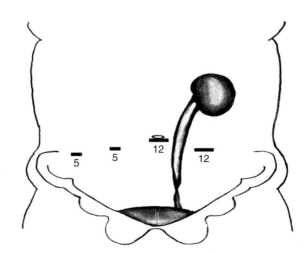

Fig. 23.2 Port position for a left laparoscopic Boari flap (Reprinted with permission, Cleveland Clinic Center for Medical Art & Photography © 2010. All Rights Reserved)

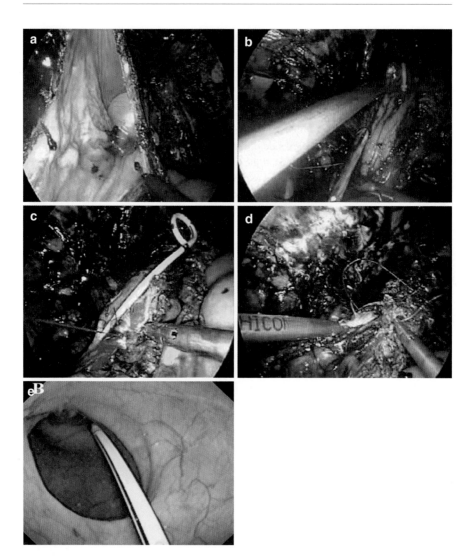

Fig. 23.3 (**a**) The bladder is opened, revealing the catheter balloon and a flap is created. (**b**) The ureter and flap are brought together to ensure that the anastomosis will be tension free. (**c**) After spatulation, the posterior wall of the ureter is sutured to the bladder mucosa. Once the posterior anastomosis is completed, a ureteral stent a placed. (**d**) Completed anastomosis. (**e**) Appearance at cystoscopy. (**f**) Intravenous pyelogram detailing outline of the Boari flap

Fig. 23.3 (continued)

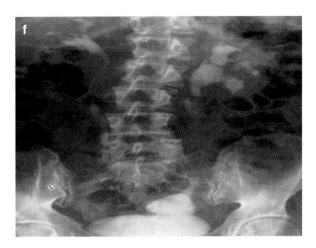

Retzius. If necessary, the superior and middle vesical arteries on the contralateral side of the diseased ureter can be divided to gain additional bladder length and mobility.

A U-shaped flap is outlined on the anterior aspect of the bladder with the flap base being wider than the apex. The base of the flap should be at least 3 cm and the apex should be at least 2 cm. The apex of the flap should be at least 2 cm away from the bladder neck. Intraoperatively, a ureteral stent serves as a benchmark and can be measured in order to determine the length of the required flap. In view of tissue contraction, flap length should be 1.5 times longer than the defect to be bridged.[4]

The posterior wall of the ureter-flap anastomosis is constructed by using interrupted full-thickness 4-0 Vicryl™ sutures (Ethicon, Inc., Somerville, NJ). After the posterior anastomosis is completed, a stent is inserted. To aid with guidewire passage and stent insertion, a 2-mm needlescopic port can be placed just superior to the pubic symphysis. A 0.038 in. diameter guidewire is advanced through the port and, using a laparoscopic grasper, guided into the ureter and kidney. After the wire is positioned, a double J stent is advanced over the wire.[4] Full-thickness interrupted sutures are used to complete the ureter-flap anastomosis. A U-stitch can be used as the final anastomotic suture anteriorly and is passed through one side of the flap then through the ipsilateral side of the ureter, followed by the contralateral side of the ureter and finally the contralateral side of the bladder flap. The remainder of the bladder defect is then closed with a running absorbable suture.

A nonrefluxing anastomosis can be created by making a 2-mm to 3-cm midline incision in the mucosa at the apex of the flap. The mucosa is then undermined 1 cm laterally on each side of the incision. Then the ureter sutured to the apex of the mucosal incision while the flap edges are sutured to the edges of the ureter circumferentially. The midline of the mucosal incision is then closed over the ureter, thus creating a tunneled anastomosis (Fig. 23.4).[4] However, since the ratio of ureteral length to diameter should be at least 4:1 to prevent reflux, use of this technique is limited to situations in which a long ureteral length is present. It is the preference of the authors to create refluxing anastomoses as nonrefluxing maneuvers may increase the risk of postoperative ureteral obstruction. If required to ease tension on the anastomosis, the bladder dome can be fixed to the ipsilateral psoas muscle.

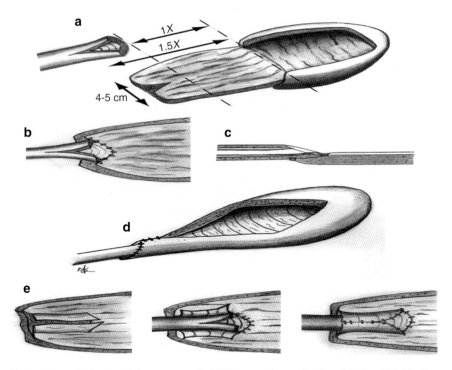

Fig. 23.4 Non refluxing Boari flap anastomosis. (**a**) The ureter is spatulated, and the Boari bladder flap is raised followed with incision of mucosa at the apex to raise mucosal flaps. (**b**) The spatulated ureter is sutured to the bladder flap edges. (**c**) Side view of anastomosed ureter to bladder flap. (**d**) Outside view of bladder closure after the ureteral bladder anastomosis. (**e**) Inside view illustrating first raising the bladder mucosa, followed by anastomosis of ureter to bladder flap and finally bladder mucosal flap closed over the ureteral bladder anastomosis as antireflux mechanism. (Reprinted with permission, Cleveland Clinic Center for Medical Art & Photography © 2010. All Rights Reserved)

The integrity of the closure and anastomosis is then tested by filling the bladder, and a drain and Foley catheter are left in place. The drain is removed when output is less than 50 cc/24 h, whereas the Foley catheter is left for 7–10 days and is removed when a cystogram shows no extravasation. The ureteral stent is removed 4–6 weeks postoperatively.

A modification to the above technique includes making a transverse incision along the anterior bladder wall, one third distal to the dome. The mid portion of the flap is sutured to the spatulated end of the ureter. After completion of the lateral and medial anastomosis, the bladder is closed in a Heineke-Mikulicz fashion.[5] Additionally, use of the *da Vinci*® robot (Intuitive Surgical, Inc., Sunnyvale, CA) positioned between the patient's legs with a similar port configuration makes intracorporeal suturing decidedly easier.

Discussion

Several reports detail experience with laparoscopic Boari flap. Fugita et al. reported three cases of which none demonstrated ureteric obstruction on postoperative imaging.[6] Castillo et al. reported their experience with laparoscopic Boari flap in eight patients with ureteral strictures 4–7 cm in length.[3] There was no intraoperative complication and at mean follow up of 17.6 months, all patients were symptom free and had a nonobstructive intravenous urogram.

Modi et al. described a case report of a Boari flap performed after iatrogenic ureteral injury.[7] They reported no complications and the patient was asymptomatic at 1 year follow up.

Ramalingam et al. reported three ureteroneocystostomy procedures with a laparoscopic Boari flap.[8] They described no intraoperative or postoperative complications. With a range of 6 months to 3 years of follow up, all patients were asymptomatic and CT urogram at 6 months postoperatively showed improved drainage for the entire cohort.

Simmons et al. retrospectively compared their experience with laparoscopic reconstruction and open reconstruction.[9] This included five laparoscopic ureteroureterostomies, four laparoscopic ureteroneocystostomies, and three laparoscopic Boari flaps. The laparoscopic group had less blood loss and a shorter hospital stay. At a mean follow up of 23 months, ureteral patency was 100% in the laparoscopic group. One patient who underwent a laparoscopic Boari flap developed a postoperative urinoma. This was treated by bladder catheter drainage.

Rassweiler et al. reported ten cases of laparoscopic psoas hitch procedures performed with ($n=4$) and without ($n=6$) a Boari flap.[10] These ten patients were retrospectively compared with ten patients treated via an open approach. They noted that, compared with the open group, blood loss, analgesic requirement and convalescent time were significantly shorter in the laparoscopic group. Conversely, in the laparoscopic group the operative time was significantly longer.

Symons et al. retrospectively reviewed their cases of laparoscopic reconstructive surgery.[11] This included direct reimplantation in three patients and Boari flap in three patients. They reported no complications; intravenous urogram at 3 months showed prompt excretion in all patients.

Psoas Hitch

In the adult population, ureteroneocystostomy is most often performed as a result of ureteral obstruction or fistula. When ureteral length is inadequate for a tension free anastomosis, or if a nonrefluxing anastomosis is desired, a psoas hitch is a useful adjunctive procedure.

Technique

Positioning and Port Placement

Positioning and port placement is similar to that of the laparoscopic Boari flap (Fig. 23.5).

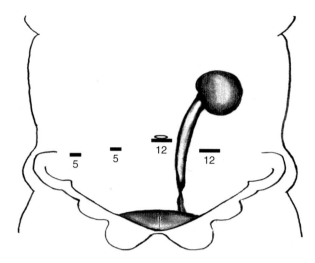

Procedure

The colon is mobilized and the ureter identified as in a laparoscopic Boari flap. After ureteral mobilization, the diseased segment of ureter is excised (Fig. 23.6). Attention is then turned to the bladder. The bladder is filled with normal saline. The peritoneum overlying the bladder is incised and the space of Retzius is developed. After bladder mobilization, the need for a psoas hitch is assessed. If the ureter can be brought down to the bladder under no tension, then a cystotomy is made in the side of the dome ipsilateral to the ureter and a primary anastomosis can be performed.

If a psoas hitch is required, often the contralateral bladder pedicle must be divided. The bladder dome is then anchored to the psoas muscle using at least two separate 2-0 Vicryl™ sutures.

If a refluxing anastomosis is preferred, an incision is made in the bladder to expose the mucosa. The ureter is then spatulated and anastomosed to the bladder mucosa using 3-0 Vicryl™ suture in an interrupted or running fashion. After completing the initial three interrupted sutures of the anastomosis at the apex of the spatulation, a ureteral stent is inserted as is described for the Boari flap and the remainder of the anastomosis is completed.

If desired, a nonrefluxing anastomosis can be performed by various techniques. Frequently, a Lich-Gregoir onlay procedure is performed. Puntambekar et al. also describe an intravesical nonrefluxing anastomosis[12] whereas Chung et al. describe a cystoscopy-assisted technique for creation of the submucosal tunnel.[13] However, the antireflux mechanism is likely less important in adults than for children and may increase the risk of postoperative ureteral obstruction.

After completion of the anastomosis, a closed suction drain is placed. The Foley catheter is left in place for 7 days and is removed when a postoperative cystogram shows no leakage. The suction drain is removed when the output is less than 50 cc/24 h. A ureteral stent is left in place for 4 weeks. Additionally, use of the *da Vinci*® robot positioned between the patient's legs with a similar port configuration makes intracorporeal suturing decidedly easier.

Fig. 23.6 Ureteroneocystostomy with psoas hitch. (**a**) After mobilization, the anterior wall of the bladder is brought to the psoas muscle. (**b**) The bladder is fixed to the psoas muscle. (**c**) The ureter is extended to the bladder to ensure that there is no tension on the anastomosis. (**d**, **e**): After spatulation, the ureter is anastomosed to the bladder. After the initial three sutures are placed at the apex of the spatulation, a ureteral stent is inserted. (**f**) Completed anastomosis. (**g**) Cystographic appearance after repair

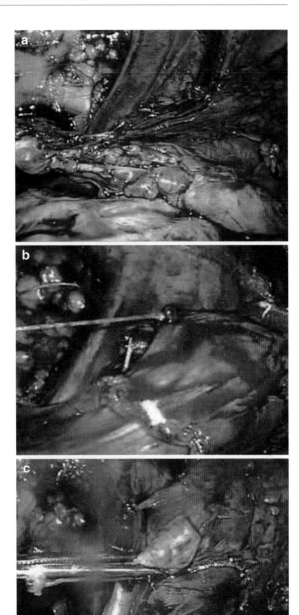

Fig. 23.6 (continued)

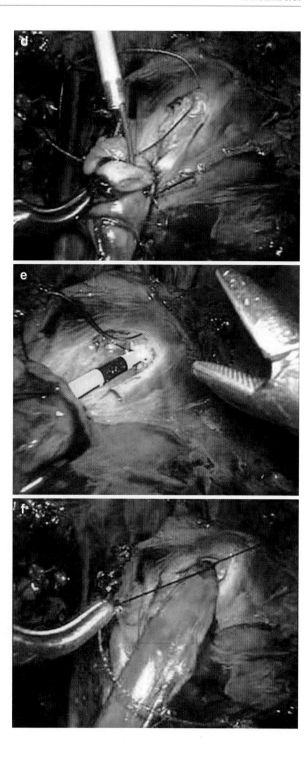

Fig. 23.6 (continued)

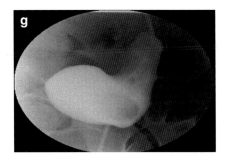

Discussion

Nezhat et al. reported on six patients who underwent a laparoscopic psoas hitch procedure for endometriosis.[14] No postoperative complications occurred and all patients had normal imaging at 1 year follow up. Rouprêt et al. described six patients who underwent laparoscopic distal ureterectomy and direct reimplantation with ($n=2$) and without ($n=4$) a psoas hitch for low-grade transitional cell carcinoma (TCC).[15] At a mean follow up of 32 months, two recurrences were documented, one patient recurred in the bladder and required a cystectomy and ileal conduit while another patient had tumor recurrence in the renal pelvis treated by percutaneous ablation. The authors state that during the ureteral dissection: (1) contact with the tumor should be avoided, (2) the ureter should be ligated proximal and distal to the tumor before transaction, and (3) intraoperative frozen sections to assess margin status are imperative before reimplantation.

Modi et al. reported 18 patients who underwent ureteroneocystostomy with a psoas hitch secondary to ureterovaginal fistula that occurred as a result of iatrogenic injury sustained during hysterectomy.[16] According to their report, 17 cases were successfully completed laparoscopically while 1 procedure was aborted due to intraoperative arrhythmia. At a mean follow up of 26 months, all patients were free of obstruction on postoperative excretory urography.

Ileal Ureter

Ileal interposition is indicated in the management of both benign and malignant ureteral stricture disease (Fig. 23.7). It is reserved for situations in which the defect cannot be bridged by other methods. Contraindications to ileal ureter include renal insufficiency ($Cr > 2$ mg/dL), bladder dysfunction, inflammatory bowel disease, and radiation enteritis.

Technique

Positioning and Port Placement[17] (Fig. 23.8a, b)

Bowel preparation is given the day before surgery. Preoperatively antibiotics for bowel and urinary tract surgical prophylaxis are also administered. The patient is placed in a

Fig. 23.7 Ileal ureter. The
ureter is anastomosed to a
loop of ileum in a side to
side fashion. The distal end
of ileum is sutured to the
bladder (Reprinted with
permission, Cleveland
Clinic Center for Medical
Art & Photography
© 2010. All Rights
Reserved)

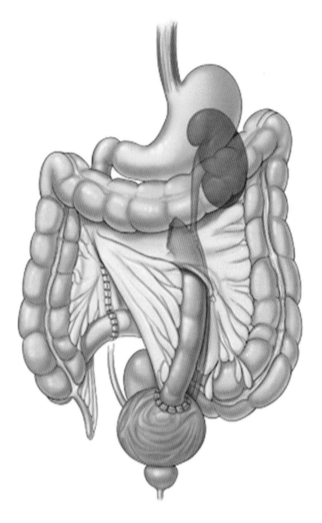

modified flank position for the upper tract portion of the procedure and then in lithotomy
with the table in full Trendelenburg position for the lower tract portion. However, the
procedure can be completed without repositioning of the patient.

Once pneumoperitoneum is established, a 12-mm port is placed at the lateral border of
the rectus muscle 3–4 cm below the umbilicus. In right-sided ileal interposition during the
upper tract dissection, this will serve as the left-hand port. Conversely, when the lower
tract dissection is performed, it will be used as the right-hand port and used for dissection/
anastomosis. In left-sided ileal interposition, it will be used as a right-hand port during
kidney/upper ureter dissection and as a left-hand port during bladder dissection. A second
12 mm port is placed at the lateral border of the rectus, 2 cm below the costal margin. In
right sided procedures, this will also be used for the upper tract dissection. In the case of a
left-sided procedure, this should be a 5 mm port and will be used by the left hand for the
upper tract dissection.

Fig. 23.8 Port placement for laparoscopic ileal ureter (**a**) right side and (**b**) left side (Reprinted with permission, Cleveland Clinic Center for Medical Art & Photography © 2010. All Rights Reserved)

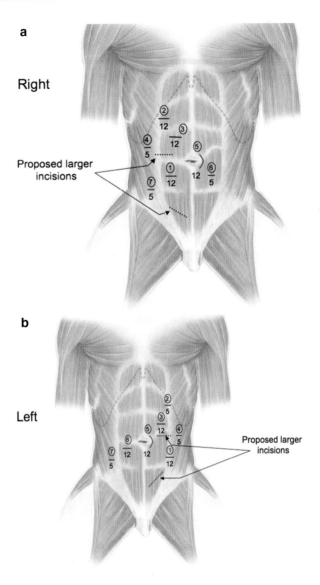

A third 12-mm port is placed midway between the two previous ports. In both right- and left-sided procedures, it serves as the camera port during the upper tract portion of the procedure, whereas it can be used as a retraction port during the lower tract dissection. A fourth 5-mm port is placed below the ribs at the level of the anterior axillary line. In both right and left procedures, it serves as a retraction port during the upper tract portion of the procedure. A fifth 12-mm port at the umbilicus will be used as a camera port during the bladder dissection in both right and left procedures. A sixth port should be placed 3–4 cm below the umbilicus on the contralateral side of the ileal interposition. In right-sided procedures, a 5-mm port will suffice and this will serve as the left-hand port during the bladder dissection. In left ileal interposition, a 12-mm port is required as this will be used by the right hand during the lower tract dissection A 5-mm assistant port will be placed two to three fingerbreadths medial to the anterior superior iliac spine.

A 3-mm to 7-cm open incision is made at the level of the ureteropelvic junction or the ureterovesical junction. This incision will serve as the site for ileal isolation, open ureteral dissection and for completion of one of the final two anastomoses. In cases for which the excision of a cuff of bladder is required, the incision is positioned in the pelvis. The incision is positioned in the ipsilateral upper quadrant when dense proximal ureteral strictures are anticipated.

Procedure

The line of Toldt is incised and the colon is reflected medially. The ureter is identified and traced superiorly to the renal pelvis (Fig. 23.9). Distally, the ureter is mobilized up to the

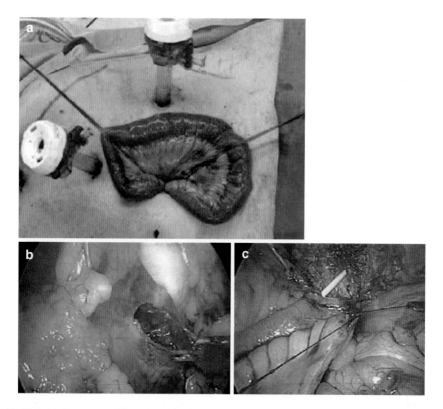

Fig. 23.9 (**a**) A segment of ileum is exteriorized. The required length of ileum is isolated and bowel continuity restored. The distal staple line is excised and an incision is made on the antimesenteric side near the proximal end. The ileum is vigorously irrigated and a stent placed through and through and secured in place. (**b**) A window is created within the mesentery of the ascending colon. (**c, d**) Distal end of Ileum is anastomosed to bladder in an isoperistaltic fashion. (**e, f**) After the proximal ileum is brought through a window in the large bowel mesentery, it is anastomosed to the renal pelvis. (**g**) Cystographic appearance of an ileal ureter

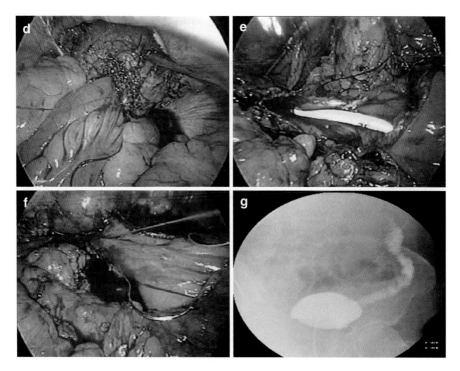

Fig. 23.9 (continued)

point of entry into the bladder. A 15-mm to 18-cm segment of ileum is identified approximately 15 cm from the ileocecal valve. The selected ileal segment is then exteriorized through the preselected incision site. Alternatively, Ramalingam et al. describe a transportal technique to exteriorize the bowel.[18] Instead of using a 12-mm port or a 3-mm to 7-cm incision, a 20-mm port is used. The bowel can then be brought out through the port for extracorporeal manipulation. This has the advantage of resulting in a smaller abdominal incision, but will not aid in ureteral or bladder dissection or anastomosis.

Using standard open techniques with gastrointestinal staplers, the segment of ileum is isolated and bowel continuity restored. The distal staple line of the isolated ileal segment is removed. The proximal staple line is not excised. An incision is then made on the proximal antimesenteric border of the bowel segment for the pyeloileal anastomosis. An anastomosis in this area is felt to result in less tension on the pyeloileal suture line.[17] The bowel segment is then copiously irrigated, a JJ stent placed through and through and secured in place. The intestinal loop is subsequently returned to the abdomen and the incision is then closed.

The diseased segment of ureter is transected and the proximal end spatulated. If performed for TCC, a cuff of bladder should be excised and the complete ureter extracted and frozen sections obtained to confirm negative margins. The bladder is then mobilized. The bladder is distended and a cystotomy is created at the dome.

In preparation for the anastomosis, care must be taken to orient the bowel segment in an isoperistaltic configuration. On the right side, this often requires twisting the segment 180°

on its mesentery. On the left side, a defect is created in the sigmoid mesentery just caudal to the level of the ureteropelvic junction and the interposed segment is positioned through the defect. This places less tension on the proximal anastomosis and allows for a more direct course of the ileal ureter.[17] If the mesenteric defect cannot be created safely, the ileal ureter can be passed anterior to the sigmoid colon. In this circumstance, consideration should be given to placing interrupted sutures through the ileal mesentery and the mesentery of the colon to obliterate the potential space in order to prevent potential bowel entrapment.[19] The distal end of the ileum is then anastomosed to the bladder in a mucosa-to-mucosa fashion with two running stitches of 3-0 or 4-0 Vicryl™ suture, each in a semicircular configuration. If there appears to be tension, interrupted sutures should be placed to reinforce the anastomosis. A similar procedure is performed for the proximal pyeloileal anastomosis. The proximal anastomosis should be performed to the renal pelvis to avoid a theoretically higher risk of stenosis.[17]

The anastomoses are then tested by distending the bladder to ensure a watertight seal. Two closed suction drains are placed, one near the pyeloileal and the second near the ileovesical anastomosis. The drains are removed once the output is less than 50 cc/24 h. The Foley catheter is removed after 7 days after a cystogram shows no leakage. The ureteral stent is left in place for 4 weeks.

Discussion

Reported experience with laparoscopic ileal interposition is limited. Gill et al. describe the initial case of a laparoscopic ileal ureter performed in a patient with TCC.[20] They reported no intraoperative or postoperative complications. Castillo et al. performed two cases because of extensive stenosis secondary to stone disease.[21] Patients were asymptomatic at a median of 18.5 months and postoperative urogram showed prompt drainage. They reported no complications. Kamat and Khandelwal reported their experience in two patients who underwent surgery for multiple tuberculous strictures. Short-term follow up showed good patency of the ileal loop. Complications included ileus and entrapment of the bowel by the ileal loop mesentery.[19]

Stein et al. reviewed seven cases of laparoscopic ileal substitution and compared them with seven open procedures in a retrospective fashion.[17] They noted a significantly decreased narcotic requirement and faster convalescence in the laparoscopic group. Complications included enteric anastomotic leak in one patient requiring reoperation. This occurred after a completely intracorporeal technique was used to isolate the ileum. Since this complication occurred, they state that in subsequent procedures that bowel harvesting was performed through a small open incision. Desai et al. also described a single port ileal ureter.[22] They described no intraoperative or postoperative complications.

Transureteroureterostomy

TUU is indicated in the treatment of lower ureteral lesions when ureteroneocystostomy, with or without a psoas hitch or Boari flap, is not feasible. The main concern with TUU is the potential for putting a normal ureter at risk with the intervention.

Technique

Positioning and Port Placement

The patient is given a dose of antibiotic preoperatively. The technique described is that reported by Piaggio and González.[23] The patient is initially placed in lithotomy position for cystoscopy and stent insertion into the recipient ureter. After stent placement, the patient is repositioned in the supine position. Pneumoperitoneum is established and working ports are placed in the hypogastrium and right and left flank at the level of the umbilicus in children and higher in older children. After port placement, the table is placed in Trendelenburg position and the table rotated so that the donor ureter side is elevated 30–40°.

Procedure

The ureter is identified at the level of the pelvic brim. The peritoneum overlying the ureter is incised and the ureter dissected as close to the bladder as possible. The ureter is then ligated and transected in an oblique fashion. Subsequently, the ureter is mobilized proximally, taking care to preserve the periureteral blood supply.

The surgeon then changes sides and the surgical table is repositioned to elevate the side of the recipient ureter. The peritoneum over the recipient ureter is incised at the level of the pelvic brim, but the ureter is left in situ. A tunnel through the rectosigmoid mesentery is created, joining the two peritoneal windows. The donor ureter is brought to the recipient side with care, ensuring no kinking of the ureter has occurred and no tension is present.

A longitudinal incision is made on the medial side of the recipient ureter. The donor and recipient ureter are anastomed with 6-0 reabsorbable monofilament suture and an abdominal drain is placed. The Foley catheter is removed on postoperative day number 1 or 2. The indwelling stent is left in place for 2–4 weeks.

Discussion

Dechet et al. described the feasibility of TUU in a swine model[24] but Piaggio and Gonzalez were the first to report the procedure in humans.[23] They reported their results with three cases of laparoscopic transureteroureterostomy performed in children. At 6 months follow up, all patients had normal kidney function and blood pressure. There was no conversion to open surgery. The only complication reported was a transient urinary leak. Additional complications reported by Dechet et al. included anastomotic stricture, urinary tract infection, and ileus.

Augmentation Cystoplasty

Enterocystoplasty effectively provides an increased vesical storage capacity and compliance by anastomosing an adequately sized, well-vascularized patch of bowel to the urinary bladder. The morbidity and postoperative discomfort due to the incision associated with the open technique may prolong hospital stay, increase the metabolic needs for wound healing, and delay postoperative recovery. The laparoscopic approach, albeit limited because of technical complexity, tries to mimic the steps of the well-established open technique with the advantages of a minimally invasive procedure.

Technique

Positioning and Port Placement

Preoperative preparation includes a low residue and a clear liquid diet for two days prior to surgery (Fig. 23.10). A bowel preparation is given the day before surgery. Preoperative antibiotics for bowel and urinary tract surgical prophylaxis are given.

The patient is placed in a low lithotomy position and pneumatic compression stockings are applied to both legs. Cystoscopically, single-J ileoureteral stents (7F, 90 cm, Circon-Surgitek, Santa Barbara, CA) are inserted into the renal pelves bilaterally. The external ends of both stents are secured to a Foley catheter. A four-port transperitoneal laparoscopic approach is used: 12-mm port at the superior umbilical crease, 5-mm or 12-mm port at the lateral border of the right rectus muscle at the level of the umbilicus, 5-mm port at the lateral border of the left rectus muscle at the level of the umbilicus, and 5-mm port at the level of the left anterior superior iliac spine.

Procedure[25]

The bladder is distended with saline and circumferentially mobilized laparoscopically. After mobilization, the bladder is decompressed. Depending on the preoperative choice of

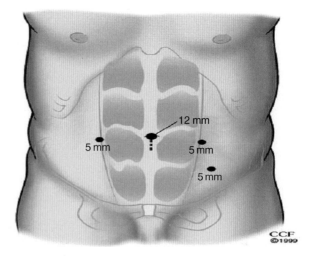

Fig. 23.10 Port placement for laparoscopic enterocystoplasty (Reprinted with permission, Cleveland Clinic Center for Medical Art & Photography © 2010. All Rights Reserved)

Fig. 23.11 Umbilical port incision is enlarged for bowel exteriorization (Reprinted with permission, Cleveland Clinic Center for Medical Art & Photography © 2010. All Rights Reserved)

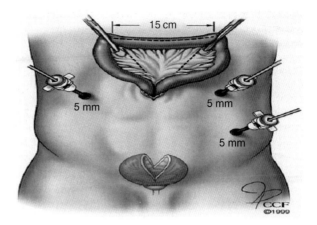

the specific bowel segment (ileum, right colon, or left colon), an appropriate 15-cm length of bowel is identified using two primary criteria. First, the bowel segment should reach the area of the bladder neck without tension, and second, a well-defined arterial arcade in its mesentery should be present. The distal end of the selected bowel segment is marked with a superficial electrocautery burn for identification.

The preselected loop of bowel is delivered outside the abdomen through a 2-cm extension of the umbilical port incision (Fig. 23.11). During laparoscopic bladder augmentation, the authors elect to perform bowel reconstruction extracorporally for the following reasons:

1. Bowel mesentery can be precisely incised after ensuring good vascularity.
2. Bowel reanastomosis can be performed using open surgical technique.
3. Irrigation of the excluded bowel loop can be performed without any peritoneal spillage, thereby limiting the potential for subsequent pelvic abscess formation.
4. Detubularization and construction of complex enteric pouches can be performed expeditiously by open suturing.
5. If the mesenteric length allows the segment of bowel to be delivered outside the anterior abdominal wall without evidence of bowel ischemia, it is also likely to reach the bladder without tension.
6. This approach allows considerable savings in overall operative time.

Using open technique, the appropriate bowel segment with its mesenteric pedicle is isolated, bowel continuity is reestablished, and the mesenteric window is closed (Fig. 23.12).

The isolated bowel segment is meticulously cleansed by irrigation and detubularized along its antimesenteric border. No additional reconstruction is necessary if the sigmoid colon is used. For the ileum, a U-shaped plate is created by side-to-side anastomosis using continuous absorbable suture (2-0 Vicryl™). When using the cecum and the proximal ascending colon, they are detubularized, and an appendectomy is performed.

Fig. 23.12 Bowel
reanastomosis is performed
cephalad to the excluded
segment of bowel
(Reprinted with permission,
Cleveland Clinic Center for
Medical Art & Photography
© 2010. All Rights
Reserved)

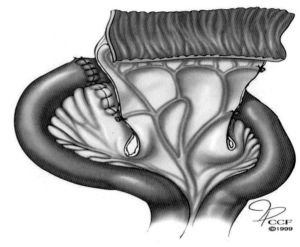

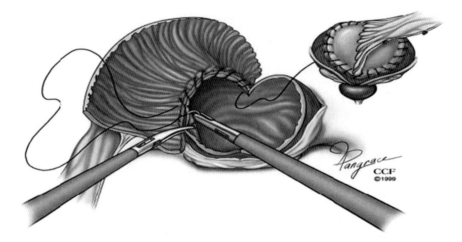

Fig. 23.13 Enterovesical anastomosis (Reprinted with permission, Cleveland Clinic Center for
Medical Art & Photography © 2010. All Rights Reserved)

An orientation suture is placed at the cephalad end and at the caudal end of the bowel
patch to facilitate subsequent laparoscopic identification. The bowel is then returned to the
abdominal cavity, and the infraumbilical incision is closed around the reinserted 12-mm
umbilical port. A 15-cm anteroposterior cystotomy incision is created using electrosurgical scissors. The preplaced stay sutures on the bowel segment are oriented properly, and
the mesenteric pedicle is inspected to rule out torsion. Circumferential, continuous, full-
thickness, single-layer anastomosis of the bowel mucosa and muscularis with the bladder
wall is created by laparoscopic suturing (Fig. 23.13).

Discussion

The surgical technique of enterocystoplasty has the following basic prerequisites:

1. Bladder mobilization with creation of an adequate-sized cystotomy (in some cases, subtotal cystectomy)
2. Selection of an optimal segment of bowel based on a broad, well-vascularized mesenteric pedicle
3. Isolation of the bowel segment
4. Reestablishment of bowel continuity and closure of mesenteric window
5. Detubularization and appropriate fashioning of the bowel segment without peritoneal soiling from bowel contents
6. Performance of a tension-free, watertight, full-thickness, circumferential, mucosa-to-mucosa anastomosis of the bowel to the bladder
7. Establishment of adequate urinary drainage

On the basis of the authors' experience, laparoscopic enterocystoplasty appears to adequately and efficaciously achieve all these objectives.

Conclusions

Minimally invasive techniques are being applied with increasing frequency to complex reconstructive procedures.

- The laparoscopic approach attempts to duplicate the principles of open surgery while offering minimal morbidity, decreased hospitalization and blood loss, and enhancing cosmesis.
- All techniques described are evolving. The prolonged operative time reflects an initial laparoscopic learning curve.
- Careful case selection and planning is important. However limited data reported in the literature tend to support the safety and efficacy of a laparoscopic approach.
- Boari flap, ileal interposition, and enterocystoplasty remain more challenging and are highly advanced techniques.

References

1. Hasan ST, Marshall C, Robson WA, Neal DE. Clinical outcome and quality of life following enterocystoplasty for idiopathic detrusor instability and neurogenic bladder dysfunction. *Br J Urol.* 1995;76:551-557.
2. Mundy AR, Stephenson TP. "Clam" ileocystoplasty for the treatment of refractory urge incontinence. *Br J Urol.* 1985;57:641-646.

3. Castillo OA, Litvak JP, Kerkebe M, Olivares R, Urena RD. Early experience with the laparoscopic Boari flap at a single institution. *J Urol*. 2005;173:862-865.
4. Simmons MN, Gill IS, Fergany AF, Kaouk JH, Desai MM. Technical modifications to laparoscopic Boari flap. *Urology*. 2007;69:175-180.
5. Lima GC, Rais-Bahrami S, Link RE, Kavoussi LR. Laparoscopic ureteral reimplantation: a simplified dome advancement technique. *Urology*. 2005;66(6):1307-1309.
6. Fugita OE, Dinlenc C, Kavoussi L. The laparoscopic Boari flap. *J Urol*. 2001;166:51-53.
7. Modi P, Goel R, Dodia S, Devra A. Case report: laparoscopic Boari flap. *J Endourol*. 2006;20(9):642-645.
8. Ramalingam M, Senthil K, Pai MG. Laparoscopic Boari flap repair: report of 3 cases. *J Laparoendosc Adv Surg Tech A*. 2008;18(2):271-275.
9. Simmons MN, Gill IS, Fergany AF, Kaouk JH, Desai MM. Laparoscopic ureteral reconstruction for benign stricture disease. *Urology*. 2007;69:280-284.
10. Rassweiler JJ, Gözen AS, Erdogru T, Sugiono M, Teber D. Ureteral reimplantation for management of ureteral strictures: a retrospective comparison of laparoscopic and open techniques. *Eur Urol*. 2007;51(2):512-522.
11. Symons S, Kurien A, Desai M. Laparoscopic ureteral reimplantation: a single center experience and literature review. *J Endourol*. 2009;23(2):269-274.
12. Puntambekar S, Palep RJ, Gurjar AM. Laparoscopic ureteroneocystostomy with psoas hitch. *J Minim Invasive Gynecol*. 2006;13:302-305.
13. Chung H, Jeong BC, Kim HH. Laparoscopic ureteroneocystostomy with vesicopsoas hitch: nonrefluxing ureteral reimplantation using cystoscopy-assisted submucosal tunneling. *J Endourol*. 2006;20(9):632-639.
14. Nezhat CH, Malik S, Nezhat F, Nezhat C. Laparoscopic ureteroneocystostomy and vesicopsoas hitch for infiltrative endometriosis. *JSLS*. 2004;8(1):3-7.
15. Rouprêt M, Harmon JD, Sanderson KM. Laparoscopic distal ureterectomy and anastomosis for management of low-risk upper urinary tract transitional cell carcinoma: preliminary results. *BJU Int*. 2007;99:623-627.
16. Modi P, Gupta R, Rizvi SJ. Laparoscopic ureteroneocystostomy and psoas hitch for post-hysterectomy ureterovaginal fistula. *J Urol*. 2008;180:615-617.
17. Stein RJ, Turna B, Patel NS, et al. Laparoscopic assisted ileal ureter: technique, outcomes and comparison to the open procedure. *J Urol*. 2009;182:1032-1039.
18. Ramalingam M, Senthil K, Pai MG. Modified technique of laparoscopy-assisted surgeries (transportal). *J Endourol*. 2008;22(12):2681-2685.
19. Kamat N, Khandelwal P. Laparoscopy-assisted ileal ureter creation for multiple tuberculous strictures: report of two cases. *J Endourol*. 2006;20(6):388-393.
20. Gill IS, Savage SJ, Senagore AJ, Sung GT. Laparoscopic ileal ureter. *J Urol*. 2000;163(4):1199-1202.
21. Castillo OA, Sanchez-Salas R, Vitagliano G, Diaz MA, Foneron A. A laparoscopy-assisted ureter interposition by ileum. *J Endourol*. 2008;22(4):687-692.
22. Desai MM, Stein R, Rao P, et al. Embryonic natural orifice transumbilical endoscopic surgery (E-NOTES) for advanced reconstruction: initial experience. *Urology*. 2009;73(1):182-187.
23. Piaggio LA, González R. Laparoscopic transureteroureterostomy: a novel approach. *J Urol*. 2007;177:2311-2314.
24. Dechet CB, Young MM, Segura JW. Laparoscopic transureteroureterostomy: demonstration of its feasibility in swine. *J Endourol*. 1999;13(7):487-493.
25. Gill IS, Rackley RR, Meraney AM, Marcello PW, Sung GT. Laparoscopic enterocystoplasty. *Urology*. 2000;55(2):178-181.

Difficulties in Laparoscopic Ureterolysis and Retroperitoneal Lymph Node Dissection

24

Mohamed A. Atalla, Eboni J. Woodard, and Louis R. Kavoussi

Laparoscopic Ureterolysis

Retroperitoneal fibrosis (RPF) is a chronic progressive disease process characterized by inflammation and fibrosis in the retroperitoneum that may lead to compression of vital structures, including the ureters. RPF primarily affects patients between 40 and 60 years of age, with an estimated incidence of 1:200,000 to 1:500,000 per year. Most cases are deemed idiopathic with drugs, such as methysergide and other ergot alkaloids, accounting for a significant portion of cases with identifiable causes. In some instances, RPF can be attributed to retroperitoneal malignancies or prior exposure to retroperitoneal radiation therapy.[1]

The retroperitoneal fibrotic mass generally centers near the distal aorta at the level of L4–L5 and may extend from the mediastinum to the iliac vessels. The mass can encase the ureters, leading to hydronephrosis and a functional obstruction via extrinsic compression and interference with ureteral peristalsis.[2] Patients often present with pain in the lower back or flanks. Other presenting symptoms include weight loss, anorexia, nausea, malaise, fever, hypertension, and oliguria. Compression of the inferior vena cava (IVC) may result in deep venous thrombosis or lower extremity edema. Symptoms related to compression of other organs are rare. Symptoms are typically present for 4–6 months before the diagnosis of RPF is made. Laboratory evaluation may reveal an elevated erythrocyte sedimentation rate, moderate leukocytosis, and mild anemia. Historically, 50% of patients have uremia of variable degrees.[3]

Medical management of RPF consists mainly of immunosuppressants, such as mycophenolate mofetil, and corticosteroids, or a combination thereof.[4] Clinical response rates of up to 80% have been reported with resolution of pain and constitutional symptoms, reduction in mass size, and improvement in ureteral obstruction and IVC compression. However, medical management has been shown to be most effective in the proliferative phase. For patients who have failed medical therapy or for definitive primary therapy, surgery is the mainstay of treatment.

M.A. Atalla (✉)
The Arthur Smith Institute for Urology, Hofstra University Medical School, North Shore LIJ Health System, New Hyde Park, New York, USA
e-mail: atalla@att.net

A.M. Al-Kandari and I.S. Gill (eds.), *Difficult Conditions in Laparoscopic Urologic Surgery*, 343
DOI: 10.1007/978-1-84882-105-7_24, © Springer-Verlag London Limited 2011

Historically, pyelography was the radiographic study of choice for cases of suspected RPF, and typical findings included hydronephrosis and medial deviation of the ureters.[2] Today, radiographic diagnosis has largely been dominated by computed tomography (CT) with or without contrast, depending on the patient's renal function. CT can be used to evaluate the degree of obstruction, as well the extent of the retroperitoneal mass and its relationship to surrounding anatomy. In patients with significant renal impairment, retrograde pyelography can demonstrate findings similar to those seen on intravenous pyelography. MRI and MR urography may also be of assistance in differentiating RPF from other causes of hydronephrosis. Diuretic nuclear renography is the best modality to quantify obstruction, and also assesses differential renal function, which is useful in planning treatment for unilateral RPF.

The main principles of operative therapy include careful dissection of the ureter with preservation of the periureteral blood supply, and isolation of the ureter from the fibrotic process. Although open ureterolysis was the traditional method for surgical management, laparoscopic ureterolysis in the hands of an experienced surgeon has been shown to be a safe and effective approach. The first laparoscopic ureterolysis was reported by Kavoussi and associates in 1992, and later reproduced by others with similar success.[5] When compared with open surgery, laparoscopic ureterolysis has equivalent results including operative time, estimated blood loss, length of hospital stay, complication rates, transfusion requirements, and success rates. For cases of idiopathic RPF, laparoscopy has the advantage of a shorter hospital stay and reduced transfusion requirement.[6] The difficulties encountered with laparoscopic ureterolysis usually correlate with the degree of fibrosis, owing to a more difficult dissection.

Technique and Tips

Preoperative antibiotics are administered intravenously. If stents are not in place, they should be placed prior to the procedure. Long stents should be used to avoid pulling the distal end proximally into the ureter by traction during the dissection. It is helpful to prep the genitalia into the operative field in the event the stent needs to be exchanged intraoperatively. The patient is secured to the operating table in a supine postion. The procedure is performed through a transabdominal approach. After insufflation with a Veress needle, three trocars are placed in the midline, starting at the subxyphoid position spaced 8–10 cm apart. A fourth trocar can be placed lateral to the rectus abdominus muscle at the level of the umbilicus. After inspecting the bowel for inadvertent injury during trocar placement, the bowel is moved medially to expose the white line of Toldt. The white line is then incised from the inferior margin of the kidney to the level of the iliac vessels. The colon is reflected medially to expose the renal hilum and fibrotic retroperitoneal process.

The ureter should be identified outside the mass or area of involvement. In cases of primary pelvic involvement, it is helpful to identify the kidney and renal pelvis and work distally. When the upper ureter is involved, an incision is made medial to the medial umbilical ligament and the ureter is identified as it courses posterior into the bladder. If the ureter cannot be identified, it may be helpful to exchange the stent for a super stiff guidewire. Gentle manipulation of the wire can demonstrate bowing of the ureter. Occasionally, lighted stents may be helpful, although the fibrotic process can block transmission of bright light.

Before excising the mass, biopsies should be obtained for the frozen section to exclude obvious malignancy. The ureter sometimes will peel off the fibrotic process. Many times there is a loss of distinction between the ureteral wall and surrounding tissue. In these cases, sharp dissection is required. After dissecting the ureter free of the fibrotic mass, the ureter should be carefully inspected and any ureterotomies should be primarily repaired.

There is a temptation to try to bluntly pull the ureter away from the surrounding tissue. Unfortunately, the normal elasticity of the ureter is compromised by this process, making the ureter liable to tearing or avulsion. Small tears may be oversewn and a drain left adjacent. In cases of avulsion, ureteral reimplantation may be needed. If it is high, alternatives such as bowel interposition, autotransplantation, or even nephrectomy should be entertained. These scenarios should be discussed preoperatively with the patient.

Intraperitonealization of the ureter is helpful to avoid reincorporation within the fibrotic process. The lateral edge of the peritoneum posterior to the ureter should be secured to the psoas fascia or area of prior peritoneal incision at the line of Toldt. Care needs to be taken to ensure that pockets for internal herniation are obliterated. Alternatively, a piece of omentum can be placed around or posterior to the ureter and secured to itself or the sidewall. The ureter should not be kinked or placed under any tension during this process. Assess that the internal stent has not migrated and conclude the procedure in a standard manner. Drains are unnecessary unless a ureteral injury is suspected.

Postoperatively, patients are allowed clear liquids and are advanced to a regular diet as tolerated. They are transitioned from intravenous to oral pain medication. The Foley catheter is removed on postoperative day 1. Patients are typically ready for discharge on postoperative day 2. The ureteral stent can be removed in 3 weeks. Two weeks after stent removal, laboratory tests and imaging are obtained to evaluate renal function and resolution of obstruction.

Difficulties

Exposure and Port Placement

Improper positioning and port placement can result in a difficult dissection, inadvertent bowel injury, and a higher incidence of complications. As with all laparoscopic surgery, proper port placement is essential to providing adequate working space and sufficient access to the surgical field. Trocar placement should be determined by the proximal and distal extent of the fibrotic process and the length of ureter involved. Rotating the bed 45° toward the surgeon and placing the patient in the Trendelenburg position helps to displace the bowel medially and superiorly and away from the operative field. This helps decrease the risk of inadvertently injuring the bowel during trocar placement. When incising the white line of Toldt, maintaining a generous lateral sleeve of peritoneum on the bowel facilitates later intraperitonealization of the ureter.

Bowel Injury and Internal Hernias

Careful dissection should be exercised around the colon and small bowel. Avoid thermal dissection within a centimeter of any bowel. Bowel injuries are best repaired shortly after their occurrence, and, therefore, recognition is vital. Mesenteric defects resulting from colon reflection are often caused inadvertently. These defects are important to recognize intraoperatively and should be closed primarily using clips or absorbable suture to avoid the high risk of small bowel obstruction resulting from internal herniation.

Vascular Injuries

Any laparoscopic surgery of the retroperitoneum carries the risk of vascular injury. Renal, gonadal, and lumbar vessels are most commonly afflicted. When such an injury occurs, imprudent application of clips and staples should be avoided. Instead, begin compression with a blunt instrument or a mini laparotomy tape introduced through a 12-mm trocar. This allows time for careful planning to control the hemorrhage. Clips or sutures are then used to control or repair the bleeding vessels.

Major vascular injuries, such as those involving the IVC, should be approached in a similar manner. Venous lacerations will usually stop bleeding after pressure is applied. After adequate compression using a mini laparotomy tape, an additional trocar should be placed, if needed. The trocar can be used for introduction of a laparoscopic Satinsky clamp or another vascular clamp. Apply the clamp beyond the laceration while it is repaired using a fine Prolene™ (Ethicon, Inc., Somerville, NJ) suture.

Ureteral Injury and Stricture Formation

Ureteral injury is more likely to occur during ureterolysis due to the associated inflammatory process, making the dissection more difficult. Preoperative ureteral stent placement will facilitate identification and dissection of the ureter and may help reduce the incidence of ureteral injury.

When dissecting the ureter from the fibrotic mass, dissection directly along the ureter should be avoided to prevent devascularization of the ureter and an increased risk of postoperative stricture formation. Excessive dissection also increases the risk of ureterotomy. Additionally, judicious use of electrocautery is important to reduce the risk of thermal injury to the ureter. The entire ureter should be carefully inspected after the dissection is complete, and any ureterotomies should be repaired primarily with a fine, absorbable suture.

The ureter also could be injured or kinked during intraperitonealization. The lie of the proximal ureter should be inspected carefully to avoid kinking of the ureter and subsequent obstruction.

Laparoscopic Retroperitoneal Lymph Node Dissection

Patients with stage I nonseminomatous germ cell tumors (NSGCT) have several treatment options, including surveillance, chemotherapy, and retroperitoneal lymph node dissection (RPLND).[7] The primary, and often only, site of metastasis in NSGCT is the retroperitoneal lymph nodes. Left untreated, retroperitoneal lymph node metastasis is usually fatal. Despite improvement in radiographic techniques, 15–40% of patients are clinically understaged. Open RPLND is the standard of care for staging and treatment. With advances in surgical technique, perioperative morbidity and mortality have been minimized, but up to 70% of patients undergoing RPLND receive no therapeutic benefit.[8] This outcome makes a minimally invasive approach a sensible option.

Laparoscopic RPLND first emerged as a diagnostic and staging tool. With advances in imaging technology, the development of automated suturing devices, the advent of hemostatic agents, and the increasing skill level of surgeons, laparoscopic RPLND has evolved into a therapeutic operation that upholds all the necessary oncologic principles that open surgery provides.[9] Nevertheless, laparoscopic RPLND is a technically challenging procedure that should be reserved for experienced laparoscopic surgeons who are also comfortable performing open RPLND and applying advanced vascular skills as necessary.

The indications for RPLND in low-stage NSCGT are clinical stage I or IIA, negative serum tumor markers, and the absence of comorbidities that would preclude safe surgery. More recently, laparoscopic RPLND has also been offered to patients with residual masses following primary chemotherapy. In the hands of an experienced laparoscopic surgeon, the benefits of laparoscopic RPLND include shorter convalescence, more favorable cosmetic results, less postoperative pain and morbidity, and reduced operative blood loss and length of hospital stay.[10]

Postchemotherapy laparoscopic RPLND is more technically demanding due to the resulting desmoplastic reaction, and should be performed in centers with experience in primary laparoscopic RPLND. Permpongkosol et al. reported on 16 consecutive patients who underwent postchemotherapy laparoscopic RPLND by a single surgeon, with 14 dissections successfully completed.[11] Seven patients (43.8%) developed complications and two (12.5%) required open conversion. All intraoperative complications were vascular injuries. Underscoring the importance of surgeon experience, all operative complications occurred during the first half of the series. Retrograde ejaculation is severalfold more common in postchemotherapy than in primary laparoscopic RPLND.[12] No perioperative mortality has been reported with either procedure.

Technique and Tips

Patients undergo a mechanical bowel preparation the day before surgery and take only clear liquids until midnight. Broad-spectrum antibiotics are administered preoperatively, and sequential antiembolic pneumatic boots are placed on the lower extremities. With the patient in the supine position, the arms are padded and secured to the patient's sides. The patient should be secured to the table to allow safe rotation of the table. After placement of an orogastric tube and a Foley catheter, the abdomen is insufflated with a Veress needle. Four 12-mm trocars are placed in the midline, equally spaced, beginning 2 cm inferior to the xiphoid process and extending to the symphysis pubis (Fig. 24.1).

Reflection of the colon is carried out differently, depending on the side that is approached. On the left side, incise the white line of Toldt from the level of the spleen to the iliac vessels. Incise the splenocolic and colorenal ligaments for added mobility. On the right side, incise the peritoneum superior to the hepatic flexure and medially to Winslow's foramen. The Kocher maneuver is performed to the second portion of the duodenum to expose the IVC.

When incising the posterior peritoneum, avoid incising lateral to Gerota's fascia, which would release the lateral attachments of the kidney, allowing it to fall into the operative field. Avoid using electrocautery near the bowel to prevent inadvertent thermal injury. When mobilizing the colon, if a hole is made in the mesentery, it should be repaired immediately. If left unrepaired, it can be a source of bleeding and lead to the formation of an internal hernia postoperatively.

The spermatic cord is first dissected (Fig. 24.2). The camera is placed in the second lowest port and a retractor is placed in the subxyphoid port. Identify the cord at the internal

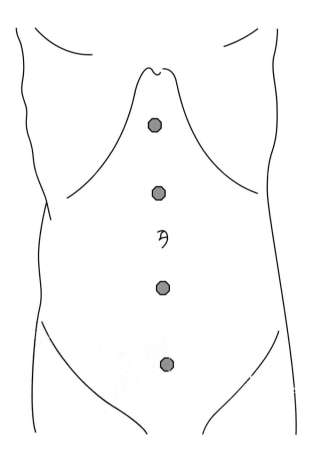

Fig. 24.1 Port placement for laparoscopic RPLND

Fig. 24.2 Dissection of the spermatic cord at the internal inguinal ring

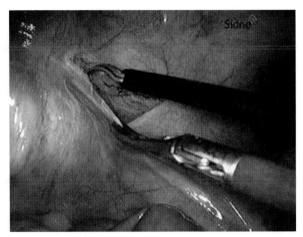

ring and dissect it toward the IVC on the right and the renal vein on the left. This can be the most physically challenging aspect of the dissection. Placement of a lateral trocar at the level of the umbilicus in the mid-axillary line may facilitate the dissection. The roof of the internal ring may be opened, but care must be taken to avoid injury to the inferior epigastric vessels. Clips should be placed on the cord to prevent bleeding if the cord is inadvertently avulsed. Dissect distally until the orchiectomy suture is encountered.

The cord is traced proximally to identify the IVC (right), left renal vein (left), and aorta. The cord is adherent to the lower pole of Gerota's fascia and dissection with ligation is needed to free the cord in this area. It is important to identify the ureter early to avoid inadvertent injury. Ligate and transect the proximal end of the packet and remove the specimen in a retrieval bag.

Once the cord is dissected, the camera is shifted to the second uppermost port. A paddle retractor is placed in the lowest port. The renal vessels are identified next and clips are used generously to gather lymphatics and prevent a postoperative lymphocele. Following these vessels medially will identify the great vessels. On the right side, the lymphatic tissue is split from the surface of the IVC and bluntly dissected both medially and laterally. Care should be taken about the insertion of the clipped gonadal vein to avoid bleeding. On the left side, the left renal vain is traced to the IVC and the tissue is rolled medially off the IVC to help create the inter-aortocaval package.

Score the anterior lymphatic tissue, and use blunt dissection to separate the tissue from the anterior surface of the great vessels. Lift the lateral tissue and, using the suction irrigation device, separate this tissue from the underlying psoas fascia. Lumbar vessels and lymphatics should be meticulously clipped. Observe the distinction between the sympathetic chain and prominent lymphatic channels: the former should be left intact. Observe for accessory lower pole renal vessels. Excise the inter-aortocaval lymphatic tissue with great caution to avoid major vascular injury. When the dissection follows the surface of the aorta, care must be taken to avoid avulsing the gonadal arteries or injuring the inferior mesenteric artery. However, in some instances, it may be necessary to divide the inferior mesenteric artery.

Fig. 24.3 Retrocaval
dissection completed

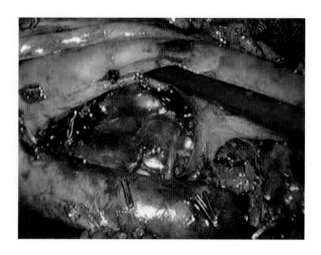

The retrocaval and retroaortic nodes are the last to be dissected. Using atraumatic forceps and an irrigation suction device, develop a plane between the posterior lymphatic
tissue and the great vessels. With the great vessels retracted anteriorly, tease the nodal
packet off the undersurface of the great vessels in a "split-and-roll" technique (Fig. 24.3).
Finally, laterally transpose and excise the nodal packet. Each packet should be placed in a
separate retrieval bag and removed.

At the conclusion of the dissection, inspect the abdomen carefully for bleeding or injury
to the surrounding viscera. Remove all trocars under direct vision and close the port sites
with a wound closure device.

Postchemotherapy laparoscopic RPLND presents special challenges when compared to
primary laparoscopic RPLND.[11] To be considered for such a procedure, patients with Stage
II or III disease should have negative tumor markers and should have demonstrated a
response to prior therapy, as evidenced by a decrease in size of the initial mass. Desmoplastic
tissue changes following chemotherapy may make standard templates difficult to follow
(Fig. 24.4). Nevertheless, a bilateral RPLND is performed in addition to removing the
residual tumor mass. Fine bipolar grasping forceps can be helpful and hemostatic agents
may be used.

Postoperatively, patients can be managed on a standard patient care unit. The Foley
catheter is usually removed on postoperative day 1. Diet can be advanced on postoperative
day 1, as bowel function usually returns within 24 h. Early ambulation is encouraged.
Patients are usually ready for discharge on postoperative day 2.

Difficulties

Exposure and Port Placement

The patient must be safely secured to the operating table with the arms tucked. This allows
ample rotation during the course of dissection. All four 12-mm ports must be adequately

Fig. 24.4 Dissection of a precaval residual mass following chemotherapy for testis cancer

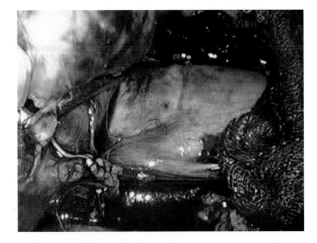

spaced in the midline, regardless of relation to the umbilicus, to prevent limitation in instrument mobility. The fourth port that is not in use by the working instruments or laparoscope should be used by the assistant for retraction of the bowel to aid in exposure. A paddle retractor is helpful in this instance.

Bleeding

Intraoperative bleeding is the most frequent complication of laparoscopic RPLND. Troublesome bleeding can occur from lumbar, gonadal, or mesenteric vessels, as well as from the vasa vasorum of the aorta. Most bleeding of this type can be controlled with electrocautery, clips, and hemostatic agents such as fibrin glue or Surgicel® (Ethicon, Inc., Somerville, NJ). Intracorporeal suturing may be required for persistent bleeding.

Significant bleeding can occur due to laceration of renal or lower pole accessory renal vessels. Every effort should be undertaken to repair injuries to these vessels without their division. Compression with mini laparotomy tapes should therefore be the first step, followed by repair using fine Prolene™ suture and clips.

IVC or aortic injuries usually occur while controlling tributaries or branches. When ligating lumbar vessels, leave a long stump on the aortic or caval side to facilitate their control in the event that a clip is dislodged. If a lumbar vessel retracts into the psoas muscle, uncontrolled bleeding can be managed with indirect pressure or a figure-of-eight stitch placed deep in the muscle. Lacerations of the IVC can often be controlled with prolonged, pinpoint direct pressure and, if necessary, hemostatic agents. It is important not to re-explore these lacerations after hemostasis is achieved, as the forming clot may be inadvertently dislodged. Laceration of the aorta can be managed initially with direct pressure, but usually requires intracorporeal suturing or open conversion. An Endo Stitch™ (Covidien, Dublin, Ireland) with a Lapra-Ty (Ethicon Endo-Surgery, Inc., Cincinnati, OH) on the end can accelerate suturing.

Organ Injury

Bowel injury is rarely reported (1–2%), but is potentially catastrophic, particularly if unrecognized. Sharp injuries can be primarily repaired, but thermal injuries require excision and often segmental resection. Particular care should be taken while mobilizing the duodenum, as these injuries are usually detrimental.

The ureters can also be inadvertently injured sharply using thermal energy, or by excessive skeletonization and devascularization. Care in dissection is the main preventive technique. Postchemotherapy RPLND patients may benefit from preoperative ureteral catheter placement if the residual mass intimately involves one of the ureters.

In the upper abdomen, the pancreas, gall bladder, spleen, and liver are rarely injured. Intraoperative pancreatic injury should be repaired promptly, and a drain should be placed. Injury to the gallbladder may require cholecystectomy. Splenic and liver injuries can usually be conservatively treated with argon beam coagulation and hemostatic agents.

Organ injury can also result from vascular injury. Irreparable renal vascular injury may necessitate nephrectomy. Accessory renal vascular injury should not lead to nephrectomy. These vessels are often injured when their course is anomalous or during the inter-aortocaval, retroaortic, or retrocaval dissections. Inferior mesenteric artery or vein injury should not have a deleterious effect. Superior mesenteric artery injury, on the other hand, is detrimental, and requires open reconstruction and possible bowel resection if infarction occurs.

Ejaculatory Dysfunction

Operative template modification has allowed preservation of antegrade ejaculation in most patients.[13] Sympathetic chain injury can result in ejaculatory dysfunction in 5% of cases. This is best avoided by careful dissection of lymphatics posterior to the IVC and distinction from sympathetic chain fibers, which they can closely resemble. Due to the risk of ejaculatory dysfunction, patients should be encouraged to undergo preoperative sperm banking.

Chylous Ascites

Chylous ascites and lymphocele development are delayed postoperative complications.[14] These can be avoided by liberal clipping of lymphatic channels during dissection. Preoperatively, to reduce the risk of chylous ascites, patients are started on a low-fat diet 1–2 weeks before surgery, which they continue up to 2 weeks postoperatively. Ultimate management may require reexploration to identify the site of leakage with clip placement. Lymphangiography has also been helpful in identifying and sealing a leak.

Small Bowel Obstruction

Bowel obstruction can result from fascial hernial defects stemming from improper closure of port sites. Internal hernias can also result in bowel obstruction if mesenteric defects caused during dissection are not appropriately closed. These defects should be closed with absorbable suture or clips.

Conclusion

Laparoscopic ureterolysis and laparoscopic RPLND are both challenging surgeries requiring advanced laparoscopic skills to duplicate the success seen with their open counterparts. The most important skill necessary to master these procedures is the ability to recognize potential difficulties and complications and take appropriate steps to minimize these risks before they result in an adverse event. Being able to anticipate such complications allows the surgeon to be mentally prepared to respond effectively and expeditiously and have the necessary instruments available ahead of time. Finally, complications will occur, but having a high level of suspicion for both common and unusual events will allow the surgeon to minimize the most catastrophic sequelae.

References

1. Vaglio A, Salvarani C, Buzio C. Retroperitoneal fibrosis. *Lancet.* 2006;367(9506):241-251.
2. Cronin CG, Lohan DG, Blake MA, et al. Retroperitoneal fibrosis: a review of clinical features and imaging findings. *AJR Am J Roentgenol.* 2008;191(2):423-431.
3. van Bommel EF. Retroperitoneal fibrosis. *Neth J Med.* 2002;60(6):231-242.
4. Scheel PJ Jr, Piccini J, Rahman MH, et al. Combined prednisone and mycophenolate mofetil treatment for retroperitoneal fibrosis. *J Urol.* 2007;178(1):140-143.
5. Kavoussi LR, Clayman RV, Brunt LM, et al. Laparoscopic ureterolysis. *J Urol.* 1992;147(2): 426-429.
6. Srinivasan AK, Richstone L, Permpongkosol S, et al. Comparison of laparoscopic with open approach for ureterolysis in patients with retroperitoneal fibrosis. *J Urol.* 2008;179(5):1875-1878.
7. Bosl GJ, Bajorin DF, Sheinfeld J. Cancer of the testis. In: DeVita VT, Hellman S, Rosenberg SA, eds. *Cancer, Principles & Practice of Oncology.* 7th ed. Philadelphia: Lippincott Williams & Wilkins; 2005:1491-1518.
8. Lashley DB, Lowe BA. A rational approach to managing stage I nonseminomatous germ cell cancer. *Urol Clin North Am.* 1998;25(3):405-423.
9. Allaf ME, Bhayani SB, Link RE, et al. Laparoscopic retroperitoneal lymph node dissection: duplication of open technique. *Urology.* 2005;65(3):575-577.
10. Janetschek G, Hobisch A, Peschel R, et al. Laparoscopic retroperitoneal lymph node dissection for clinical stage I nonseminomatous testicular carcinoma: long-term outcome. *J Urol.* 2000;163(6):1793-1796.
11. Permpongkosol S, Lima GC, Warlick CA, et al. Postchemotherapy laparoscopic retroperitoneal lymph node dissection: evaluation of complications. *Urology.* 2007;69(2):361-365.
12. Kenney PA, Tuerk IA. Complications of laparoscopic retroperitoneal lymph node dissection in testicular cancer. *World J Urol.* 2008;26(6):561-569.
13. Donohue JP, Thornhill JA, Foster RS, et al. Retroperitoneal lymphadenectomy for clinical stage A testis cancer (1965 to 1989): modifications of technique and impact on ejaculation. *J Urol.* 1993;149(2):237-243.
14. Link RE, Amin N, Kavoussi LR. Chylous ascites following retroperitoneal lymphadenectomy for testes cancer. *Nat Clin Pract Urol.* 2006;3(4):226-232.

Difficulties in Laparoscopic Management of Vesicovaginal Fistula

25

Shrenik Shah

Introduction

Vesicovaginal fistula (VVF) is an abnormal fistulous connection extending between the bladder and the vagina that allows the continuous involuntary discharge of urine into the vaginal vault (Fig. 25.1). It is the most common acquired fistula of the urinary tract, and has been known since ancient times. In addition to the medical sequelae from these fistulas, they often have a profound effect on the patient's emotional well-being.

History of the Procedure

The first basic surgical principles for the repair of VVFs were described in 1663 by Hedrik von Roonhuyse by denuding the fistula margin of the bladder wall, with reapproximation of the edges using stiff, sharpened swan quills. Later, using Roonhuyse's technique, Johann Fatio documented the first successful VVF repair in 1675. In 1838, by use of leaden suture, John Peter Mettauer was the first U.S. surgeon to claim successful VVF repair. James Marion Sims published his famous discourse on the treatment of VVF in 1852. Sims achieved success on his 30th surgical attempt and emphasized the importance of good exposure, adequate resection of the fistula and scarred vaginal edges, and the critical importance of continuous postoperative bladder drainage. The first successful transabdominal approach to VVF repair was reported by Trendelenburg in 1888. The concept of interpositional flap was first proposed by Martius in 1928, using the labial fat pad. In 1950, O'Conor and Stovsky popularized the transabdominal approach and also proposed the use of electrocoagulation as an initial treatment modality in women with VVFs of 3.5 mm or less, citing a 73% success rate.

S. Shah
Department of Urology, Civil Hospital and B J Medical College, Ahmedabad, India
e-mail: drshreniks@gmail.com

A.M. Al-Kandari and I.S. Gill (eds.), *Difficult Conditions in Laparoscopic Urologic Surgery*, **355**
DOI: 10.1007/978-1-84882-105-7_25, © Springer-Verlag London Limited 2011

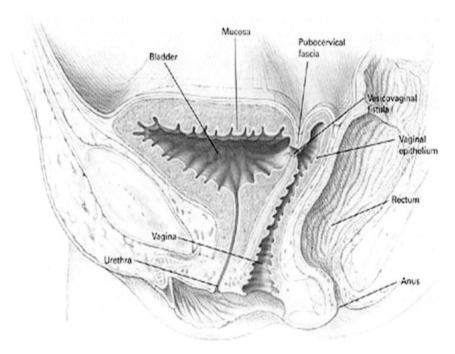

Fig. 25.1 Anatomy of VVF (From Shah.[16] Reprinted with permission from Mary Ann Liebert, Inc.)

Incidence

Vesicovaginal fistula has been a social and surgical problem for centuries. In the developed world, 90% of cases are caused by inadvertent injury to the bladder during gynecological, urological, and other pelvic surgery. Of the 190 consecutive patients at the Mayo Clinic, VVF resulted following gynecological surgery (82%), obstetric procedures (11%), malignant diseases (7%) and trauma (3%).[1] The incidence of fistula after hysterectomy is estimated to be approximately 0.1–0.2%. It occurs as a result of incidental unrecognized, iatrogenic cystotomy near the vaginal cuff.[2] In developing countries, the predominant cause of VVF is prolonged obstructed labor (97%). VVFs are associated with marked pressure necrosis, edema, tissue sloughing, and cicatrization. Incidence of obstetric fistula in developing countries is estimated to be 0.3–0.4% of total deliveries.

Clinical Presentation

- The uncontrolled leakage of urine into the vagina is the hallmark symptom of patients with VVF.
- Increase in vaginal discharge following pelvic surgery or pelvic radiotherapy with or without antecedent surgery.

- The patient may become a social outcast due to constant discharge of urine which causes strong repulsive odor and soakage of clothing.

Physical Examination

- *Per vaginal examination*: Pelvic examination by bivalved speculum usually provides a precise assessment of VVF including the location, size, and number. A full vaginal inspection is essential and should include assessment of tissue mobility; accessibility of the fistula to vaginal repair; determination of the degree of tissue inflammation, edema, and infection; and possible association of a rectovaginal fistula.
- *Local changes*: There may be associated skin excoriation and features of ammoniacal dermatitis.

Workup

Diagnosis and Evaluation

- *Urine culture sensitivity*: Urine should be collected for culture and sensitivity, and patients with positive results should be treated prior to surgery.
- *Cystoscopy*: Endoscopic examination is performed preoperatively for confirmation, and for proper preoperative planning. Mature fistula have smooth margin with variable size opening, whereas a bullous edema without a distinct opening suggests immature fistula. It is important to note the relation of fistula with the ureteric orifice, size, and its position in relation to the trigone (Fig. 25.2).
- *Cystogram* may confirm the presence and location of the fistula. Upon filling the bladder with contrast material, the vagina begins to opacify almost immediately, confirming the presence of VVF. A cystogram can also make an assessment of the bladder capacity, which is important in patients with prior history of radiotherapy, cystocele, bladder neck competence, and vesicoureteral reflux. The presence of any of these conditions will have an impact on the operative repair and postoperative outcome.

Optional Tests

Imaging Studies

- *Intravenous urogram (IVU)*: An IVU may be necessary to exclude ureteral injury or fistula because 12% of VVFs have associated ureteral fistulas.[3]
- *Retrograde pyelography*: If suspicion is high for a ureteral injury or fistula and the IVU findings are negative, retrograde ureteropyelography (RGP) should be performed at the time of cystoscopy and examination under anesthesia.

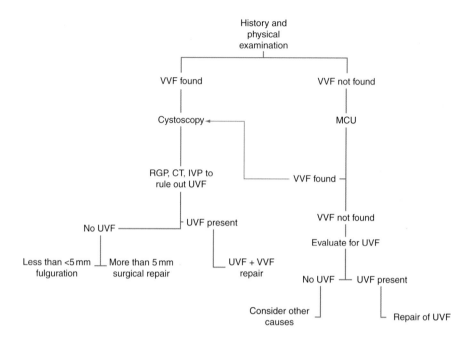

Fig. 25.2 Algorithm for diagnosis and management of VVF

- *Computed tomography (CT) scan*: A CT scan with intravenous contrast or a CT cysto-gram can be performed to isolate the bladder. A tampon placed pervagina during CT scan may improve the sensitivity for finding the small or occult VVF with an otherwise a normal evaluation.
- *Biopsy*: Biopsies are usually only performed in patients with a history or suspicion of local malignancy to exclude recurrent disease.

Treatment

Rapid cessation of urine leakage and preservation of normal voiding and sexual functions are the goal of the VVF repair. Immediate placement of a bladder catheter will decrease/stop the continuous urinary leakage and odor, which temporarily improves the patient's well being, decreases the burden of continuous wetness and odor, and helps restore the patient's self-confidence and esteem. If VVF is diagnosed within the first few days of surgery, a transurethral catheter should be placed and maintained for up to 2–3 weeks along with anticholinergic medications as spontaneous healing may occur.[4]

Timing of Surgery

It is generally recommended that for VVFs resulting from obstructed labor, a 3–6 month delay is required before the definitive repair is taken.[5,6] The waiting period allows reduced tissue edema and inflammation and better pliable tissue for a tension-free repair. In rare cases when VVF presents within 24–48 h postoperatively, an immediate repair can be attempted.

VVF Classification

1. Type I: Less than 5 mm
2. Type II: More than 5 mm
   (a) Supratrigonal
   (b) Trigonal
   (c) Infratrigonal
3. Type III: Involvement of ureteric orifice irrespective of location and size
4. Type IV: Radiation induced and previously failed surgery (ReVVF)

   Type I: A small fistula (3–5 mm) that has already epithelized can be treated with electrofulguration of the fistulous tract, along with anticholinergic medications with prolonged catheterization. This approach was advocated by O'Conor and Sokol for small and highly situated fistula.[7] Other conservative management, such as curettage of the fistulous tract or application of fibrin sealant, may be attempted with varied success rate in small fistulas. For small VVF less than 5 mm, cystoscopy and electrofulguration of the fistula followed by placement of a perurethral catheter for 4 weeks can be attempted. The patient should also be given anticholinergic drugs to prevent bladder spasms.

   Type IIa: Options include laparoscopic transvesical/extravesical surgery, open abdominal surgery, robotic and single port surgery (laparoendoscopic single-site surgery (LESS)). The optimal approach can be either abdominal or vaginal. Of uncomplicated postgynecologic procedures, VVF repair is usually the most successful in the individual surgeon's hand.

   Type IIb and IIc: The vaginal approach is usually preferred, however, fistula high (at the level of hysterectomy cuff) in a deep narrow vagina may be best managed by an abdominal approach. The abdominal approach may be either laparoscopic or open, depending on the surgeon's choice and expertise.

   Type III: Fistula involving the ureteric orifice or nearby requires ureteric reimplantation in addition to VVF repair.

   Type IV: Meticulous dissection and respect of vascularity with interposition of vascularized tissue is the key to success in these cases.

Summary of Surgical Principles

1. *A water-tight, tension-free repair should be performed.* This can be accomplished by various means of adequate mobilization of the tissue.
2. *Fistulous tract excision is not necessary.* Routine excision of the fistulous tract is not always necessary: In their experiences, Raz et al. and Margolis and Mercer note that routine excision of the fistula tract is not mandatory.[8,9] They emphasize the risks of increasing the size of the fistula tract with attempts to resect it. Additionally, these

surgeons contend that the fibrous ring of the fistula may add to the strength of the repair and prevent postoperative bladder spasms.

3. *Good hemostasis* should be achieved at the end of the procedure.
4. *Interposition of various tissues*, such as omentum, peritoneum, a bladder flap (taken from a site away from the fistula) or an epiploic appendix (taken from the sigmoid colon).
5. *Proper selection of the suture material*: An absorbable suture with adequate strength to hold the edges together without any tension should be used. The author uses 4–0 polyglactin for repair with good results.
6. *Efficient postoperative bladder drainage*: Adequate bladder drainage along with anticholinergics is of paramount importance in patient postoperative care. The author does not routinely apply suprapubic catheterization to drain the bladder.

Laparoscopic Approach

This chapter will mainly concentrate on the laparoscopic approach. The laparoscopic approach provides all the benefits of the open transabdominal transvesical approach; in addition, it also gives an excellent view deep inside the pelvis, with shorter stay and better cosmesis. Today, VVF post hysterectomy is a common occurrence, with a rate of 1 in 1,800 hysterectomies, resulting in many adhesions within the pelvis. An excellent view is required to dissect around this area, which is aided by the laparoscope.

Instruments Required

No high-end equipment is required to perform this surgery. Basic laparoscopic instruments such as a 30° laparoscope, camera, Maryland forceps, Allis forceps, curved endoscissors, needle holder, and suction cannula are the only instruments required.

Technique

1. *Cystoscopy* is done with bilateral ureteral catheterization, using 5 F ureteral catheters to help identify and protect the ureters during surgical dissection. A 4 F ureteral catheter of a different color is passed through the fistula and taken out through the vagina. A urethral Foley catheter is placed.
2. *Ports*: A primary (camera port) 10-mm port is inserted in the midline infraumbilically. A 10-mm port (working port) is inserted in the midpoint of the right spinoumbilical line and another 5-mm port is inserted on the midpoint of the left spinoumbilical line (Fig. 25.3).
3. *Adhesiolysis*: Adhesions are lysed in the pelvis, and the uterus and the bladder are identified. The peritoneum between the bladder and the vagina is incised with cautery. Using laparoscopic scissors and gentle countertraction, a plane is developed between the bladder and the vagina.

Fig. 25.3 Port placement with midline scar

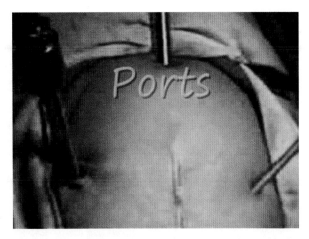

4. *Vertical cystotomy*: The vertical cystotomy is created with laparoscopic scissors, starting at the dome and continuing down to the fistula site posteriorly as described by O'Conor and Sokol.[7] Flaps of bladder wall are dissected free from the vagina until the fistula is separated completely from the vagina. Some surgeons do not open the bladder, instead they dissect the fistulous tract extravesically. Dense adhesions may be encountered during this maneuver, which may result in a difficult dissection.

5. *Dissection of fistula*: Adequate bladder margins are exposed on all sides of the fistula by further dissecting the bladder from the underlying vagina.

6. *Closure of the vaginal wall*: The edges of the fistula opening into the vagina are trimmed back to healthy tissue and are sutured with interrupted 4–0 polyglactin sutures in a single layer.

7. *Interposition of tissue*: Once the vagina is sutured, the omentum, pericolic, or mesenteric fat is mobilized and anchored to the vagina with two more sutures so that it covers the vaginal suture line.

8. *Closure of the bladder*: The defect in the bladder is then sutured in single layer with 4–0 polyglactin intracorporeal sutures, followed by anterior cystotomy closure.

9. *Drain and catheter placement*: An abdominal drain is placed and a 16 F urethral Foley catheter is left in place. The authors do not place a suprapubic catheter after surgery for bladder drainage. The vagina is packed with roller gauze soaked in betadine ointment at the end of the procedure (Fig. 25.4).

Sotelo et al. demonstrated a 93% cure rate in the laparoscopic repair of vesicovaginal fistulas in 15 selected patients who had clear indications for abdominal approach surgical treatment.[10] Between June 2003 and July 2009, 30 patients with VVF were treated laparoscopically at the author's institute. Of the 30 patients who underwent laparoscopic surgery, 3 patients were converted to open surgery because of dense adhesions. Average operative time was 133 min, average blood loss was 140–160 mL, and average hospital stay was 4.3 days. Of the 27 cases completed laparoscopically, 24 (88.88%) were successful. Nezhat

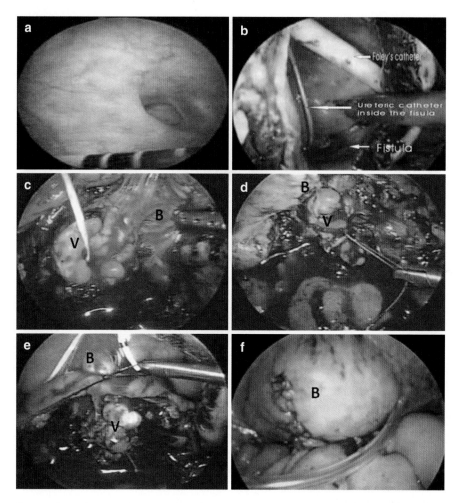

Fig. 25.4 Operative steps: (**a**) Cystoscopy showing fistula with ureteric catheter in situ, (**b**) anterior cystotomy with ureteric catheter inside the fistula and Foleys in situ, (**c**) dissection of fistulous tract, (**d**) closure of vaginal wall, (**e**) closure of the bladder wall over the vaginal repair, (**f**) completed closure with drain in situ. *B* bladder, *V* vagina wall

and colleagues assessed the laparoscopic closure of intentional and unintentional bladder lacerations in a series of 20 cystotomies. In this study, the only complication noted was a single VVF that required reoperation.[11]

Laparoscopy is an alternative to abdominal approach for VVF repair. All the advantages of a minimally invasive procedure can be extended to the repair, which includes magnification during the procedure, hemostasis, decreased postoperative pain and a shorter hospital stay with more rapid recovery and earlier return to normal activities.

Postoperative Details

1. *Bladder drainage*: Continuous, postoperative bladder drainage is vital for successful VVF repair. A large-caliber catheter minimizes the potential for catheter blockage by blood clots, mucus, and calcareous deposits.
2. *Control of postoperative bladder spasms*: Anticholinergics are effective in controlling postoperative bladder spasms.
3. *Antibiotic therapy*: The authors administer oral antibiotic prophylaxis postoperatively to patients who have undergone VVF repair until the Foley catheter is discontinued.
4. *Catheter removal*: At 14 days after surgery, patients are assessed by cystography to confirm complete bladder integrity. During cystography, methylene blue is injected into the bladder and any leakage into the vagina is detected by inserting gauze. If there are any doubts about bladder integrity, the urethral catheter is kept in for an additional week.

Troubleshooting

1. *Supratrigonal, trigonal, or infratrigonal fistula*: In the author's practice, the preferred approach for a supratrigonal fistula is abdominal (laparoscopic), and a vaginal approach is preferred in infratrigonal fistula (Fig. 25.5). Lee et al. recommend an abdominal approach for certain indications, namely: (1) inadequate exposure related to a high or retracted fistula in a narrow vagina, (2) close proximity of the fistulous tract to the ureter, (3) associated pelvic pathology, and (4) multiple fistulas. An abdominal approach is also useful in those cases requiring augmentation cytoplasty or ureteral reimplantation. Infratrigonal fistula may involve the bladder neck or urethra, so these are easily amenable to vaginal repair.[12]
2. *Preoperative cystogram*: A cystogram performed on a full bladder is an excellent indicator of bladder capacity, which is very important, especially in cases of radiation-induced VVF. A small capacity bladder may require augmentation cystoplasty.
3. *Previous surgery*: As many of these patients have history of previous surgery, the Hasson open technique of initial trocar placement may be required and preferred in patients with a midline suprapubic scar to avoid bowel insufflation by Veress needle and bowel injury during blind primary port placement. Alternatively, Veress needle insertion in the left hypochondrium can be performed.
4. *Adhesions*: Adhesions may be present due to prior surgery, which may preclude reaching the bladder or dissection of the fistulous tract. Patience is the key during this scenario; careful blunt and sharp dissection may help in obtaining the correct plane. In patients with previous hysterectomy, the small bowel may be adherent in the pelvis, so careful dissection is necessary.
5. *Maintaining pneumoperitoneum*: At times it may be difficult to maintain pneumoperitoneum in patients with VVF. In this case, application of mild traction on the Foley catheter along with the placement of petroleum jelly-soaked gauze in the vagina may

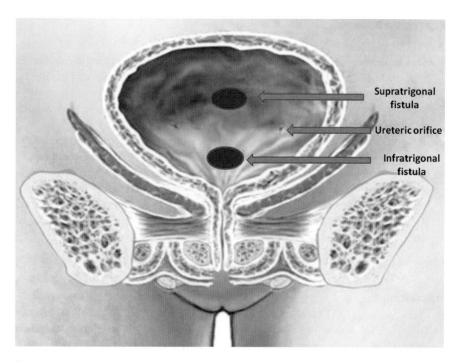

Fig. 25.5 Location of the supratrigonal and infratrigonal fistula and their relation to the ureter

help in minimizing the leakage of air. A pressure of 15 mm Hg should be maintained intraabdominally.

6. *Absence of omentum*: In cases where omentum is not available for interposition or cannot be adequately mobilized (especially in ReVVF repair), a peritoneum flap or epiploic appendixes of sigmoid colon can be used. It may be difficult to bring the omentum down to the pelvis when the patient is in the Trendelenburg postion; in this case the omentum can be mobilized early and kept in the paracolic gutter.

Difficult Scenarios

1. *ReVVF repair*: It is challenging to reoperate on a previous VVF repair as there are questions of vascularity, dense adhesions, vaginal length, and the size of the bladder. It is very important to achieve a good dissection with healthy margins of the fistula, which is opposed in a tension-free manner. In this case, tissue interposition (either the omentum or the peritoneal fold) is essential.
2. *Large VVF*: Large infratrigonal fistula involving the urethra or the bladder neck may require a vaginal approach or a combined abdominal and vaginal approach.
3. *Associated ureteral involvement or fistula near the ureteric orifice*: Cystoscopy and identification of the ureteric orifice and its relation is mandatory in order to avoid any

on table surprises and to determine if ureteric reimplantation should be performed. Approximately 12% of VVF can be associated with ureterovaginal fistula, and these cases may require additional ureteric reimplantation. Ureteric reimplantation can be done laparoscopically along with the VVF repair. The following steps should be added in case ureteric reimplantation is needed:

(a) During dissection of the ureter, the lower end of the healthy ureter is identified and its lower distal end is clipped.

(b) The bladder is filled with water to distend it; this may require vaginal packing with petroleum jelly-soaked gauze.

(c) The detrusor muscle on the proposed site of the ureteric reimplantation is incised with the help of the electrocautery until the bluish bladder mucosa protrudes and enough tunnel can be reconstructed. This may not be necessary if the fistula is nearby.

(d) Fix the lower end of the ureter with the bladder by taking first posterior stitch with an interrupted 4–0 polyglactin suture.

(e) A double J stent can be placed.

4. *Urinary diversion*: In cases where VVF repair is not possible or in cases of multiple failed surgical attempts, urinary diversion may be required. Urinary diversion can be implemented with a urinary conduit or a continent reservoir or a ureterosigmoidostomy can be considered.[13]

5. *Poor surgical candidates*: Fistula in patients who are not candidates for surgical intervention may be managed by permanent ureteral occlusion and permanent nephrostomy.[14,15]

Complications

Integral to all major surgeries are risks of infection; hemorrhage; injury to other organs, particularly the ureters; surgical failure of fistula repair; possible new fistula formation; thromboembolism; and death. Patients should be informed preoperatively of the possibilities of sexual dysfunction or dissatisfaction, new-onset incontinence, and the progression of preexisting urge and/or stress incontinence symptoms.

References

1. Massee JS, Welch JS, Pratt JH, Symmonds RE. Management of urinary-vaginal fistula: ten-year survey. *JAMA*. 1964;190:902-906.

2. Kursh ED, Morse RM, Resnick MI, Persky L. Prevention of the development of a vesicovaginal fistula. *Surg Gynecol Obstet*. 1988;166(5):409-412.

3. Goodwin WE, Scardino PT. Vesicovaginal and ureterovaginal fistulas: a summary of 25 years of experience. *J Urol*. 1980;123(3):370-374.

4. Davits RJ, Miranda SI. Conservative treatment of vesicovaginal fistulas by bladder drainage alone. *Br J Urol*. 1991;68(2):155-156.

5. Wein AJ, Malloy TR, Greenberg SH, Carpiniello VL, Murphy JJ. Omental transposition as an aid in genitourinary reconstructive procedures. *J Trauma*. 1980;20(6):473-477.

6. O'Conor VJ Jr, Sokol JK, Bulkley GJ, Nanninga JB. Suprapubic closure of vesicovaginal fistula. *J Urol*. 1973;109(1):51-54.

7. O'Conor VJ, Sokol JK. Vesicovaginal fistula from the standpoint of the urologist. *J Urol*. 1951;66:579-585.

8. Raz S, Bregg KJ, Nitti VW, Sussman E. Transvaginal repair of vesicovaginal fistula using a peritoneal flap. *J Urol*. 1993;150(1):56-59.

9. Margolis T, Mercer LJ. Vesicovaginal fistula. *Obstet Gynecol Surv*. 1994;49(12):840-847.

10. Sotelo R, Mariano MB, García-Segui A, et al. Laparoscopic repair of vesicovaginal fistula. *J Urol*. 2005;173(5):1615-1618.

11. Nezhat CH, Seidman DS, Nezhat F, Rottenberg H, Nezhat C. Laparoscopic management of intentional and unintentional cystotomy. *J Urol*. 1996;156(4):1400-1402.

12. Lee RA, Symmonds RE, Williams TJ. Current status of genitourinary fistula. *Obstet Gynecol*. 1988;72(3, pt 1):313-319.

13. Kisner CD, Kesner KM. Use of the transverse colon conduit for vesicovaginal fistula in late-stage carcinoma of the cervix. *Br J Urol*. 1987;59(3):234-238.

14. Kinn AC, Ohlsén H, Brehmer-Andersson E, Brundin J. Therapeutic ureteral occlusion in advanced pelvic malignant tumors. *J Urol*. 1986;135(1):29-32.

15. Farrell TA, Wallace M, Hicks ME. Long-term results of transrenal ureteral occlusion with use of Gianturco coils and gelatin sponge pledgets. *J Vasc Interv Radiol*. 1997;8(3):449-452.

16. Shah SJ. Laparoscopic transabdominal transvesical vesicovaginal repair. *J Endourol*. 2009;23(7):1135-1137.

Difficulties in the Laparoscopic Treatment of Female Genital Prolapse

Ahmed E. Ghazi and Günter Janetschek

Principles of Correction

To understand the nature of pelvic floor dysfunction, one must understand both the fundamentals of pelvic anatomy and the dynamics of the pelvic floor. This chapter describes the laparoscopic technique used to correct most defects in the pelvic support that contribute to pelvic floor dysfunction and prolapse. It also gives a brief prospective of certain concepts of the structures involved in pelvic support and how harmony among these structures contribute to normal function of the pelvic organs.

Pelvic anatomy may be defined as those bones, muscles, ligaments and organs that contribute to normal pelvic floor function. The pelvic organs, urethra, vagina, and rectum have no inherent form, structure, or strength. These organs attain these characteristics through the synergistic action of their surrounding ligaments, fascia, and muscles. Normal function of the pelvic organs is directly dependent on the integrity of the pelvic floor structure and any disturbance in this structure leads to dysfunction.

To understand how damage of pelvic floor structures lead to dysfunction of the pelvic organs, the pelvis is divided into three zones as described by Petros[1]:

The **anterior zone** extends from the external urethral meatus to the bladder neck and contains three structures that may be damaged: the pubourethral ligament (PUL), the suburetheral hammock, and the external urethral ligament (EUL).

The **middle zone** extends from the bladder neck to the cervix or hysterectomy scar and also contains three structures that may be damaged: the pubocervical fascia (PCF), the arcus tendineus fasciae pelvis (ATFP), and the anterior cervical ring.

The **posterior zone** extends from the cervix or hysterectomy scar to the perineal body. The ureterosacral ligament (USL), the rectovaginal fascia (RVF), and the perineal body (PB) are the key structures that may be damaged.

A.E. Ghazi (✉)
Department of Urology, Krankenhaus der Elisabethinen Linz, Linz, Austria
e-mail: ahmed_ghazimd@yahoo.com

A.M. Al-Kandari and I.S. Gill (eds.), *Difficult Conditions in Laparoscopic Urologic Surgery*, **367**
DOI: 10.1007/978-1-84882-105-7_26, © Springer-Verlag London Limited 2011

Defects at Each Zone and the Resulting Dysfunction

Anterior Zone

The **PUL** acts to stabilize the urethra forward. Weakness or laxity of the PUL or suburethral hammock causes symptoms of stress urinary incontinence. Isolated weakness of the suburethral hammock would create a urethrocele.

The **EUL** anchors the external urethral meatus to the anterior surface of the descending pubic ramus. Laxity of this ligament leads to an open or everted mucosa of the external urethral meatus.

Middle Zone

There are no transverse ligaments in the middle zone, therefore the PCF is the main supporting structure. The fibromuscular layer of the vaginal wall (PCF) is attached laterally to the ATFP and posteriorly to the cervical ring. Contractions of pelvic muscles stretch the PCF, providing support to the bladder base.

Three potential sites of damage are present in the middle zone: (1) a midline defect at the central part of PCF would create a mid cystocele; (2) dislocation of the attachment of the PCL to the cervical ring would create a high cytocele or even an anterior cystocele; and, finally, (3) dislocation of the ATFP from the ischial spine would create a paravaginal (lateral) defect. Central and lateral defects may coexist.

Posterior Zone

Uterine prolapse is caused by weakened USL or cardinal ligaments that cause descent of the uterus; this is often accompanied by weakness of the PCF and RVF that collapse the upper vaginal walls. These defects result in prolapse of the uterus into the upper vagina, therefore simple suspension of the uterus by reinforcing only the USLs may not be sufficient to restore the prolapse. Additional reinforcement of the PCL and RVF to strengthen the upper vaginal walls would be required to sufficiently correct the prolapse.

Vault prolapse is essentially intussusceptions of the vaginal wall into itself. The cervix and its attaching ligaments (which are a key anchoring point of the proximal vaginal membrane), are lost following total hysterectomy, leaving the vaginal vault supported by the anterior PCF and posterior RVF. Any defects in this support lead to vault prolapse, which is frequently accompanied by traction enterocele, high cystocele, and rectocele. Therefore, correction of a prolapsed vault would require not only tension of the vaginal apex, but also correction of the PCF and RVF defects.

Damage to the RVF would lead to lateral displacement of the fascia as well as their attached cardinal and ureterosacral ligaments. The anterior wall of the rectum may balloon anteriorly resulting in a rectocele.

Cervical ring defect: The cervical ring acts as a bridge between the two cardinal ligaments. A cervical ring tear not only causes lateral displacement of the cardinal ligaments (leading to uterine retroversion and downward displacement of the uterus and/or vaginal apex), but it also dislocates the attachment of the PCF to cause a high cystocele. Therefore, both defects should be addressed during surgical correction.

Symptoms Due to Defects in Pelvic Support

Laxity of the vagina or its supporting ligaments may not allow the muscles to tension the vaginal membrane causing symptoms of lower urinary tract symptoms (LUTS). During bladder filling, the pelvic muscles stretch the vaginal membrane, which supports the hydrostatic pressure exerted by the urine column on the stretch receptors at the bladder base. Laxity in the ligaments or in the vagina may not transmit forces applied to the vagina by the muscles, so the vagina cannot be adequately stretched. The stretch receptors may fire off at a lower hydrostatic pressure (smaller bladder volume) and the cortex interprets this as urgency. In this case, a passive barrier to reinforce the vagina (passive mesh) alone would not restore function, unless the natural tension of the fascia is restored as well (tensioned mesh).

Laxity and stretch of the USLs in cases of uterine prolapse may result in the stretching of the unmyelinated afferent fibers present within their substance, causing referred abdominal and sacral pain.

Laparoscopic Sacrocolpopexy

Disorders of the pelvic floor are interconnected and frequently coexist, as discussed previously. Therefore, in approaching a case of pelvic organ prolapse, the surgeon must seek to correct coexisting defects occurring at different zones of the pelvis. The surgeon must also take into consideration that reinforcement without tension, or vice versa, is usually not sufficient to correct most defects. A combination of both is usually required.

The pelvic viscera involved in genital prolapse constitute a block in which the structures are closely associated with each other. If the support and anchoring systems are defective, the uterus, bladder, and rectum can bulge abnormally through the urogenital opening. The aim of an operation would be (1) to suspend the uterus, returning it to a physiologically normal line; (2) reconstruction of the posterior vaginal support by restoration of a strong anchorage point low down (level with the levator ani muscles) and a higher point of traction to bring the vagina back into a normal anatomic position; and (3) support of the posterior bladder wall.

Laparoscopic sacrocolpopexy not only provides a minimally invasive approach to correct various pelvic floor defects but also addresses both anterior and posterior vaginal defects. The ventral mesh supports and reinforces the anterior vaginal defects and the dorsal mesh reinforces posterior vaginal defects. Both the ventral and dorsal mesh are fixed to the sacral promontory, restoring the natural tension lost by fascia defects or laxity in supporting ligaments. The dorsal mesh is also fixed to the USLs, providing the additional mechanical support needed for reduction of the prolapse. Therefore, laparoscopic sacrocolpopexy can efficiently and completely correct most defects occurring at the middle and posterior zone. The only exception would be a lateral defect in the PCF (which would need a concomitant Burch suspension).

The main disadvantage of laparoscopic sacrocolpopexy is the fact that the procedure does not address anterior zone defects and can exacerbate preexisting ones by restoring anatomical relation of displaced pelvic organs with the development of new symptoms. Therefore, coexisting anterior zone defects are corrected using a suburetheral sling via a vaginal approach.

For further reading regarding pelvic anatomy and the dynamics of the pelvic floor, please refer to *The Female Pelvic Floor: Function, Dysfunction and Management According to Integral Theory* by Peter Petros.[1(pp1–167)]

Operative Setup

The patient is placed in a supine position, with the legs spread apart. The Trendelenburg position is applied progressively to move the bowel away from the pelvis (Fig. 26.1). The vagina and the abdomen are prepared and draped in a sterile fashion. The vagina, including the apex, is thoroughly prepared with povidone-iodine solution. A 2-way, 14 F Foley catheter is placed to drain the bladder and is pulled as far back as possible to help the identification of the bladder neck. The surgeon stands on the left of the patient, with the nurse to the surgeon's right. The assistants stand on the opposite side. The laparoscopic cart is placed between the patient's legs.

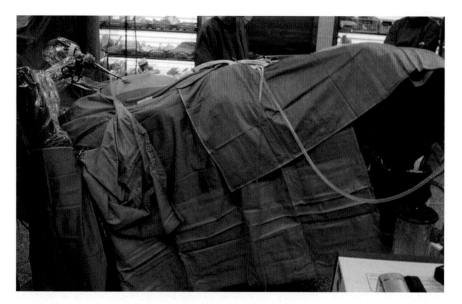

Fig. 26.1 Patient position for laparoscopic sacrocolpopexy

Instruments

Laparoscopic instruments used are listed below:

Aesop® 3000 robot (Intuitive Surgical, Inc., Sunnyvale, CA) (used for laparoscope support)

Trocars: one 12 mm, one 5–11 mm and two 5 mm

30° (degree), 10-mm laparoscope

Harmonic scalpel

5-mm grasping forceps

Suction irrigator

Two needle drivers (non-self-righting)

Bipolar forceps

Endoscissors

Sponge-holding forceps

Mesh (Parietex Prosup, Tyco Healthcare France, Les Ulis, France; both ventral and dorsal mesh are supplied in a sterilized package)

Access and Trocar Position

The surgeon uses four trocars: one 11-mm trocar at the site of Veress needle introduction (for the 0°, 10-mm optic lens); a 12-mm trocar in the midline, midway between the umbilicus and symphysis pubis (for introduction of the mesh and needles); two 5-mm trocars placed midway between the anterior superior iliac spine and the umbilicus (Fig. 26.2). After the pneumoperitoneum is established with a Veress needle (via an infra-umbilical incision), the initial trocar is placed through the same incision and the optic introduced for

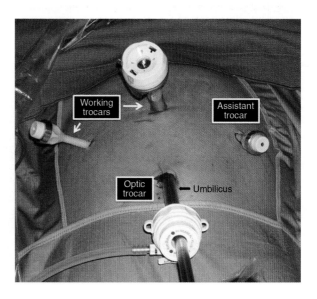

Fig. 26.2 Four trocar arrangement

visualization of the pelvis. The remaining trocars are then placed under visualization; any adhesions that may hinder trocar application are freed beforehand.

Surgical Technique

Initial landmarks that should be identified include: sacral promontory, right ureter, sigmoid colon, uterus, and bladder (Fig. 26.3). In cases where the sigmoid colon hinders visualization, a figure-of-eight stitch is placed through a tenia coli of the sigmoid colon using a 0-PDS™ suture (Ethicon, Inc., Somerville, NJ) on a straight needle. It is brought through the left side of the abdominal wall and tied over a pad to retract the colon away from the area of dissection. The uterus is also suspended upward, toward the anterior abdominal wall (Fig. 26.4).

Presacral Dissection

This begins with incision of the peritoneum in the midline to the right of the sigmoid mesocolon and medial to the right ureter. The fat is dissected off the sacral promontory until the bone is exposed. Care is taken not to shear the presacral veins by excessive blunt dissection. The posterior prevertebral parietal peritoneum is incised vertically along the sigmoid mesocolon until the base of the broad ligament on the right side. During incision of the peritoneum, it is essential to create sufficient retroperitoneal space to later harbor the mesh used for support (presacral tunnel) (Fig 26.5).

Dissection of the Rectovaginal Space

A hand-held vaginal retractor is used to elevate the vagina to widen the space during dissection. The peritoneal incision at the base of the broad ligament is extended (in a hockey stick

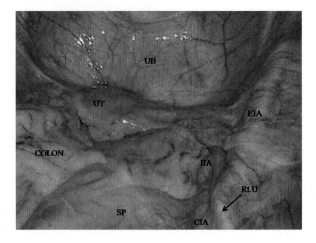

Fig. 26.3 Initial landmarks to be identified include. *SP* sacral promontry, *UT* uterus, *UB* urinary bladder, *COLON* sigmoid colon, *Rt. U* right ureter, *CIA* common iliac artery, *EIA* external iliac artery, *IIA* internal iliac artery

Fig. 26.4 Uterus suspended toward anterior abdominal wall

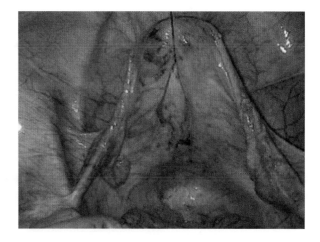

Fig. 26.5 Peritoneal incision exposing the sacral promontory and creation of the presacral tunnel within the retroperitoneal space. *CIA* common iliac artery, *EIA* external iliac artery, *Rt. Ureter* right ureter

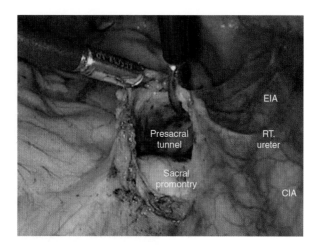

manner) over the posterior peritoneal reflection at the rectovaginal space overlying the vaginal apex. Both blunt (sponge stick) and sharp dissection (monopolar scissors and bipolar forceps) are used to dissect the plane between the posterior vaginal surface and the rectum, which is a relatively bloodless field. Once the rectum is visualized, the pelvic floor muscles (levator ani) are exposed on either side of the rectum (Fig. 26.6). This dissection should be performed as distal (toward the introitus) as possible to maximize the support given by the Y-shaped dorsal mesh. During this dissection, the USLs on both sides should be also identified and dissected, as they form an integral part of the posterior support (Fig 26.7). Once this area (bounded superiorly by the posterior vaginal wall, inferiorly by the rectum, on either side by USLs) is dissected, the Y-shaped mesh can be introduced for fixation. The Y-shaped mesh (15 × 4.5 cm, with a Y-shaped limb and an opposite horizontal limb; Parietex Prosup, Tyco Healthcare France, Les Ulis, France) is introduced through the 12-mm trocar and positioned so that the Y-shaped limb is facing the pelvic floor. The Y-shaped mesh is fixed

Fig. 26.6 Dissection of the
rectovaginal space.
Intraoperative site: the
pelvic floor muscles (levator
ani) exposed on either side
of the rectum

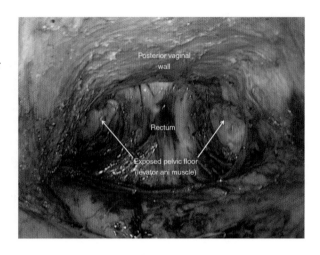

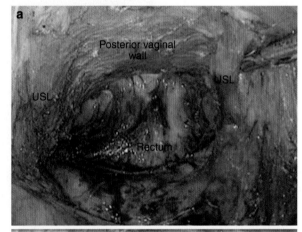

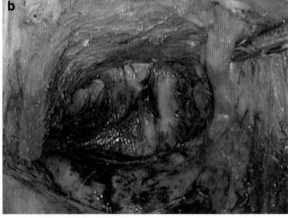

Fig. 26.7 Dissection of the
rectovaginal space. (**a**)
Intraoperative site:
identification of the
uterosacral ligaments on
both sides. (**b**) Outline of
utero-sacral ligaments. *USL*
utero-sacral ligaments

Fig. 26.8 The dorsal
Y-shaped mesh fixed to the
pelvic floor

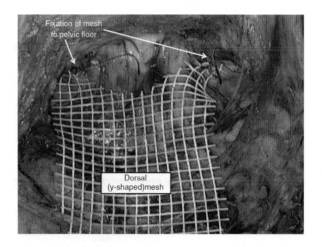

Fig. 26.9 Fixation of the
dorsal mesh to the
uterosacral ligaments.
USL = uterosacral ligaments

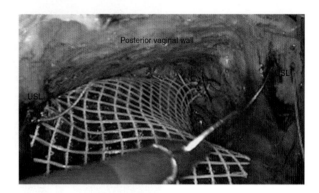

to the dissected pelvic floor muscles on either side (Fig. 26.8) and to the previously dissected USLs (Fig. 26.9), using a 2-0 Ethibond suture (Ethicon, Inc., Somerville, NJ). Six to eight knots are needed for a firm anchorage point. The authors prefer not to fix the mesh in the midline to the rectum in order to prevent the risk of transfixation of the rectal wall and its consequences. The peritoneal reflection is then approximated in running manner, up to the point of passage of the posterior (Y-shaped) into the presacral tunnel. A 3–0 Vicryl™ suture (Ethicon, Inc., Somerville, NJ) tapered on a 5/8 needle and secured at its free end with a PDS locking clip (Lapra-Ty™, Ethicon Endo-Surgery, Inc., Cincinnati, OH) is used with another clip to secure the thread after the peritoneal ends are opposed to avoid the need for intracorporeal suturing. The remaining tread is left in place to continue closure of the peritoneum over the presacral tunnel after securing the anterior mesh (Fig. 26.10).

Passage Through the Mesosalpinx (Formation of a Tunnel to Retroperitonalize the Ventral Mesh)

This step is essential in order to retroperitonalize the ventral mesh within the presacral tunnel. With the uterus still suspended upward, dissection starts through an opening made

Fig. 26.10 (**a**) Final position of the dorsal mesh in the rectovaginal space and presacral tunnel. (**b**) Approximation of the peritoneal reflection overlying the rectovaginal space. *SP* sacral promontory

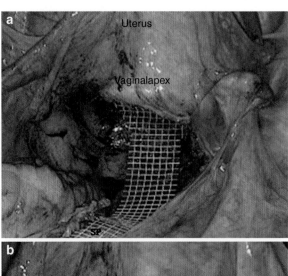

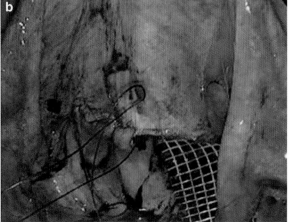

in the posterior peritoneum of the mesosalpinx on the right side (Fig. 26.11). An opening is made by cutting firmly into an area of dissected peritoneum, after which simple traction in opposite directions is usually sufficient to enlarge the opening. The anterior peritoneum of the mesosalpinx is then open to complete the tunnel created between the rectouterine and the vesicovaginal spaces (Fig. 26.12).

Dissection of the Vesicovaginal Space

The suspended uterus is returned to its original position and the opening created in the anterior peritoneal covering of the mesosalpinx is extended anteriorly over the vaginal apex (Fig. 26.13). Downward traction of the vagina (via the vaginal retractor), together with upward traction of the bladder (via grasping forceps) aids in dissecting the plane between the anterior vaginal surface and the bladder, using a combination of both sharp

Fig. 26.11 Creation of a tunnel through the right mesosalpinx. The *arrow* demonstrates the direction of dissection

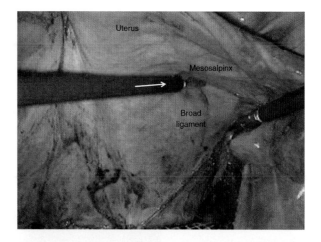

Fig. 26.12 Passage of an instrument through the tunnel created between the rectouterine and vesicovaginal spaces. *FT* right fallopian tube, *MS* right mesosalpinx

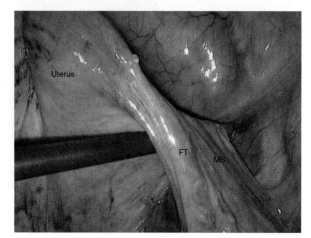

Fig. 26.13 Dissection of the vesicovaginal space. Peritoneal incision over the vaginal apex anteriorly

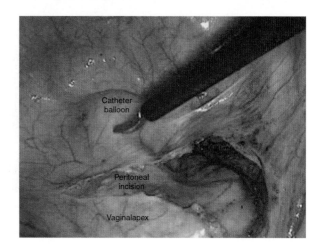

and blunt dissection. The dissection is continued deep to the bladder neck, identified by the traction balloon of the placed urinary catheter (Fig. 26.14). The ventral mesh (rectangular in shape with a tapered end, 15×2.5 cm, Parietex Prosup) is introduced and its tapered end is fixed to the anterior surface of the vagina at five points: three distal, at the deepest point of dissection (one in the midline and two lateral stitches), and two proximal, at the vaginal apex (both lateral) (Fig. 26.15). The cranial (free) end of the ventral mesh is passed through the tunnel created in the mesosalpinx and placed in the presacral tunnel alongside the posterior mesh (Fig. 26.16). The edges of the peritoneal reflection at the vesicovaginal space are approximated.

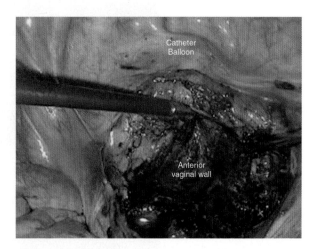

Fig. 26.14 Dissection of the vesicovaginal space toward the bladder neck

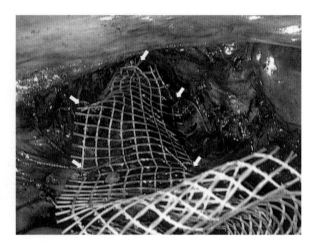

Fig. 26.15 The ventral mesh fixed to the anterior vaginal wall. The *arrows* indicate the five points of fixation

Fig. 26.16 Passage of the mesh from the vesicovaginal space to the presacral tunnel

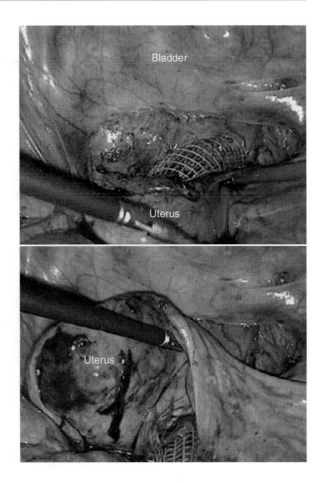

Fixation of the Mesh to the Sacral Promontory

The ventral and dorsal meshes together in the presacral canal are fixed to the exposed sacral promontory, using a 0 Vicryl™ suture tapered to a 1/2 circle needle (Fig. 26.17). Slight tension on the mesh is ideal for the mechanical benefit from this procedure. The passage of the needle must be shallow – indeed, transparent – to avoid any risk for spondylodiscitis. It should take up solely the fibrous layer of the aponeurosis and avoid any perforation of the disk substance. Excess mesh is cut and the posterior peritoneum is then approximated to completely retroperitonealize the mesh and allow the integration of the prosthetic material into the peritoneum (Fig. 26.18).

At the end of the operation (with both meshes totally isolated), the sigmoid colon is returned to its correct position. Hemostasis is checked and the peritoneum washed out. No drains need to be placed.

Fig. 26.17 (**a**) Passage of the needle through the periosteum of the sacral promontory. (**b**) Both ventral and dorsal meshes in the presacral canal, fixed to the exposed sacral promontory

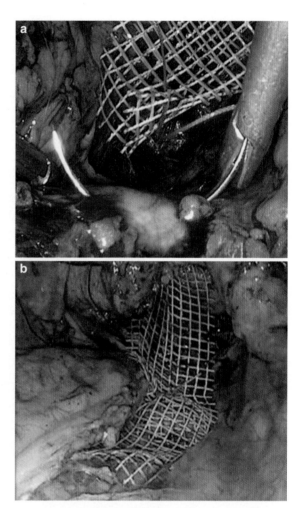

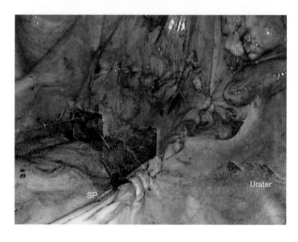

Fig. 26.18 Final outcome following approximation of the posterior peritoneum and the mesh completely retroperitonealized. *SP* sacral promontory

Technical Caveats

Peritoneal Incision over the Presacral Tunnel

Both during incising the peritoneal incision (extending from the sacral promontory to the base of the broad ligament on the right side) and during its closure, the surgeon should be cautious not to injure the right ureter which is covered by posterior peritoneum.

Vaginal Retractor

A handheld vaginal retractor is of great assistance during this operation; however, its position varies during each step of the operation. During dissection of the rectovaginal space, it is pushed toward the pelvic cavity and held upward in a horizontal position, allowing identification of the posterior vaginal wall along which the dissection is performed. During dissection of the vesicovaginal space, it is pushed inward and down. In both of these situations, this maneuver widens the space to be dissected. During fixation of the mesh to the sacral promontory, the vagina retractor is pushed inward horizontally, stretching the vaginal wall and providing the appropriate tension required.

Dissection of the Rectovaginal Space

The correct plane of dissection is in the fatty tissue just deep to the posterior vaginal wall. This dissection should be extended laterally to the uterosacral ligaments to create enough space for positioning and fixation of the dorsal mesh to the levator ani muscle. During exposure of the pelvic floor muscles (prior to fixation of the dorsal mesh), the dissection should be limited to the pararectal space. If dissected more laterally, the middle rectal arteries may be encountered and injured. Nevertheless, dissection in close proximity to the rectum may injure the rectal nerves and cause problems during defecation.

Fixation of the Dorsal Mesh to the USL

The dorsal mesh should be fixated to the uterosacral ligaments at the closest point to the posterior vaginal wall. This positions the dorsal prostatic mesh away from the rectal wall, avoiding functional problems of the rectum. In addition to providing the mechanical support needed for reduction of the prolapse, it also reinforces the posterior vaginal wall when fixed in this position.

Dissection of the Vesicovaginal Space

This dissection can be difficult in cases of previous surgery or recurrent urinary tract infections.

It may be useful to fill the bladder with 150 cc of saline during the dissection to identify the borders of the bladder. In case of any injuries to the vagina or bladder, the edges are approximated using a 3–0 Vicryl™ suture tapered on a 5/8 needle and secured at its free end with a PDS locking clip. It is also wise to rinse the pelvic cavity with diluted betadine solution following injury to the vagina.

After Hysterectomy

Following hysterectomy, the dorsal and ventral mesh are fixed in a similar manner; the exception is that the ventral mesh is passed into the presacral tunnel by joining of both peritoneal incisions over the rectovaginal and vesicovaginal spaces over the vaginal apex. Following positioning and fixation of both the ventral and dorsal meshes together in the presacral canal, the peritoneal gap is closed by approximation of the posterior lip of peritoneum at the rectovaginal space to the anterior lip of peritoneum overlying the vesicovaginal space to completely retroperitonealize both meshes. Care should be taken when dissecting the vesicovaginal space, as the plane is usually distorted following hysterectomy.

Reference

1. Petros P. *The Female Pelvic Floor: Function, Dysfunction and Management According to the Integral Theory*. 2nd ed. Heidelberg, Germany: Springer Medizin Verlag; 2007:1-167.

Difficulties in Pediatric Laparoscopic Urologic Surgery

Angus G. Alexander and Walid A. Farhat

Introduction

The experience of surgical difficulties is highly subjective and is primarily dependent on the nature of the procedure, however, training, aptitude, and the natural ability of an individual surgeon contribute significantly to a "difficult" procedure. As a result, no text can be all inclusive and therefore, this chapter is not written exclusively for experts. This chapter will attempt to cover issues that many have mastered, as well as those subtleties that continue to frustrate the most accomplished laparoscopist.

The chapter is divided into a general discussion on difficulties applicable to all pediatric laparoscopy. It will then focus on individual procedures commonly performed in urology.

Common Difficulties

The following section is divided into seven parts, each discussing common problems unique to laparoscopic surgery: (1) patient selection, (2) counseling and consent, (3) equipment and staff, (4) port positioning and insertion, (5) ergonomics, (6) insufflation, and (7) maintaining the pneumoperitoneum.

Patient Selection

As laparoscopists have developed in skill and confidence, the authors have seen a decrease in the contraindications to minimally invasive surgery. Cardiac and pulmonary pathology, intolerant of the physiological impact of the pneumoperitoneum, remain contraindications.

Beyond this, surgical discretion should guide patient selection. In the case of an infant, an open dismembered pyeloplasty would use a 2- to 3-cm muscle separating wound and an

A.G. Alexander (✉)
Department of Pediatric Urology, The Hospital for Sick Children, Toronto, ON, Canada
e-mail: angus.alexander@sickkids.ca

A.M. Al-Kandari and I.S. Gill (eds.), *Difficult Conditions in Laparoscopic Urologic Surgery*, DOI: 10.1007/978-1-84882-105-7_27, © Springer-Verlag London Limited 2011

extraperitoneal approach. Compare this with the laparoscopic approach that alters physiology, breaches the peritoneal cavity and takes longer to perform. Would the patient benefit from this approach?

Counseling and Consent

Endoscopic surgery is better termed "minimal access surgery" as its invasiveness is only minimized at the somatic insertion site.

The consent for a laparoscopic approach requires more time and explanation, as the procedure has more variables and possible complications. One of the fundamental principles of taking consent is to manage the patients' and/or parents' expectations of surgery. If this is done well, the patient or parent becomes empowered as part of the team, and is alerted to possible complications. In this way, complications are viewed as inherent in the procedure rather than an indictment of the surgeon and the procedure performed. The conversion of a laparoscopic procedure to an open one is always an option. However, this should not be seen as a complication, but rather a wise maneuver to achieve better access if difficulties are encountered.

Equipment and Staff

Endoscopic surgery can be rewarding, but at times is the source of huge frustrations. Aside from the technical abilities of the surgeon and the inherent demands of the procedure, there are many other factors that influence the course of the operation that are not necessarily present in open surgery. Three factors stand out in the ability to frustrate even the most patient endoscopist: (1) mechanical and electronic equipment failure, (2) an unsteady, inaccurate camera operator, and (3) nursing personnel that are unfamiliar or poorly trained in endoscopic procedures.

Solutions to minimize these frustrations include regular training and updates on the procedures performed, and scheduled maintenance of equipment.

Regarding camera operators, a comfortable position and arm stabilization are helpful. Getting the camera operator to sit will often accomplish both of these with the added advantage of providing the surgeon with more space in which to maneuver. Simultaneously rotating the camera and the lens can optimize visualization. Pulling back on the camera to increase the visual field is preferable to lateral "tracking movements" at close range.

Port Positioning and Insertion

The pediatric abdomen is highly distensible and allows for significant distortion. Care should be taken when port sites are to be used for permanent stomas or catheters and these sites should be chosen on the undistended abdomen.

Ergonomics

Laparoscopic surgery on children encounters many ergonomic challenges. Some of them have been offset by the design and development of smaller ports and instruments. This has been an ergonomic advancement, but visibility and applicability are arguably compromised as a result of this miniaturization.

The pediatric abdomen is small and relatively close to the bed. This leaves little space for port placement and maneuverability. Novel approaches to positioning can have a major impact on ergonomics. Effort should be made to shorten the table or place the infant in an oblique or transverse position. This will improve both ergonomics and optics.

Infant patients whose procedures require low-lying instruments can be elevated partially or completely off the table with lateral bolsters or gel pads. Moving the child close to the edge of the table can be equally effective.

Cables and tubing are an added consideration of endoscopic surgery. Their placement should be well thought out. In order to declutter the operating field, all leads and cables should be grouped together in several places as they circuit the patient. The length of insufflation tubing should be just enough to reach the port tasked with inducing the pneumoperitoneum. Items less likely to be used during the procedure, like the suction irrigation and hand held diathermy, can be tucked into pockets to keep them out of the operating arena until they are required.

Insufflation

The pediatric abdomen has a smaller volume and consequently fills more rapidly with standard flow rates. Rapid insufflation can be dangerous and often compromises physiology more than low-flow, low-pressure insufflation. Target pressures should be just sufficient for adequate exposure, tailored to the physiology of the child, and crudely represented by weight and age.

Maintaining the Pneumoperitoneum

Poor visibility may either be the result of a "light" patient who has begun to contract their abdominal wall musculature or a loss of pneumoperitoneum. The difficulty with both of these circumstances is that they can be subtle enough to go unnoticed, yet frustrate a procedure because of poor exposure.

Educate your anesthetists and communicate with them throughout the operation. Many laparoscopists insist on paralysis as a routine, but this is not always necessary, provided adequate exposure is maintained.

Loss of pneumoperitoneum should trigger an ordered search for the cause. This search is best started with the patient and ended with the carbon dioxide gas supply in a sequence of troubleshooting.

- Observe the flow rate in comparison to the pressure of the pneumoperitoneum. This is a good indication of where the problem is: poor supply, increased demand, or a light patient.
- Insertion of ports should be meticulous. Incisions must be appropriately matched to the size of the ports. Big incisions allow mobility of the port that can cause gas leakage or repeated extubation of the port during instrument withdrawal. If the incision is too big, it will need to be occluded using a purse string-type occlusion suture. If this suture can be placed into the sheath it can be used for closure at the end of the procedure.
- Check that the insufflation taps are closed and that the internal valves are the right size, the right way around, and are not damaged. The offending port can be localized by dropping water onto the aperture and looking for bubbles. This same technique can be used at the skin level.
- Many instruments have a cleaning port that must be capped to prevent air leaks.
- Check that insufflation taps have not been partially closed during the procedure.
- Exclude kinked tubing.
- Check that the carbon dioxide cylinder is not empty.

Procedure-Specific Difficulties

Partial Nephrectomy

Partial nephrectomy in the pediatric population is most often indicated for the removal of the upper, dysplastic moiety of a duplex kidney. The approach can be either transperitoneal or extraperitoneal. The best approach is the one the laparoscopist is most familiar with.

In the retroperitoneal approach, it is important to preserve the integrity of the parietal peritoneum. Holes allow gas into the peritoneal space, which can compress the perinephric neocavity, obscuring visibility. If the peritoneum is breached, a transcutaneous angiocath can be placed into the peritoneum to decompress it, or alternatively, the tear can be sutured.

Complete mobilization of the kidney in either approach is contraindicated because of the potential for the remaining moiety to undergo torsion.

Retrograde stenting of the normal ureter is a foolproof method of avoiding inadvertent injury. Stenting is essential when dealing with a lower pole nephrectomy as neither ureter is dilated and identifying the correct ureter intraoperatively is difficult. This is in contrast to the upper pole nephrectomy, where the pathological ureter is very ectatic and easily identified (Fig. 27.1).

Once the ureter is isolated and transected, it should be used as a traction and orientation tool.

The polar vessels must never be transected until the supply is clearly delineated (Fig. 27.2). If clarity cannot be achieved, then it is an indication for conversion. Staying close to the renal capsule as much as possible will avoid inadvertent damage to the remaining moieties' vessels. Once the vessels have been secured, clamping them will show demarcation without the irreversibility of transection. If it does not, consider an alternative supply, incomplete dissection, or incorrect vessel.

Fig. 27.1 Extraperitoneal
dissection demonstrating the
dilated, pathological upper
pole ureter

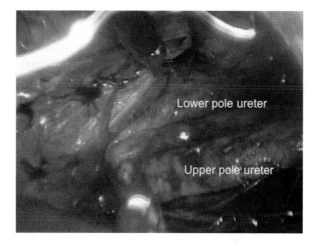

Fig. 27.2 Meticulous
perirenal dissection reveals
the hilar vessels supplying
the normal lower pole

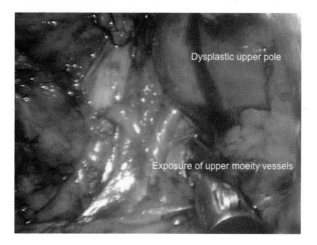

If bleeding is encountered from the renal pedicle, place the pedicle on tension by elevating the kidney. This maneuver will stop or slow the bleeding for adequate assessment and conversion to open surgery if necessary.

Transection of the renal parenchyma should be performed within the ischemic tissue of the demarcation line to ensure a safe amputation. If a pelvis of uncertain origin is opened, blue dye infused into the normal ureter can reassure the surgeon that the pelvis of the normal moiety has not been breached. Some surgeons deliberately open the pelvis in order to safely transect the pole. Once this is done, the parenchyma can be trimmed according to the demarcation line.

If diathermy smoke obscures visibility, it is helpful to allow a leak from one of the ports and increase the gas flow in order to vent this smoke.

The polar tissue is easily extracted through one of the port sites as it is usually dysplastic and has little bulk.[1]

Pyeloplasty

The results of laparoscopic surgery should be equivalent to those of open surgery. The results of open pyeloplasty are excellent and, in order to justify performing the procedure laparoscopically, surgeons need to match that success.

In a child under the age of two, an open standard dismembered pyeloplasty is done through a 2- to 3-cm muscle separating incision, is retroperitoneal, and is highly success-ful. In this age group, there is no clear benefit to laparoscopy – it requires a breach of the peritoneal cavity and is technically more demanding than the open approach. In older children, the authors use a 5-mm camera port with two, 3-mm working ports. A fourth trocar can be useful in retracting tissues or maintaining tension on the sutures. With experi-ence, this extra instrument can be abandoned (Fig. 27.3).

The suture material used by the authors for laparoscopic pyeloplasty in children is an absorbable, braided 5/0 suture. Small needles can be passed down the 3-mm port. Larger needles can be straightened or passed directly through the abdominal wall. The latter maneuver can prove problematic in well-nourished patients.

The renal pelvis is frequently rotated posteriorly. In order to deliver the pelvis, the pelvic traction suture takes on the additional roles of a derotation and stabilization. This pelvic suture is passed through the abdominal wall and secured extracorporeally.

When spatulating the ureter, care should be taken to open it laterally and avoid spiraling the incision, as both of these mistakes can twist the ureter and affect drainage.

The authors use a double-J stent, which is passed through the abdominal wall muscula-ture using a 12-gauge angiocath (Fig. 27.4). The length of the ureteral stent should be chosen carefully, as too long a stent can cause discomfort to the child, negating the principle benefit of the laparoscopic approach. If in doubt, use fluoroscopy to guide the stent placement.

Difficulty can be experienced passing any stent into the bladder in an ante-grade fashion. In order to overcome this, a transanastomotic nephrostomy or pyelostomy (Salle) stent may be used. Preoperative retrograde placement of the ureteral stent is another solution but it can cause difficulties when suturing the anastomosis as it obscures the posterior suture line.[2–4]

Bladder Augmentation

Although pure laparoscopic enterocystoplasty in children is an advanced procedure that is technically demanding, it is feasible and gaining popularity. Extensive experience with

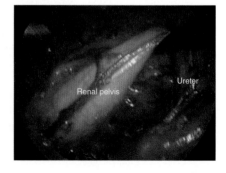

Fig. 27.3 Isolation of the pathological ureteropelvic junction using the transperitoneal approach

Fig. 27.4 An angiocath is used to place the guidewire in a percutaneous, antegrade manner

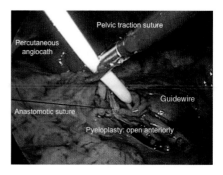

laparoscopy is necessary before attempting this procedure, since superiority over conventional open techniques has not yet been demonstrated. Difficulties unique to this procedure are discussed below in sequence as they arise during the operation.

- It is often difficult to identify the ureteric orifices laparoscopically. Bilateral ureteric stents are an essential presurgical procedure.
- A Foley catheter is inserted and the bulb pulled down onto the bladder neck to ensure the ability to create a pneumovesicum.
- Transcutaneous traction and stay sutures will facilitate exposure without impacting on space. This relatively simple maneuver keeps the proper orientation and tension on the ileum and secures the anatomic structure of interest to prevent kinking and twisting of the mesentery. It also has the advantages of easy relocation and facilitates changes in the angle of dissection.
- Measurement of the required bowel lengths is difficult with the magnification of the laparoscopic telescope. This is easily overcome with the introduction of a premeasured silk 1/0 suture (Fig. 27.5).
- Selection of the loop to be used is based on a 15-cm segment of bowel that has a good vascular pedicle and that is of sufficient length to allow the antimesenteric border to reach the bladder neck.

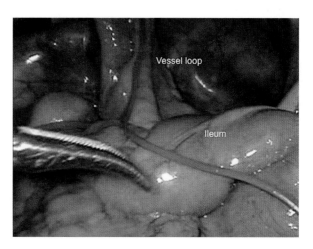

Fig. 27.5 A vessel loop of known length, used to measure the bowel segment required for the bladder augmentation

- Transection of the bowel and reanastomosis can be effected intracorporeally or extra-corporeally depending on the preference and experience of the surgeon. Endo-staplers have greatly enhanced the ease with which the intracorporeal anastomosis can be performed.
- Intensive suturing and intracorporeal tying are required and are often the most difficult and time-consuming steps in this procedure. Shortening the suture will greatly facilitate intracorporeal handling of the suture material.[5-8]

Appendicovesicostomy

The appendix is a near perfect catheterizable conduit. However, its presence, location, length, and relationship to the cecum are not consistent and this can present surgical and decision-making difficulties.

Understanding that the cecum can be poorly fixed or incompletely descended is crucial to finding the appendix and planning surgery. In order to consistently locate the appendix, the cecum should be located first. Once this is found, the tenia should be traced distally. The three tenia of the colon will always converge at the base of the appendix on the bulb of the cecum. Identification of the base of the appendix will aid mobilization of the body and tip of the appendix, which is usually retrocecal.

Preservation of the mesoappendix is obviously essential to the success of the operation and dissection must be done with this in mind. In order to facilitate this dissection, a traction suture can be placed into the tip of the appendix to unfurl it and expose the mesentery.

Dissection of the vessels should, as far as possible, be done without diathermy. Where hemostasis is required, clips can be used. In the absence of clips, cutting diathermy gives adequate hemostasis without the collateral damage of coagulation diathermy.

The vessels to the appendix are terminal branches of the ileocecal vessels. Mobilization of the cecum will allow mobility of the appendix in the form of a "tissue flap." This added mobility is essential to accurate positioning of the conduit and a tension free anastomosis.

Division of the appendix stump should be performed as close to the base as possible. Stapling devices can be used to transect and staple this stump; alternatively, it can be suture-ligated with intracorporeal sutures.

When positioning the bladder anastomosis, it should aim to drain the most dependent part of the bladder, allow for an adequate tunnel, and define a gentle arc that allows easy catheterization.

If possible, the conduit should be brought out in the umbilicus and careful thought should be given to the incision in order to create a skin flap to prevent the anastomosis from stenosing.[9]

Peritoneal Dialysis Catheter

Peritoneal dialysis catheter insertion is a life-preserving procedure that, if done well, can maintain renal failure patients for many years without the complications associated with hemodialysis.

Laparoscopy has been used as both an insertion technique and as a salvage procedure. When used as an insertion technique, it is effective at assessing the suitability of the peritoneal cavity, removing the omental curtain, holding the fimbria out of the pelvis, and accurately placing the catheter.

Difficulties encountered include poor catheter placement because of insertion sites being based on an insufflated abdominal wall. Always mark boney landmarks or intended insertion sites prior to insufflation.

Omentectomy is best performed via the umbilical wound. An endosuction device is placed into the peritoneal cavity to retrieve the omentum. It is then resected in a piecemeal fashion. Always be sure to replace the tied-off stalk before embarking on the next piece of omentum; multiple ties may create a bulk that is difficult to return to the abdomen. Bleeding from a poorly tied omentum can be very problematic in the renal failure patient once dialysis has started. A 10-mm port will certainly facilitate the omentectomy, but is not necessary in small children as the omental curtain is usually fine and easily delivered in stages through a 5-mm port.

Gentle, blunt dissection of fibrous adhesions within the peritoneal cavity may be appropriate provided the adhesions are not dense, there is minimal serosal and peritoneal trauma, and that dialysis is started relatively soon to maintain this regained cavity space.

The ovaries can be pexied out of the pelvis in order to prevent the fimbria getting stuck in the tubing, another common source of potential blockage of the catheter. The suturing should be tension free and involve the ovary, not the fimbria.

The catheter should be measured prior to insertion. The tubing should reach from the intended cuff site to the pubic bone. The tunnel for the supraperitoneal catheter should be created in such a way as to run obliquely through the muscle wall and fascia. This will help ensure that the tip remains in the pelvis and avoid migration to nondependent parts of the peritoneum. The catheter tip may or may not be sutured in to the pelvis depending on the intraperitoneal environment and lie of the catheter. If it is sutured into the pelvis, it should be with a nonabsorbable suture and as a result include a relatively shallow bite of pelvic tissue to facilitate removal (Fig. 27.6).

Leaks and hernias can prove problematic where dialysis is started early, before the peritoneum has had time to seal. Where acute dialysis is required, all port sites should be closed with the creation of a watertight seal in mind. This is best accomplished with a multilayered closure. The use of low volumes of dialysate can further contribute to avoiding leaks in the immediate postoperative period.

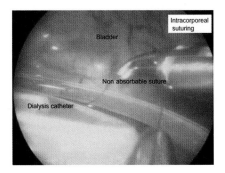

Fig. 27.6 The peritoneal dialysis catheter is fixed to the pelvic peritoneum using a loop of nonabsorbable suture

Laparoscopy can further contribute to peritoneal dialysis catheter management in the form of identifying the reason for catheter malfunction or nonfunction. Very often the problem is easily corrected with laparoscopy.[10, 11]

Orchidopexy

The use of laparoscopy in the cryptorchid child is both diagnostic and therapeutic. In terms of diagnosis, laparoscopy is superior to ultrasound, and considering the need for anesthesia is more appropriate than computed tomography (CT) or magnetic resonance imaging (MRI) in that therapeutic intervention can follow immediately. Initially, difficulties come in the form of decision-making:

- What should be done with the peeping testicle?
- When should a primary orchidopexy be done as opposed to a staged procedure?
- Should the testicular vessels be divided or maintained?

The peeping testicle is resident in the abdominal compartment but can be passed through the internal ring. This diagnosis can be made by examination under anesthesia prior to surgery and is amenable to the open approach with a high retroperitoneal dissection. If discovered at laparoscopy, it is equally well dealt with by a single laparoscopic mobilization and scrotopexy via the inguinal canal or through Hesselbach's triangle.

The decision to stage the surgery can be made based on two questions:

1. Are the vessels going to be too short for primary orchidopexy?

- If the testis reside more than 2 cm from the internal ring, the answer is usually "yes."

2. Once the vessels have been divided, is it safe to proceed with scrotopexy given the tenuous vesicular blood supply?

- There is evidence to suggest that dividing the vasculature and proceeding to orchidopexy is associated with a higher testicular atrophy rate. Dissection of the peritesticular tissue should be as superficial as possible, as the peritoneum is all that is required to adequately mobilize the vas and vessels. Deep dissection can often be bloody, and runs the risk of damaging ureter and iliac vessels.

Assessing sufficient length for a tension free orchidopexy can be done by attempting to place the mobilized testicle on the contra lateral internal ring.

Passage of the mobilized testis can be anatomical or nonanatomical. If sufficient length of cord structure exists, then the inguinal canal can be used. If the length is insufficient, then a more direct passage through Hesselbach's triangle can be created medial to the epigastric vessels. The neo-canal can be either medial or lateral to the median umbilical ligament.[12-14]

Conclusion

Laparoscopic surgery has advanced pediatric urology and become a well-established method of surgical intervention. The risk inherent in this new and challenging field is that patient care may be compromised as the surgeon attempts to find the limits of the minimally invasive approach. Significant skill and experience are prerequisites for anyone who is going to push these limits. This is especially true of those procedures that have open surgical approaches that are simple, successful, and have stood the test of time.

References

1. Leclair MD, Vidal I, Suply E, Podevin G, Heloury Y. Retroperitoneal laparoscopic heminephrectomy in duplex kidney in infants and children: a 15-year experience. *Eur Urol.* 2009;56(2):385-391.
2. Braga LH, Pippi-Salle J, Lorenzo AJ, Bagli D, Khoury AE, Farhat WA. Pediatric laparoscopic pyeloplasty in a referral center: lessons learned. *J Endourol.* 2007;21(7):738-742.
3. El-Ghoneimi A. Laparoscopic management of hydronephrosis in children. *World J Urol.* 2004;22(6):415-417.
4. Farhat W, Afshar K, Papanikolaou F, Austin R, Khoury A, Bagli D. Retroperitoneal-assisted laparoscopic pyeloplasty in children: initial experience. *J Endourol.* 2004;18(9):879-882.
5. Elliott SP, Meng MV, Anwar HP, Stoller ML. Complete laparoscopic ileal cystoplasty. *Urology.* 2002;59(6):939-943.
6. Lorenzo AJ, Cerveira J, Farhat WA. Pediatric laparoscopic ileal cystoplasty: complete intracorporeal surgical technique. *Urology.* 2007;69(5):977-981.
7. Meng MV, Anwar HP, Elliott SP, Stoller ML. Pure laparoscopic enterocystoplasty. *J Urol.* 2002;167(3):1386.
8. Rackley RR, Abdelmalak JB. Laparoscopic augmentation cystoplasty: surgical technique. *Urol Clin North Am.* 2001;28(3):663-670.
9. Hsu TH, Shortliffe LD. Laparoscopic Mitrofanoff appendicovesicostomy. *Urology.* 2004;64(4):802-804.
10. Numanoglu A, McCulloch MI, Van Der Pool A, Millar AJW, Rode H. Laparoscopic salvage of malfunctioning Tenckhoff catheters. *J Laparoendosc Adv Surg Tech A.* 2007;17(1): 128-130.
11. Numanoglu A, Rasche L, Roth MA, McCulloch MI, Rode H. Laparoscopic insertion with tip suturing, omentectomy, and ovariopexy improves lifespan of peritoneal dialysis catheters in children. *J Laparoendosc Adv Surg Tech A.* 2008;18(2):302-305.
12. Godbole PP, Najmaldin AS. Laparoscopic orchidopexy in children. *J Endourol.* 2001;15(3): 251-256.
13. O'Brien MF, Hegarty PK, Healy C, DeFrietas D, Bredin HC. One-stage Fowler-Stephens orchidopexy for impalpable undescended testis. *Ir J Med Sci.* 2004;173(1):18-19.
14. Sharifiaghdas F, Beigi FMA. Impalpable testis: laparoscopy or inguinal canal exploration? *Scand J Urol Nephrol.* 2008;42(2):154-157.

Difficulties in Single-Port Laparoscopic Procedures

28

Raj K. Goel and Jihad H. Kaouk

Introduction

Single-port laparoscopic surgery has revolutionized the minimally invasive approach to urological disorders. Originally conceptualized in 1999,[1] single-port surgery has recently expanded due to instrument modification and growing experience in laparoscopy. In specialized centers, reconstructive and extirpative single-port procedures have been performed.[2-5] At this time, single-port surgery holds great promise in reducing patient morbidity, although its exact role in urologic oncology and reconstruction is still pending. Thus far, the authors' experience at their center in single-port laparoscopy has identified various limitations to both renal and pelvic surgery. Herein, a description of both technical and surgical challenges will be described and various modifications used to overcome such challenges.

Single-Port Laparoscopic Surgery: Instrumentation

Classically, laparoscopic surgery utilizes multiple single channel ports spaced on the abdominal wall to provide triangulation to the respective organ being dissected. Single-port or single-site surgery amalgamates all trocar sites to one entry point in order to minimize abdominal wall trauma. In either method, limited trocar entry sites hopefully translate into reduced patient morbidity. Initial attempts at single site surgery utilized preexisting laparoscopic ports placed at a single anatomical location. These bulky ports do not immediately allow for an adequate range of motion and "scissoring" of ports is common. Continued research and development to provide an ergonomically designed surgical port that can accommodate various sized instruments is currently under way. The authors' experience using two commercially available ports will be described in this chapter.

R.K. Goel (✉)
Department of Urology, University of Western Ontario Schulich School of Medicine, Windsor, ON, Canada
e-mail: rajgoel24@hotmail.com

A.M. Al-Kandari and I.S. Gill (eds.), *Difficult Conditions in Laparoscopic Urologic Surgery*, 395
DOI: 10.1007/978-1-84882-105-7_28, © Springer-Verlag London Limited 2011

Fig. 28.1 Uni-X Single Port
Trocar (P Navel Company,
Brooklyn NY, USA).
Three 5-mm port sites
are available with one
site acting dually for
insufflation (With kind
permission from Springer
Science+Business Media:
Romanelli JR, Roshek TB
III, Lynn DC, Earle DB.
Single-port laparoscopic
cholecystectomy: initial
experience. *Surg Endosc.*
2010;24:1374–1379,
Figure 3)

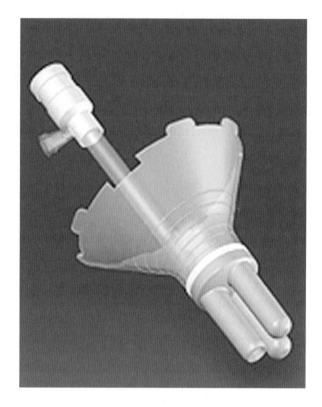

The Uni-X™ Single Port Trocar (Pnavel Systems, Inc., Cleveland, OH) is designed
similarly to a single blunt-tipped Hasson trocar with a conical shaped sheath (Fig. 28.1).
Stay sutures placed within the abdominal fascia are used to anchor the port to prevent air
leakage during its use. Instruments inserted through the channels maintain pneumoperitoneum using a valved system. The port itself is comprised of three 5-mm channels with one
that is elongated, which functions dually as a camera and an insufflation port. Some of the
world's first urological single-port surgeries were made possible via this multichannel
port. Advanced laparoscopic surgery, including radical cystectomy, prostatectomy, and
abdominal sacrocolpopexy, were possible without the incorporation of additional ports.[5]
An immediate limitation of this surgical port was the absence of a 10-mm entry site. When
and if 10-mm instruments were required, they were often placed alongside the port to
maintain the single-site principle. This ensuing air leak during renal and pelvic procedures
posed a challenge; however, endoscopic staplers and ultrasound probes were successfully
used without compromise. Unfortunately, the valved system lacked durability as frequent
instrument exchange resulted in significant damage that required port exchange.

Limitations of channel size have been overcome by a multichannel gel port designed by
Advanced Surgical Concepts, which utilizes two 5-mm and one 12-mm channels (ASC
TriPort, Ireland). The ASC TriPort's design is analogous to a laparoscopic hand-assist gel
port (Fig. 28.2). It is comprised of an external and internal plastic ring, which is delivered
intraabdominally through a 1.5-cm to 1.8-cm periumbilical incision. The internal ring

Fig. 28.2 The Triport trocar comprises of three gel-valved port sites (one 12 mm and two 5 mm), which provide more resilience during single-port procedures (Image courtesy of Advanced Surgical Concepts. Used with permission)

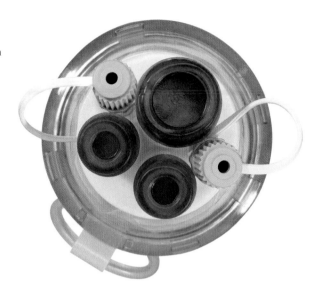

secures the port and maintains an air seal, obviating the need for stay sutures while maintaining pneumoperitoneum. Although not formally tested, clinical experience has demonstrated greater channel resilience of the ASC TriPort during repeated instrument exchange. A significant advantage of the gel port design is the flexibility of individual channels and the ability to accommodate a larger laparoscopic instrument, such as an ultrasound probe or an endovascular stapler. Despite addressing the limitations of the valved system, external clashing is minimized, but not entirely eliminated with the ASC TriPort. However, this conflict may not be entirely dependent on port design.

Given the proximity of channels during single-port surgery, triangulation is lost with straight laparoscopic instruments. The abdominal wall functions as a pivot for laparoscopic instrumentation, therefore, adequate external range of motion directly relates to reduced internal mobility. Instrument modifications were necessary to address these mechanical barriers. The EndoEYE™ system (Olympus America Inc., Center Valley, PA) is a 5-mm laparoscope consisting of a low-profile handle with in-line placement of both optical and power cords. The 0° optical tip is steerable via controls located at the base allowing the assistant to position him/herself away from the surgeon while still maintaining internal visibility (Fig. 28.3).

Flexible laparoscopic instruments have now been developed to address the space constraints inherent to single-port laparoscopy. By moving the fulcrum of the laparoscopic instruments proximally, the flexible tip can be angulated with wrist action, thereby reducing external conflict. Although initially counterintuitive, the learning curve to acquire routine dissection skills using articulating instruments is short. However, more complex skills, such suturing and knot tying as in regular laparoscopy, require more expertise. Currently, articulating laparoscopic needle drivers, monopolar scissors, and hooks are available for clinical use.

Although equipment flexibility limits external clashing, it does not eliminate it. The external design of clinically available laparoscopic instruments is bulky, which competes

Fig. 28.3 EndoEYE system
(Olympus America Inc.,
Center Valley, PA), offers an
articulating 5 mm digital
laparoscope which reduces
external conflict during
single-port procedures
(Image courtesy of
Olympus America Inc.)

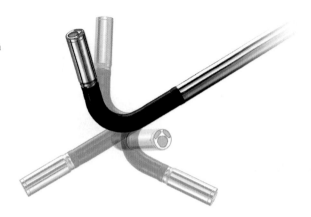

for the limited space surrounding the single multichannel port. Also, the internal flexibility of articulating instruments does not provide adequate rigidity for blunt dissection or retraction. To circumvent this obstacle, straight and articulating instruments are used in conjunction to maximize dissecting capabilities during single-port surgery. At times, stay sutures are placed into tissue and anchored to the abdominal wall to provide fixed exposure during laparoscopic dissection. Despite these technical constraints, various single-port renal and pelvic procedures have been performed and will be discussed further.

Single-Port Laparoscopic Renal Surgery

The authors' initial experience with the single-port laparoscopy involved various renal procedures. To provide a virtually "scarless" approach, the port was placed at the level of the umbilicus. The instruments traversed the distance from the umbilicus to their respective left or right upper quadrants during renal dissection. In addition to the space constraints mentioned above, obese patients added to this distance and currently elongated articulating instruments are unavailable. Reflection of the colon away from Gerota's fascia also impacted visibility. Despite lateral rotation of the patient, the colon was further displaced medially but not completely. The steerable laparoscope that provided visibility to the upper quadrant had to be oriented cranially and then deflected posteriorly, placing torque on the single port. As in most surgery, thinner patients without previous abdominal or renal surgery prove ideal candidates for single-port renal operations.

Thus far, an array of single-port renal procedures has been performed, ranging from cyst decortications to more complex procedures, such as partial nephrectomy. The authors' initial published series of single-port procedures included renal cryoablation.[4] Single-port access renal cryoablation (SPARC) offers an attractive introduction to single-port laparoscopy as the procedure involves minimal dissection and reconstruction. SPARC has been successfully performed via transperitoneal and retroperitoneal approaches with minimal postoperative morbidity or complications. As previously mentioned, the

Fig. 28.4 Diagrammatic representation of single port renal cryoablation. The ultrasound probe given its size slides adjacent to the single-port trocar through the same incision to provide intraoperative guidance during cryoprobe insertion into the tumor (Reprinted with permission, Cleveland Clinic Center for Medical Art & Photography © 2008–2010)

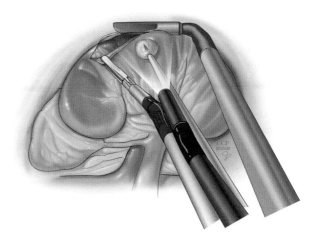

laparoscopic ultrasound probe inserted alongside the Pnavel port can result in loss of pneumoperitoneum. With bedside manipulation of the port, the pneumoperitoneum can be maintained during tumor identification and probe ablation (Fig. 28.4). All patients are currently being evaluated with regard to their oncological outcomes; however, initial results are promising. Patient selection for SPARC is essential as upper pole, large exophytic tumors or solitary kidneys are generally omitted due to surgical complexity and potential for intraoperative bleeding.

Familiarity with the single-port approach provides a platform to proceed to more complex renal operations including simple, radical, partial, and ultimately donor nephrectomy. Clearly, initial attempts at single-port renal surgery should not encompass the latter two operations, which are time-sensitive or complex. The surgeon should be adept at performing standard laparoscopic extirpative and reconstructive renal surgery prior to embarking on such procedures. Patient and tumor selection are also critical during partial nephrectomy. In addition to the aforementioned criteria, single-port partial nephrectomy without hilar control would include exophytic tumors without previous renal or abdominal surgery. Also, as in regular laparoscopy, upper pole tumors pose a challenge due to surgical exposure and adjacent solid viscera. The potential for bleeding exists, therefore surgical prowess for immediate hilar control and intracorporeal suturing should be at hand. The authors recommend that when single-port partial nephrectomy is initially performed, exophytic, anterior lower pole tumors should be selected.

Laparoscopic suturing can be a daunting task, requiring surgical persistence and patience. During regular laparoscopy, triangulation provided by port placement facilitates intracorporeal suturing and knot tying. Single-port surgery prohibits triangulation using standard laparoscopic needle drivers, therefore, the articulating variety provide the necessary angles required for intracorporeal reconstruction. Suture placement can be difficult as the flexible tip diminishes haptic feedback and thick tissue often deflects the needle driver tip. To further facilitate suturing and to minimize abdominal wall trauma, a 2-mm needlescopic grasper can reinstitute triangulation for intracorporeal suturing and knot tying. Another technique is to resort to extra-corporeal knot tying.

Overall, single-port laparoscopic and retroperitoneoscopic renal surgery has been successfully performed. An important caveat to the successful performance of all single-port renal surgery is patient selection. Patients with complicated renal pathology, previous renal surgery, or solitary kidneys were approached through traditional laparoscopic means. Given the early favorable experience with single-port procedures, now more complex operations are being performed, including single-port partial nephrectomy and donor nephrectomy. Familiarity of regular and articulating flexible laparoscopic instrumentation is essential to facilitate single-port surgery. A surgical assistant with previous laparoscopic experience is also invaluable during these complex procedures.

Single-Port Laparoscopic Pelvic Surgery

Urologists have incorporated laparoscopy in the treatment of various benign and malignant pelvic conditions for some time. Laparoscopic pelvic procedures offer certain advantages compared to renal surgery, especially during the single-port approach. When the patient is placed in lithotomy and the Trendelenburg position, it results in cranial displacement of bowel. In female patients with a uterus in situ, stay sutures through the fundus can provide cranial traction to further visualize the pouch of Douglas. In either sex, lateral displacement of the sigmoid colon can be achieved through a similar stay suture placed within the teniae coli during pelvic procedures. These maneuvers in addition to the larger working space of the pelvis provide the operator with a larger working area ideal for single-port surgery.

Laparoscopic oncologic and reconstructive pelvic surgery has been performed in various centers around the world.[6-9] Several advantages of the minimally invasive approach include shorter convalescence, less blood loss, and comparable oncological outcomes when performed by experienced surgeons.[6,10,11] Radical prostatectomy and both male and female radical cystectomies have been successfully adopted by high-volume cancer centers. Cancer control following the laparoscopic approach is still pending long-term evaluation, but early results show comparable results to that of an open series.[11] Other pelvic pathology, including pelvic prolapse, has also been successfully approached laparoscopically. Abdominal sacrocolpopexy is considered the gold standard in repair of pelvic organ prolapse. Once considered a morbid procedure, refinement in technique and the application of laparoscopy has reduced patient morbidity while maintaining surgical principle during prolapse repair.[8]

Laparoscopic abdominal sacrocolpopexy was approached through a single port to evaluate the surgical effectiveness of dissecting within the deep pelvis for a nonmalignant condition. Patients who were candidates to undergo a traditional laparoscopic repair were considered for the single-port approach. In addition, patients who had failed previous prolapse surgery or who had multiple abdominal surgeries were avoided for this new technical approach. Patients were not excluded based on a previous hysterectomy, and, in fact, a uterine preserving sacrocolpopexy was performed in this circumstance. To provide exposure to the deep pelvis, stay sutures to the tenia coli and to the uterine fundus provided lateral and cranial retraction respectively.

Perhaps the most challenging aspect of this procedure was intracorporeal suturing of the mesh to the vaginal wall. Laparoscopically suturing with traditional straight instruments was challenging given the limited external and internal range of motion as described previously. Although the articulating needle drivers facilitate suture placement, knot tying requires patience. Placement of the sacral anchor is also difficult during single-port surgery. The triangulation provided by laparoscopy allows for suture placement through the anterior spinous ligament and into the mesh. The port, when placed at its periumbilical location, places surgical instruments nearly perpendicular to the sacrum making suturing impossible. Articulating needle drivers have been utilized to provide fixation at the sacrum, however, the malleability of the instruments does not allow for sufficient purchase of the ligamentous structure. The EndoTak (Ethicon Endo-Surgery, Cincinnati, OH) provides the solution for this clinical problem. The device functions by delivering a titanium coil through the mesh and into a bony structure. Thus far, this device has been used for ten single-port laparoscopic sacrocolpopexies, and has provided excellent prolapse reduction without recurrence to date.

Single-port pelvic surgery for malignant disease has been performed at the authors' institution, including radical prostatectomy and radical cystectomy with bilateral lymph node dissection. The initial series of radical prostatectomy incorporated patients with small-volume, organ-confined disease. The technical points of laparoscopic prostatectomy were initially attempted, however, given the range of motion and surgical visibility, modifications were needed. Knowledge of performing both antegrade and retrograde radical prostatectomy is essential as both techniques were employed during the procedure. Upon completion of the prostatectomy, the urethral-vesical anastomosis was performed. Experiential use of the articulating needle drivers enabled the placement of progressively more anastamotic sutures during succeeding cases (Fig. 28.5).

Single-port cystectomy has also been approached in both male and female bladder malignancies. During laparoscopic radical cystectomy, the vascular pedicle for the bladder can be controlled by various means including endovascular staplers, Hem-o-lok® clips (Teleflex Medical, Inc., Research Triangle Park, NC) and hemosealant devices. Initially, radical cystectomy was performed using the Pnavel port and the 5-mm channels can only accommodate the Ligasure™ (ValleyLab, Boulder, CO) or the harmonic scalpel to control the vascular pedicles. At times, 5-mm Weck clips were utilized for control of substantial pedicles. Following the cystectomy, bilateral pelvic lymphadenectomy was carried out. Despite initial concerns of visibility, a mean yield of 16 ± 3 nodes were obtained amongst all three patients.[12] Negative surgical margins were obtained in all cystectomy patients.

Single-port laparoscopic surgery has challenged the field of minimally invasive surgery to further reduce abdominal trauma and surgical scarring. Although its exact role in reconstructive and oncologic surgery is pending, initial results are showing promise for replicating the standard laparoscopic approach. The ability to perform single-port laparoscopy hinges on the comfort and skill of performing standard laparoscopic procedures. Just as the introduction of the robotic platform has provided a bridge from open to minimally invasive surgery, the applicability of robotics to single-port surgery has been explored. The articulation and degrees of motion available to robotics would address the limitations encountered during single-port dissection and reconstruction. At the authors' institution, single-port robotic surgery was recently performed in both the laboratory and clinical setting.

Fig. 28.5 Illustration of
single-port laparoscopic
suturing during radical
prostatectomy. The
articulating needle drivers
provide the ability to
perform the urethral-vesical
anastamosis (Reprinted with
permission, Cleveland
Clinic Center for Medical
Art & Photography
© 2008–2010)

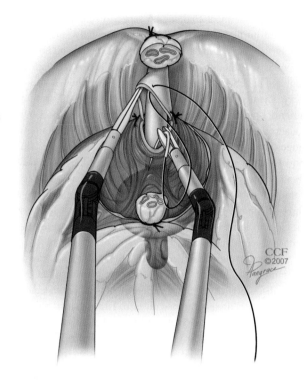

Single-Port Robotic Surgery

The current robotic platform has not been designed specifically for single-port surgery. Various technical modifications were necessary to allow the robotic arms to function in such close confinement. Adjusting robotic port placement and instrument configuration were essential to provide enough maneuverability during surgery. Thus far, both pelvic and renal procedures have been performed using the *daVinci®* S surgical robotic platform (Intuitive Surgical, Inc., Sunnyvale, CA). The ASC TriPort, with its gel-based design and 12-mm port, provided intraabdominal access and was resilient enough to tolerate the torque exerted by the robot. To allow surgical control of the camera, a 10-mm port was placed within the clasps of the robotic camera holder. The 8-mm robotic lens was easily navigated through the 12-mm channel of the ASC TriPort. Also, pediatric 5-mm trocars minimized the space occupied by the traditional 8-mm trocars. Another modification was to placing the 5-mm robotic port alongside the ASC TriPort through the same skin incision. These adjustments improved the freedom of motion from the surrounding camera arm and contralateral robotic instrument (Fig. 28.6). Thus far, single-port robotics have been successful for radical prostatectomy, radical nephrectomy, and dismembered pyeloplasty.[13] Based on the authors' early surgical experience, the robotic platform offered comparable operative results with improved range of motion during urethral-vesical and ureteropelvic anastomosis.

Fig. 28.6 Intraoperative image of single-port robotic prostatectomy. Due to space limitation, the robotic camera and arm are inserted into the trocar while one arm is placed adjacent to the trocar but through the same skin incision. This provides for improved articulation of the working arm and minimizes external conflict

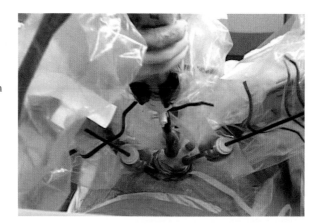

Conclusion

Single-port laparoscopy has offered a significant challenge to the minimally invasive surgical community. Currently available instrumentation designed for traditional laparoscopy is being utilized for this challenging procedure. Ongoing modification to equipment and technique has allowed single-port surgery to grow in the urological community. Experience has demonstrated various limitations of single-port surgery, however, persistence has proven itself as various renal and pelvic surgeries have been completed. To disseminate this technology into the lay public, further adjustments to preexisting instruments is necessary. Robotics may be the next step in evolution to provide a more ergonomic and user-friendly platform for single-port laparoscopy.

References

1. Piskun G, Rajpal S. Transumbilical laparoscopic cholecystectomy utilizes no incisions outside the umbilicus. *J Laparoendosc Adv Surg Tech A*. 1999;9(4):361-364.
2. Desai MM, Rao PP, Aron M, et al. Scarless single port transumbilical nephrectomy and pyeloplasty: first clinical report. *BJU Int*. 2008;101(1):83-88.
3. Gill IS, Canes D, Aron M, et al. Single port transumbilical (E-NOTES) donor nephrectomy. *J Urol*. 2008;180(2):637-641.
4. Goel RK, Kaouk JH. Single port access renal cryoablation (SPARC): a new approach. *Eur Urol*. 2008;53(6):1204-1209.
5. Kaouk JH, Haber G, Goel RK, et al. Single-port laparoscopic surgery in urology: initial experience. *Urology*. 2008;71(1):3-6.
6. Fergany AF, Gill IS. Laparoscopic radical cystectomy. *Urol Clin North Am*. 2008;35(3): 455-466.
7. Hemal AK, Kolla SB, Wadhwa P, et al. Laparoscopic radical cystectomy and extracorporeal urinary diversion: a single center experience of 48 cases with three years of follow-up. *Urology*. 2008;71(1):41-46.

8. Sarlos D, Brander S, Kots L, et al. Laparoscopic sacrocolpopexy for uterine and post-hyster-ectomy prolapse: anatomical results, quality of life and perioperative outcome-a prospective study with 101 cases. *Int Urogynecol J Pelvic Floor Dysfunct*. 2008;19(10):1415-1422.

9. Slawik S, Soulsby R, Carter H, et al. Laparoscopic ventral rectopexy, posterior colporrhaphy and vaginal sacrocolpopexy for the treatment of recto-genital prolapse and mechanical outlet obstruction. *Colorectal Dis*. 2008;10(2):138-143.

10. Canes D, Tuerk IA. Laparoscopic radical cystectomy: formidable challenge to the gold stan-dard. *J Endourol*. 2008;22(9):2069-2071. discussion 2079, 2083.

11. Berger A, Aron M. Laparoscopic radical cystectomy: long-term outcomes. *Curr Opin Urol*. 2008;18(2):167-172.

12. White WM, Haber GP, Goel RK, Crouzet S, Stein RJ, Kaouk JH. Single-port urological sur-gery: single-center experience with the first 100 cases. *Urology*. 2009;74(4):801-804.

13. Kaouk JH, Goel RK, Haber G, Crouzet S, Stein RJ. Robotic single-port transumbilical surgery in humans: initial report. *BJU Int*. 2009;103(3):366-369.

Difficulties in Urologic Laparoscopy Complications

29

Rene J. Sotelo Noguera, Camilo Andrés Giedelman Cuevas, Golena Fernández Moncaleano, and David Canes

Introduction

Urologic laparoscopy has entered the mainstream in the modern urologist's armamentarium. Minimally invasive techniques aim to reproduce the results of open surgery with lower morbidity, less postoperative pain, and shorter convalescence.[1] Laparoscopic surgery has many advantages, but its somewhat more restricted environment requires a specialized skill set, specific troubleshooting, and unique potential complications. The degree of complexity of the surgical procedure and the experience of the surgeon significantly influence complication rates.

In urological surgery, laparoscopy has seen considerable growth in the last decade. Initially limited to a few relatively simple procedures, a variety of more sophisticated surgeries were developed, allowing removal of tumors of the adrenal gland, kidney, prostate and bladder, as well as reconstructive surgery of the urinary tract.[2] The minimally invasive approach has now become a standard approach for adrenalectomy for small masses, radical nephrectomy for T1 disease, and radical prostatectomy for organ confined cancer, to name just a few. With a rise in the number and complexity of laparoscopic surgeries, inevitably there was an initial parallel increase in associated complications.[3]

In the laparoscopic environment, not all complications require immediate open conversion, but the window to expeditiously address an evolving complication is short. Complications must therefore be anticipated, such that identification of problems is swift, and the appropriate solution can be applied. Laparoscopic recognition and management of the complication can be challenging, and multiple factors including operator skill, available instrumentation, and timing of the diagnosis will determine the need for open conversion.[4]

This chapter has several goals: (1) to give a broad overview of minimally invasive surgical complications, (2) provide tips to handle and prevent complications. For each complication, the incidence of will be noted, but the reader should be aware that the published

R.J.S. Noguera (✉)
Department of Urology, Centro de Cirugía Robotica y de Invasion Minima,
Instituto Medico La Floresta, Caracas, Venezuela
e-mail: renesotelo@cantv.net

A.M. Al-Kandari and I.S. Gill (eds.), *Difficult Conditions in Laparoscopic Urologic Surgery*, 405
DOI: 10.1007/978-1-84882-105-7_29, © Springer-Verlag London Limited 2011

incidence come from high volume centers, and may not be broadly applicable. The surgeon's biggest enemy is pride, specifically we belief that complications happen to other surgeons; always keep in mind that complications can occur at any point in time, during any case.

General Preventive Measures

- Review imaging (CT scan with 3D reconstruction or MRI) for accessory renal vessels to have an exact plan.
- In difficult cases, such as retroperitoneal lymph node dissection (RPLND) or nephrectomy, prepare all the required disposables and instruments that may be needed when dealing with large vessel injury. Also, rolls of gauze should be prepared on the table, which may be required to control bleeding, if it occurs.
- Avoid working in holes. Instead, progressively extend the dissection laterally. Laparoscopy requires correct exposure to verify the vascular and other organ anatomy.
- If endovascular staplers are being used for big vessels, double-check that the correct vascular cartridge is loaded, and be prepared for malfunctions. Always try to apply the stapler a few millimeters distally, leaving a small vascular stump. This allows the surgeon to clip it further, if needed.
- In case of bleeding, increase pneumoperitoneum to 20 mmHg and try to compress with any grasper or with the suction device. If rolled gauze has been previously inserted, this also can be used for compression. With the aid of the suction, one must then decide the best way to control the bleeding, whether by metal clip, Hem-o-lok® clip (Teleflex Medical, Research Triangle Park, NC), vascular stapler, or suture ligation.
- In case of disruption of a small branch of the vena cava, clips may be applied. If clips are not effective, use sutures. Do not use bipolar or any other kind of electrical device as it will make it worse. One good trick to suture holes in major vessels is to use a big needle (the tip of small needle will be difficult to see in a pool of blood) with a Hem-o-lok® or Lapra-Ty clip (Ethicon Endo Surgery, Inc., Cincinnati, OH) at the end. After you pass the needle through, gentle traction of the suture will decrease the bleeding, facilitating the next pass and obviating the first knot (Fig. 29.1).
- If the surgeon is unable to repair an injury laparoscopically, but the bleeding has been controlled temporarily with a grasper or gauze and the patient is hemodynamically stable, placement of a hand-assisted device may be an option (provided that it is available and the surgeon is trained to use it). Otherwise, open conversion should be performed without wasting more time in order to minimize morbidity.
- Trocar sites should always be inspected under low pressure to ensure absence of bleeding after trocar removal. The 10–12-mm trocar sites should also be closed to avoid hernias.
- After controlling cases of significant bleeding, confirm hemostasis and leave a drainage tube through one of the trocar holes (Fig. 29.2).
- Training of the laparoscopic surgeon should be exhaustive and comprehensive, especially in laparoscopic suturing.

Fig. 29.1 Vena cava transected with ENDO GIA™ (Covidien, Dublin, Ireland), misidentified

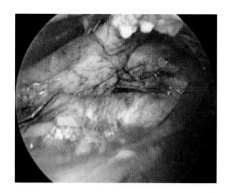

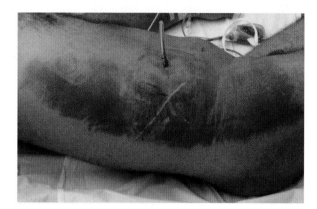

Fig. 29.2 Abdominal wall hematoma

Access-Related Complications

Care must be taken with the Veress needle as it can cause hematoma in the retroperitoneum and injury of small bowel or liver, depending on the area where it is inserted. In cases of prior open abdominal surgery, select an area away from the scar to minimize the risk of bowel injury. When in doubt, use open access.

The incidence of major vascular injuries with the first trocar is very rare, occurring in 0.05–0.26% of cases, but there is high mortality rate (8–17%) if it occurs. Therefore, care must be taken in thin and obese patients because the angle and the distance between the umbilical port and the aortic bifurcation differs. In the obese patient, the umbilical port drops with the abdominal fat, and the angle of insertion needs to be oblique (not vertical as usual). In this case, the umbilical port comes above the aortic bifurcation.[5–9]

The incidence of epigastric vessel injury during trocar insertion is 0.3–2.5%. It is surprising if this occurs during the insertion of secondary trocar, since this is supposed to occur under direct vision. Sometimes an angulated insertion of the trocar causes this injury, so a mild tilt and a more vertical insertion is a helpful trick to avoid this injury.

One of the common causes of difficulty in access is inadequate length of the skin incision, which leads to additional resistance during trocar insertion. This generates more pressure at entry so that the trocar passes through the skin with excess force. This can cause the trocar to advance more than desired, which may in turn cause intraabdominal injury. Obese patients present difficulty in reaching the fascia. In these cases, it is better to create a bigger skin incision to expose the fascia, then open the fascia, place a forceps at the lateral edges to pull up the fascia, and place the Veress needle.

It is very important to realize that there are no safe trocars. Even with newly designed trocars that have no blades (which are reported to have less incidence of hernia and less injury of the abdominal wall vessels), major vascular injuries can still occur (Figs. 29.3 and 29.4).

In case of major vascular injury, the surgeon only has seconds to evaluate and decide if it can be resolved laparoscopically or if conversion to open surgery is needed. If open conversion is chosen, the laparoscope can be used to compress the area of bleeding. An open set should always be ready for when prompt action is necessary. The anesthetist should act rapidly during resuscitation and request blood for transfusion as needed. Then the surgeon, if comfortable and confident, should work quickly by opening over the laparoscope to enter the peritoneum. In these cases, the incision should be generous since it is a life-saving procedure.

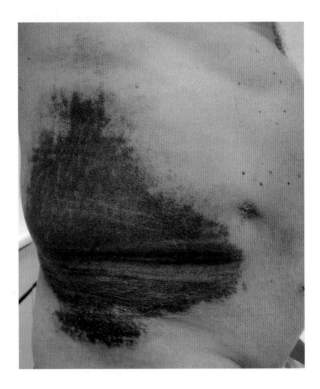

Fig. 29.3 Abdominal wall hematoma after epigastric vessel injury

Fig. 29.4 Colon injury with first trocar

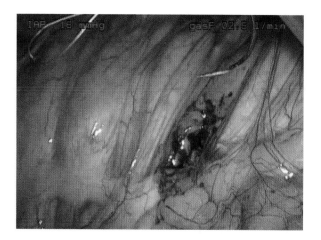

Intraoperative Complications

Regardless of the surgery that is performed, there are a number of general concepts that need to be kept in mind. The majority of the vascular and nonvascular injuries can occur due to: (1) errors during dissection; (2) inadvertent movements; (3) wrong identification of anatomical structures; and (4) instrument malfunction. The incidence of complications during laparoscopic surgery can easily be overlooked when a large series is reviewed over time. But a beginning laparoscopic surgeon should consider reports on complications in small series which reveals the real scenario.

It is important that before starting a laparoscopic procedure that all instruments for open surgery should be prepared. The laparoscopy tower must be prepared with connections for insufflators, an electrocautery set, a suction–irrigation system, and optical equipment, all ready for use before the introduction of the trocars. After introducing the first trocar, the cavity is reviewed to verify absence of injuries.

If vascular injury is encountered in the abdominal wall, then one can oversew it with a Carter-Thomason suture passer (CooperSurgical, Trumbull, CT) and then choose another site. A Foley catheter with an inflated balloon may be temporarily used for compression while preparing to manage the injury. Otherwise, one should not hesitate to open to manage bleeding. Other major intraabdominal vascular injuries require immediate conversion and compression and vascular surgeon assistance. The authors recommend a surgeon to have a laparoscopic bleeding set in a separate box identified with the color red for easy recognition. The set should contain:

- Lapra-Ty and Hem-o-lok® clips and appliers
- Two laparoscopic needle drivers
- Laparoscopic Satinski clamp
- Bulldog clamp

- Surgicel® (Ethicon, Inc., Somerville, NJ)
- Bolster of gauze
- Vicryl™ CT-1 needle (Ethicon, Inc., Somerville, NJ) 10-cm long with Lapra-Ty at the end
- Vicryl™ CT-1 needle 10 cm
- Automatic titanium clip applier

Chain of Action

- In case of bleeding, increase pneumoperitoneum to 20 mmHg, and try to compress with any grasper or with the suction device. If rolled gauze has been previously inserted, use it for compression and decide if clips or sutures should be applied.
- Decide if the suction device of 5 mm is satisfactory, or change to a 10-mm device with multiple holes at the tip. Ask the anesthesiologist for a central line if it has not been placed and request that blood be prepared.
- If the injury cannot be repaired laparoscopically, but the bleeding has been temporarily controlled with a grasper or with gauze and the patient is hemodynamically stable, the use of a hand-assisted device should be considered (if available and the surgeon has the experience to use it).
- If the bleeding is massive, then an immediate open conversion should be performed. Remember that the bleeding will worsen when the surgeon opens, so laparotomy pads should be immediately available for compression and packing.

Visceral Complications

After introduction of the first trocar, if one sees bowel contents due to an injury of the small bowel or colon, the authors recommend keeping the trocar temporarily in place which will help pinpoint the area of injury. Introduce a new trocar more than 10 cm away, as this allows the surgeon to inspect the cavity and decide if the bowel injury can be repaired laparoscopically, if the segment needs to be exteriorized for repair, or if open conversion is needed.

Early recognition of bowel injury is of utmost importance since it can usually be managed with laparoscopic or open repair. If significant fecal spillage is noted, especially without prior bowel preparation, then open conversion and either temporary colostomy or loop ileostomy may be needed. If the problem is unrecognized during surgery, it will always require open exploration since it may lead to peritonitis and all subsequent complications of intraabdominal abscess, intestinal fistula, and may eventually lead to wound dehiscence (Fig. 29.5).

Fig. 29.5 Injury of the spleen during entrapment of the specimen

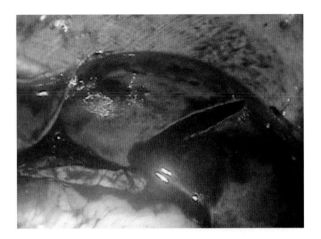

Incidence of Laparoscopic Complications in Urology

Complication rates in contemporary series of laparoscopic procedures range from 4% to 22% in both children and adults.[2,4,10] One of the largest series of urologic laparoscopic procedures was described by Perpongkolsol et al, where 2,775 laparoscopic surgeries occurring between 1993 and 2005 were reviewed for a retrospective chart analysis. They reported a total of 614 complications (22.1%). Total intraoperative and postoperative complication rates were 4.7% and 17.5%, respectively.[11] In a study of 1,085 laparoscopic urologic interventions made by Soulié, complications were described in 6.9% of cases (75 events).[12] The results of the aforementioned studies demonstrate that the case series have similar percentages of complications. (It also should be noted that the series were performed by trained and experienced urologists and in referral centers for laparoscopy.) The most common complications reported were vascular and intestinal injuries. The remaining part of this chapter will illustrate potential laparoscopic complications in each step of laparoscopic procedures.

Positioning Complications

Creating a comfortable working environment in minimally invasive genitourinary surgery, the surgeon often relies on gravity and patient positioning for optimal exposure. Patient positioning, and at times prolonged operative times, predisposes the patient to potentially painful and debilitating neuropathies if precautions are not taken. The incidence of neuromuscular injuries during laparoscopic urologic procedures is reported in some series to be 2.7%. Clinical rhabdomyolysis may be present in 0.4% of patients, the risk factors being obese patients, longer operative time (>5 h), and elderly patients.[13]

Methods to Avoid Neuromuscular Complications

Renal Surgery:

- Careful positioning and padding
- Gel pad and bean bag ("cocoon effect")
- Avoid excessive flexion of table
- Use axillary roll

Prostate Surgery:

- Arms and hands well padded
- Legs abducted on split leg operating room table
- Avoid lithotomy position; avoid table flexion
- Avoid shoulder brace

Retroperitoneal Laparoscopy

Urologists initially preferred the retroperitoneal approach because it has a direct access to a familiar space. However, the larger working space and readily identifiable landmarks have since made the transperitoneal approach more widespread. Multiple series have demonstrated its advantages.[14]

In a multi-institutional review of 1,043 retroperitoneoscopic/extraperitoneoscopic cases, Gill et al found that major complications occurred in 49 patients, related visceral injuries in 26 (2.5%). The most common visceral complications were pneumothorax (six patients), pneumomediastinum (four patients), and perforation of the urinary bladder (four patients). Vascular injuries occurred in 2.2% of cases; the most frequent blood vessels affected were the renal vein (six patients) and the inferior cava vein (four patients). The percentage of conversion to transperitoneal laparoscopy was 5.4% and to open surgery was 6.6%.[15] Meraney et al. described vascular injuries in 1.7% and bowel injuries in 0.75% in a 404 patient series.[16]

In 2006, Demey et al. presented a series of 500 patients of retroperitoneal laparoscopic procedures in the upper urinary tract with a 23% conversion due to: retroperitoneal adhesions (five patients), intraoperative bleeding (11 patients), and technical difficulties (seven patients). Revision was done in 14 patients because of: urinoma (five patients), urocutaneous fistula (two patients), deep abscesses (two patients), secondary bleeding (two patients), colostomies for gastrointestinal fistula after colonic injury (two patients), and incisional hernia (one patient).[17]

Liapis et al. presented a 10-year study on laparoscopic cases. Conversion to open surgery occurred in 4.6% of cases (28 patients) due to technical problems during dissection. Complications occurred in 5.3% (32 patients), including bleeding (12 patients) and urinomas (eight patients). Wound or deep abscesses occurred in four patients, urinary fistula in one patient and pancreatic fistula in another patient. Evisceration occurred in three patients. Postoperative complications like hyperthermia, deep venous thrombosis, pyelonephritis, pulmonary infections, pulmonary atelectasis, and transient vascular ischemic accident occurred in 4.6% of patients.[18]

In a series of 316 patients, Kumar et al. reported that minor complications occurred in 15.8% of cases; (peritoneal rent, emphysema, kidney puncture, pleural effusion, retroperitoneal collection, persistent drainage, ileus, port site infection, fever, etc.) major complications occurred in 3.5% (vascular 2.2%, visceral 0.3%, collection 0.6%, and hernia 0.3%).[19]

In a separate review of 185 cases of retroperitoneoscopic nephrectomy and nephroureterectomy for benign diseases, Hemal et al. reported conversion to open surgery in 18 cases. Complications occurred in 37 cases (16.2% were minor and 3.8% were major), and reintervention was needed in only one patient.[20] With respect to retroperitoneoscopic ureterolithotomy, Hemal et al. have reported injury to the external iliac artery in one patient.[21]

Laparoscopic Adrenalectomy

Laparoscopy has become the technique of choice for surgery of the adrenal gland. Several studies have retrospectively compared laparoscopic adrenalectomy and traditional open access, and found that the laparoscopic approach was associated with early oral intake, shorter hospitalization, less postoperative pain, and shorter convalescence.[4,22,23]

Generally, the rate of complications reported in laparoscopic adrenalectomy is low.[24] In a study of 2,407 patients by Fahlenkamp et al., 44 adrenalectomies were performed with six complications.[10] In the 350 patient series of Soulié et al., 54 underwent laparoscopic adrenalectomy, and two cases sustained vascular injury during dissection of a left renal polar artery and on the vena cava.[25]

In 2000, Terachi et al. reported on a total of 370 laparoscopic adrenalectomies, 311 procedures performed with a transperitoneal approach and 59 with a retroperitoneal approach. The intraoperative complication rate was 9% (33 patients) in total: 26/311 (8%) in the transperitoneal procedures and 7/59 (12%) in the retroperitoneoscope procedures. The postoperative complication rate was 6% in total. Open conversion occurred in 3.5% of cases.[26]

In 2006, Castillo et al. presented a series of 205 laparoscopic adrenalectomies with nine complications (4.5%). Complications were divided into intraoperative and postoperative events. Intraoperative events included vascular injuries (1.5%), pancreatic fistula (1%), retroperitoneal hematoma (1%), diaphragmatic injury (0.5%) (Fig. 29.6), and splenic injury (0.5%). A postoperative complication was trocar hernia (1.5%).[4] Conversion rate to open surgery was 0.9%.[27]

Advice to Avoid Complications

- Avoid moving the patient when ports are already in place, especially the subcostal port since it can injure the liver. Also, care must be taken during placement of the grasper for liver retraction. Use broad instrument surfaces rather than instrument tips along the liver to prevent laceration.

Fig. 29.6 Left diaphragmatic injury

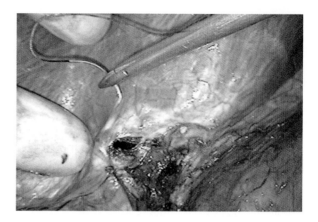

- On the left side, make sure that the spleen is completely mobilized and free. Confusion between the tail of the pancreas and adrenal tumor can be problematic, so splenic mobilization is helpful in clarifying the anatomy.
- Adrenal lesions larger than 5 cm should be approached laparoscopically only when significant expertise exists.[14]
- Keep in mind the tail of the pancreas can be confused with an adrenal tumor on the left side.

Laparoscopic Renal Cyst Ablation

Laparoscopic management of renal cystic disease is considered highly effective and safe. Simple renal cysts can be accessed either transperitoneally or retroperitoneally. Most kidney cysts are asymptomatic and do not require treatment. The indications for treatment are limited to cysts that obstruct the collecting system and compress the renal parenchyma, or cysts that bleed spontaneously, producing pain and hematuria. In addition, cysts that cause hypertension, obstructive uropathy, or are infected require intervention.

Almost all studies have demonstrated superior efficacy of the laparoscopic approach in renal cyst ablation. This is due to significant advantages, such as minimal intraoperative blood loss and minimal morbidity, short operative time and hospital stay, rapid convalescence and superior cosmesis in comparison to open surgery.[28, 29] Rubenstein et al. reported on the laparoscopic approach for drainage and ablation of symptomatic simple renal cysts. Ten patients with chronic pain (six of whom failed primary aspiration) underwent laparoscopic cyst ablation; six patients had solitary renal cysts, three patients had multiple cysts, and one patient had a peripelvic cyst. The approach was transperitoneal in nine patients and extraperitoneal in one patient. The only complication was a postoperative retroperitoneal hematoma, which was managed conservatively.[30]

Laparoscopic Radical Nephrectomy

Complications may occur in any stage of this surgery. Vascular injury during laparoscopic radical nephrectomy can be life-threatening and emergent open conversion may be needed, and so the surgeon should always confirm that the open set is available and ready.

Fig. 29.7 Inferior vena cava transected in a right retroperitoneal nephrectomy

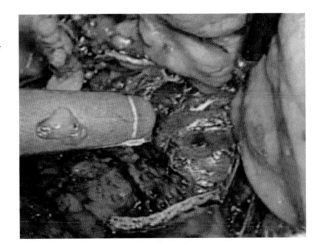

The rate of major complications varies from 3% to 15%.[31] In a series of 213 transperitoneal laparoscopic nephrectomies, the rate of conversion was 6%.[32]

Vascular injuries may include injury to the renal or gonadal vessels, inferior vena cava or lumbar vessels, adrenal vessels, splenic artery, and superior mesenteric artery. Visceral injuries may occur due to fan retractors used in laparoscopic transperitoneal approaches. Injury may occur in all adjacent organs such as the kidney, ureter, adrenal, liver, spleen, duodenum, pancreas, colon, diaphragm, or pleura. Injury can occur during the processes of dissection at the beginning, during hilar dissection, or at the completion of the case. The experienced laparoscopic surgeon should attempt to manage visceral or vascular complications laparoscopically, given that the patient's life and safety is not threatened and that the injury can be repaired – otherwise, open conversion should be done (Fig. 29.7).

Advice to Avoid Complications

- Always lift the kidney to dissect the renal pedicle. This stretches the pedicle and facilitates dissection.
- Be careful of thermal injuries to the vessels during dissection with monopolar coagulation instruments.
- Use delicate retraction during pedicle dissection and try to completely dissect the renal hilum. Separately ligate the artery and vein, dissecting its entire circumference before applying clips or the stapler. Always ligate the renal artery before the vein. In difficult situations, en bloc stapling of artery and vein can be performed, as the safety of this maneuver has been reported.
- During right laparoscopic retroperitoneal nephrectomy, always keep the psoas muscle as your horizontal line. When identifying the renal vein, verify it's direction (heading to kidney), and caliber (anticipated renal vein caliber versus larger vena cava.
- During right laparoscopic transperitoneal nephrectomy, verify that the duodenum is seen first. After the duodenum is mobilized, the cava should be visible. Make sure to

dissect the upper pole of the kidney and obtain adequate retraction of the liver to have a good view of the adrenal and cava.

- In case of bleeding, increase pneumoperitoneum to 20 mmHg and try to compress using any grasper or with the suction device. If rolled gauze has been previously inserted, use it for compression. If rolled gauze has not been inserted, consider introducing it and decide if clips or sutures need to be applied.
- In case of disruption of a small branch of the cava, try small metal clips, if these are unsuccessful, use suture. Do not use bipolar or any other kind of electrical device as it will make it worse. One good trick to suture holes in this important vessel is use a big needle (the tip of a small needle will be difficult to see in a pool of blood) with a Hem-o-lok® or Lapra-Ty clip at its end. After the needle is passed, the gentle traction of the suture will decrease the bleeding, facilitating the next pass and obviating the first knot as previously described. If bleeding cannot be controlled as described, then open conversion is needed.
- During left laparoscopic transperitoneal nephrectomy, be careful if a big artery is found first as this could be the superior mesenteric artery (generally the renal vein is found first in transperitoneal approach). It is essential to mobilize the spleen with the colon; this maneuver will move the tail of the pancreas away.
- If it is decided that staples will be used for large vessels, the surgeon should double-check that the white vascular cartilage is being used and also should be prepared for malfunctions. The stapler should always be applied few millimeters distally to leave a stump in case it needs to be grasped and secured again.
- Keep in mind that an accessory renal artery may be present. If the renal vein is still full after clipping the main artery, look for an accessory renal artery and clip it before the vein.
- Never remove the specimen without placing it in a bag as this avoids tumor spillage during specimen removal.
- The authors do not recommend kidney morcellation in malignant pathology as this minimizes the risk of tumor spillage and helps the pathologist to accurately stage and grade the tumor.
- Close the extraction incision in two layers.
- It is safer to close the fascia at trocar sites larger than 10 mm with a Carter-Thomason suture passer.
- In some high-risk obese patients, it may be safer to close the specimen extraction incision with mesh to avoid hernias.

Laparoscopic Simple Nephrectomy

The major intraoperative complications in laparoscopic simple nephrectomy are bleeding (usually from the renal vein, adrenal vein, or accessory branches), visceral injury (spleen, liver, bowel, or omentum), and vascular injury (superior mesenteric artery, aorta, and inferior cava).[32,33] It is worth mentioning that laparoscopic simple nephrectomy can generally be more difficult than radical nephrectomy due to the degree of inflammation and fibrosis of predisposing conditions like stones, infections, and obstruction. In addition, some cases may have had previous operations which cause the formation of perinephric adhesions. Postoperative complications are unusual but can occur in patients with severe inflammation of the kidney and surrounding tissue; complications are hematoma, intrabdominal abscess, pneumothorax, wound infection, and incisional hernia.[34]

Extreme care should be taken in the release of adhesions since there may be injuries to the colon and duodenum during hilar dissection. As in open surgery, the dissection may be subcapsular, which provides an easy plane. If significant difficulty is encountered and surgery is not progressing safely, then open conversion should be considered.

Laparoscopic Partial Nephrectomy

The main complication in laparoscopic partial nephrectomy is bleeding (1.3–4.3%).[35] As the hilum is dissected and prepared for clamping, tearing of a small collateral vessel may occur, so the surgeon must be very careful with the dissection and also be alert to the possibility that more than one vessel may need to be clamped. One of the postoperative complications is bleeding from area of resection or hematuria. This can be mild to moderate and is rarely severe. If the patient is hemodynamically stable, then a conservative approach with blood transfusion and close monitoring can be implemented. Otherwise, reoperation can be done laparoscopically if the patient is stable, or open if the patient is unstable. During reoperation, bleeding points can be sutured with application of hemostatic agents, otherwise radical nephrectomy is an option. In one series, reoperation was done in 2% of cases and elective laparoscopic radical nephrectomy was performed in 0.5%.[36] Vascular arterial-venous fistulas can also occur, which can be managed with endovascular embolization.

To decrease positive margin, it is important to have adequate evaluation of the preoperative images, and to use intraoperative ultrasound. In order to have appropriate vascular control for better visibility, it is important to use adequate scissors. The authors employ reusable laparoscopic scissors that have a wider opening angle but are sharp. In special situations, the authors use a laparoscopic scalpel for precise and fast resection. Spaliviero and Gill have reported their series on laparoscopic partial nephrectomy and described their technique of suturing the renal bed in order to minimize warm ischemia time. First, deep sutures of Vicryl™ on a CT-1 needle are quickly inserted in the parenchyma. Early unclamping is performed and necessary sutures are completed. Vicryl™ sutures prepared with Hem-o-lok® clips on the side are used with bolsters of Surgicel®, put into the renal bed, and closed with traction and other Hem-o-lok® clips with the addition of a hemostatic agent (FloSeal™, Baxter International Inc., Deerfield, IL).

Another complication is urine leakage which may occur in 2.1–17.4% of cases.[35] The use of an intraoperative ureteral catheter and retrograde instillation of diluted methylene blue to ensure appropriate closure of the collecting system is recommended, especially in deep tumor resections. In some difficult cases, leaving a double J stent may be necessary. The urethral catheter should be removed when the drainage is less than 30 cc in the last 12 h, then if the drainage does not increase remove it 2 or 3 days later.

A total of 592 laparoscopic nephron-sparing surgery procedures were collected from 12 centers in a report by Celia et al.; the intraoperative open conversion rate was 3.5% (21/592). Postoperative complications included bleeding in 15/592 (2.5%) and urine leakage in 13/592 (2.1%); no tumor seeding was reported.[37]

The surgical experience of Pyo et al. with 110 consecutive patients who underwent retroperitoneal laparoscopic partial nephrectomy revealed major complications in 4.5% of cases. Conversion to open surgery occurred in two cases and laparoscopic radical nephrectomy was performed in four cases. There was one incidence of local recurrence at 1 year.[38]

Laparoscopic Pyeloplasty

Laparoscopic pyeloplasty has demonstrated functional results comparable to conventional open surgery and has become, in many centers, the procedure of choice in the management of ureteropelvic junction obstruction.[4] There are reported series of laparoscopic pyeloplasty for primary and secondary ureteropelvic junction obstruction, both transperitoneal and extraperitoneal, with complication rates between 3.6% and 9.1%.[39, 40] Complications include bleeding, mechanical ileus, volvulus of the cecum, and paralytic ileus.

The management of complications of pyeloplasty is fairly simple in most cases; urinary tract fistulas are managed with double J catheter and infections are treated with antibiotic therapy and conservative measures. In the event of stent migration, the stent must be repositioned under fluoroscopy. The authors prefer to remove the urethral catheter first when the drainage in 12 h is less than 30 cc, and if the drainage does not increase 3 days later, it is removed.

The incidence of restenosis is 4%. The management of these cases depends on anatomical factors (e.g., extent of stenosis) and surgeon's preference. Most urologists choose endopyelotomy management with retrograde or antegrade endopyelotomy with success rates up to 70%. Another option is a second open or laparoscopic pyeloplasty.[14]

Advice to Avoid Complications

To counteract these complications, the surgeon should improve these technical aspects:
- Appropriate and careful dissection; the ureter should be handled without extensive devascularization or thermal injury. Adequate spatulation of the ureter is essential.
- Careful dissection of the crossing vessels.
- Precise and meticulous suture line – no tension, no eversion.

Laparoscopic Simple Prostatectomy

Laparoscopic simple prostatectomy is an alternative for patients with benign prostatic hyperplasia. Mariano et al. reported in a series of 60 patients; 41 patients developed retrograde ejaculation (68.3%), three patients developed prolonged ileus (5%), three patients developed urinary infection (5%), one patient had clot retention (1.7%), one patient prolonged bladder catheterization (1.7%), and one patient developed septicemia (1.7%).[41] Sotelo et al. reported on a series of 17 patients where complications occurred in three cases. One patient had an intraoperative blood loss of 2,500 cc during adenoma enucleation and needed transfusion. One patient had an increased drainage output due to clot obstruction of the urethral catheter, which was promptly resolved by catheter irrigation. One patient was readmitted 1 week after discharge home for upper digestive tract hemorrhage from a preexisting duodenal ulcer, and was managed conservatively.[42]

Advice to Avoid Complications

- Traction stitch in the median lobe to facilitate retraction and dissection of the adenoma; this suture can be exteriorized with a fascia closure device and kept under adequate traction by applying a grasper parallel to the skin.
- For traction of the adenoma, use a traction stitch with a big needle (CT-1) and monofilament, replacing this stitch as the dissection advances. Do not attempt to retract the adenoma with any kind of grasper since the grasper may tear the adenoma and cause difficulty in enucleation. With large adenoma more than 150 g, the prostate should be separated into two lobes; avoid separating the median lobe as it is helpful in the retraction of the lateral lobes.
- Verify hemostasis in areas with increased risk of bleeding, including the capsule in the following locations from the 4–5 o' clock positions, and through the 7–8 o'clock positions. Trigonization of the posterior prostatic fossa is crucial.
- The capsulotomy closure can be made with a running suture. Before finishing the closure, introduce the urethral catheter inside the bladder, confirm that the closure is watertight, and insert a drain.
- Postoperative saline bladder irrigation is commonly used at least in the first 12 h.[14]

Laparoscopic Radical Prostatectomy

The average reported complications for laparoscopic radical prostatectomy in some series were 12.5% and reoperation rates 3.7%. Access-related and postoperative complications are similar to other transabdominal urologic laparoscopic procedures. Thromboembolic events occur in 1.35% of cases; pulmonary infections and urinary or gastrointestinal complications are less common. Intraoperative specific complications are vascular (0–0.3%) in general, which may include bleeding from epigastric vessels, and/or bleeding from the dorsal venous complex.

Rectal Injury

Rectal injury occurs in 0.7–2.4% of cases, and may occur when the Denonvilliers' fascia is incised at the posterior aspect rather than at the base of the bladder or during the dissection of the lateral margins of the prostate. Bowel preparation for this procedure is an important point, so that it will only require primary repair at the time of injury (Fig. 29.8).[43,44]

Fig. 29.8 Rectal injury

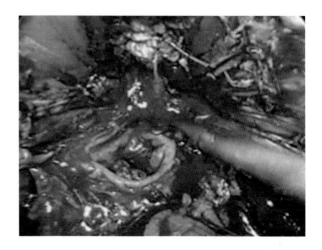

Predisposing factors for rectal injuries:

- Periprostatic fibrosis
- Previous prostate or rectal surgery
- Radiotherapy
- Locally advanced tumors
- Previous hormonal therapy
- Prostatic infection, blunt dissection
- Non-nerve-sparing radical prostatectomy (dissection close to the rectum, self-confidence in a "simpler" procedure)

Intraoperative diagnosis of rectal injury can be made with transrectal air injection in water-filled pelvis (bubbled air), transrectal balloon placement, or digital rectal examination.

Management of Rectal Injury

Close the defect in three layers (one for rectal imbrication). Check the integrity of the repair by filling the rectum with air. Air should be instilled via a rectal catheter to distend the rectal lumen and the pelvis should be filled with sterile saline to help identify air bubbles.

- Tack the rectum to the levator muscle (pulling the rectum away from anastomosis)
- Bring in a flap of omental to interpose between rectal closure and bladder/anastomosis
- A drain is placed posterior to the bladder closure, and a second drain is placed anteriorly in the space of Retzius
- Diverting colostomy (in case of tense suture line, massive fecal spillage, previous radiotherapy, or delayed diagnosis)
- Stool softeners

- Seven days of broad-spectrum antibiotics
- Cystourethrogram before catheter removal

Rectal injury may be complicated by pelvic abscess (0.1%) or by rectourinary fistula (0.1–1%).[45]

Ureteral Injury

Ureteral injury during laparoscopic radical prostatectomy was reported to occur at an incidence of 0.8%.[44, 46] This was initially described during intentional dissection of the seminal vesicles from the cul de sac (Montsouris approach). In these cases, the ureter was mistaken for the vas deferens. The other area of possible injury is the trigone, so care must be taken during the division of the posterior bladder neck. Ureteral orifices should always be identified during the dissection and during the anastomosis (Figs. 29.9 and 29.10).

Delay in diagnosis of ureteral injury takes place most often with fever and flank pain at presentation. Diagnosis is confirmed with:

- Ultrasound and/or CT scan to identify collection or hydronephrosis
- IVU-retropyelogram to see extravasation and/or obstruction
- Although rarely needed, ureteroscopy can be used to show perforation (Figs. 29.11 and 29.12)

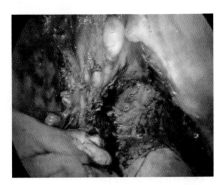

Fig. 29.9 Ureteral injury

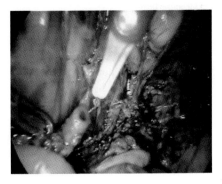

Fig. 29.10 Ureteral injury

Fig. 29.11 IV Pyelogram and CT scan. Note the presence of disruption and extravasation

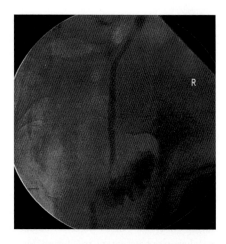

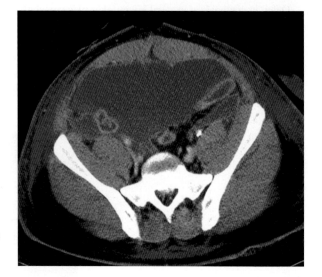

Fig. 29.12 Urinoma on CT scan from ureteral injury, with extravasation of contrast on delayed image

Management of Ureteral Injury

Intraoperative Diagnosis

- Small perforation: placement of a double J catheter
- For partial injury: suturing
- Complete transection: typically when injury occurs in the lower ureter, ureteral reimplantation is performed.

Delayed detection typically results in ureteral obstruction; in the event of short, nonobliterated strictures of less than 1 cm, these can be managed with endoureterotomy and double-J stenting. Otherwise, open or laparoscopic reconstruction of the ureter is required, including reimplantation with or without psoas hitch, or Boari flap. In longer and higher strictures, ileal interposition is an option. Kidney function is rarely compromised, however, if this complication occurs, nephrectomy may be required.

Urinary Leak

A persistent vesicourethral anastomotic leak after laparoscopic radical prostatectomy is an uncommon complication with an unclear incidence. Some series report an incidence of prolonged urethrovesical anastomotic leakage after laparoscopic radical prostatectomy to be estimated at 10%, requiring reoperation in 0.9%–2.5% of cases.[43]

Classifying the degree of leakage is based on the cystogram. If the contrast extends more than 6 cm around the anastomosis, then the leakage is considered grade 2. If the contrast extends freely into the peritoneal cavity, the leakage is considered grade 3. In grades 4 and 5, which are more severe, there was a higher incidence of anastomotic strictures.

Most urinary leaks occur in the immediate postoperative period and are usually self-limiting with prolonged retropubic drainage. Surgeons rarely encounter an anastomotic leak that does not resolve in the first 5–7 days.[47] Usually leaks close with conservative treatment, but if a leak causes irritative peritoneal symptoms, pain, and persistent ileus with significant drainage (over 1.5 L in 24 h) beyond postoperative day 6, then the surgeon should consider some of the maneuvers described below.

Several conservative treatment methods are available, including prolonged retropubic and bladder drainage, passive (rather than active) drainage, adjustment of the drain position, bladder catheter traction, and delayed bladder catheter removal. When these techniques fail, invasive techniques should be performed, including: placement of double J stent, indigo carmine to help identify the ureteral orifice for intubation, simple externalized ureteral catheter with additional side holes cut, and tunneling the externalized stent into a foley catheter. In case of ileus, abdominal pain, urinoma, or laparoscopic exploration with evacuation of the urine is required. The surgeon should irrigate and suction the bladder and replace the drain in the Retzius space; usually this last maneuver resolves the problem.

Cystoscopy will identify the dehiscence in the anastomosis and facilitate further decision-making. One possibility is laparoscopic reexploration, in which the surgeon

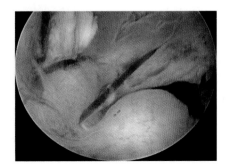

Fig. 29.13 Anastomotic dehiscence

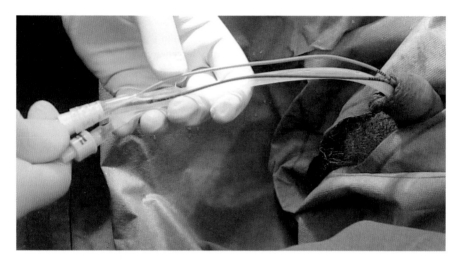

Fig. 29.14 Ureteral catheter for urine leak

attempts to place additional sutures in the anastomosis; this can be a challenging even with robot assistance. Some authors have reported successful outcomes with the placement of the bladder catheter and application of traction and adequate drainage (Figs. 29.13 and 29.14).

Symptomatic Lymphocele

The incidence of symptomatic lymphocele with laparoscopic technique is between 1.5% and 3.8%.[44, 46] The management of symptomatic lymphocele includes percutaneous drainage or laparoscopic fenestration (with a transperitoneal approach) (Fig. 29.15).

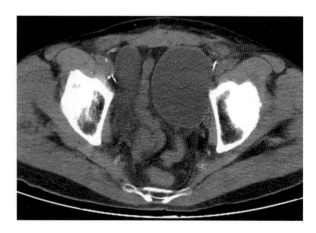

Fig. 29.15 Pelvic lymphocele

Obturator Nerve Injury and Nerve Apraxia

The incidence of obturator nerve injury and nerve apraxia has been reported to be 0.1–1% in open procedures and 0–0.3% in laparoscopic and robotic procedures.[48] Given that the obturator nerve is fixed at either end, nerve mobilization to gain additional length is not feasible. As such, in the case of nerve loss, an interposition nerve graft may be necessary.

Advice to Avoid Complications

- The first measure is the correction selection of patients for this surgery. Preoperative studies are fundamental to the adequate staging of prostate cancer that is organ confined. It is recommended for surgeons at the beginning of the learning curve to choose thin patients without previous surgery, with prostate volumes greater than 20 g and less than 50 g and preferably patients who do not wish to preserve erectile function.
- Maintain proper traction and countertraction during the opening and dissection of the Denonvilliers' fascia to avoid injury to the rectum, thus avoiding the use of thermal energy at this level.
- During the division of the urethra, keep a clear view of the prostatic apex, the neurovascular bundles, and the rhabdosphincter, and avoid unnecessary traction.
- While performing the anastomosis, verify the integrity of ureteric orifices.[14]

Laparoscopic Radical Cystectomy

Significant efforts and many contributions have been made in the execution of and research for a totally laparoscopic cystectomy. However, significant operative difficulty and increased operative times have caused many surgeons to move to a small abdominal incision where the neobladder is made in an open method with ureteral anastomosis, without losing the advantages of minimally invasive surgery. In open surgery for radical cystectomy, complications occur in up to 30% of cases. Hemal et al. reported on 11 patients undergoing laparoscopic radical cystectomy; three intraoperative complications included injury to the external iliac vein in one patient and a small rectal tear in two.[49]

Advances in laparoscopic surgery are reflected most clearly by the establishment of laparoscopic prostatectomy, with a noteworthy decrease in patient morbidity and hospital stay.[2] With regard to perioperative complications, a retrospective analysis of the National Surgical Quality Improvement Program (NSQIP) was performed on 2,538 patients and identified 774 cases (30.5%) with complications.[50] This relatively high frequency of complications is consistent with reported figures from experienced high-volume hospitals and surgeons. This retrospective analysis revealed that an ileus is the most common complication (32%), followed by urinary tract infections (7.8%), wound dehiscence (5.5%), and wound infections (5.2%).[50]

When comparing these complication rates with those of laparoscopic radical cystectomy, which is still in its infancy, it is quite clear that laparoscopic radical cystectomy must deal with the same high complication rates. Furthermore, complications unique to laparoscopy, such as hypercarbia, intraoperative bowel perforation, and subcutaneous emphysema, must be considered as well. Hemal et al. reported that three patients had intraoperative complications (rectal tear in two patients, external iliac vein injury in one patient) that were managed laparoscopically without conversion.[49]

In a study of ten patients who were candidates for salvage cystectomy or radical cystectomy, Denewer et al. found intraoperative complications consisted of one case of external iliac artery clipping, which was resected and vascular anastomosis during the open part of the procedure.[51]

The reported intraoperative complications with laparoscopic radical cystectomy included bleeding, rectal injury, and ureteral injury were similar and did not occur more than in open surgery. The complication rate is not due to the laparoscopic aspect of the procedure, since the only stage that is intraabdominal is the excision and anastomosis, which is more precise than in open surgery.

Advice to Avoid Complications

- Ureteral devascularization should be avoided; it is difficult to estimate adequate mobilization of the ureter that allows extracorporeal reimplantation, and is even more difficult in the obese patient.
- The surgeon must create an adequate incision to exteriorize the bowel and create an excellent pouch and reimplant the ureters. There are some tricks to help in the anastomosis.
- During the ureteral reimplantation, a double-J catheter should always be placed. One trick is to place a 15 cm of silk on the distal edge of the catheter, this suture will migrate toward the pouch and allow for easy removal of the catheter after the removal of the urethral catheter.
- In creating the neobladder neck, evert the mucosa as this will make it easier to recognize during intracorporeal suturing. Place a catheter in the neobladder neck and confirm it is watertight.
- To decrease the tension in the anastomosis, use the Van Velthoven technique of two needles (UR-6), two sutures of different colors, and place the first stitch with both needles in the bladder before introducing the pouch in the abdominal cavity. Reduce the Trendelenburg, and place the urethral catheter in the neobladder before entirely completing the anastomosis.
- In some situations inflate the Foley catheter and use gentle traction to help release the traction on the anastomosis.

Exit Complications

The surgeon should always be aware that getting out safely is as important as getting in. The pneumoperitoneal pressure should be lowered to 5 mmHg to check for bleeding anywhere in the work space, and special care should be taken with trocar removal.

Port-Site Hernia

Port-site hernia occurs in 0.66% cases. The most affected sites generally occur in port sites ≥10 mm and is more common at sites of multiple incisions.[52] Initially, the surgeon must determine intestinal viability with laparoscopy, and then decide if the hernia can repaired laparoscopically or with open surgery (Figs. 29.16 and 29.17).

Advice to Avoid Exit Complications

- Close all ≥10 mm port fascial defects
- Consider non-bladed or dilating trocars
- Close all ports in pediatric patients
- Routine use of Carter-Thomason suture passer

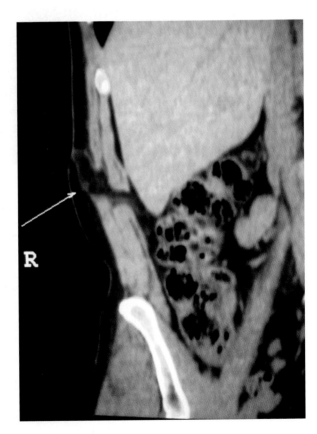

Fig. 29.16 Trocar site hernia

Fig. 29.17 Surgical repair at trocar site hernia

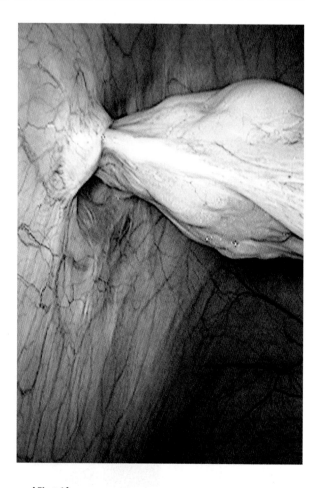

Evaluation in the Recovery Room and First 6 h

Hypotension

- Quick evaluation in the recovery room is required in order to establish whether the patient has low blood pressure because of significant blood loss during surgery (which needs replacement), or because bleeding is ongoing.
- Some effects of anesthesia cause hypotension, so accurate evaluation between the surgeon and anesthetist is essential.
- Evaluation of the drain, in terms of duration of blood filling the drainage bag is important. Accurate assessment of drainage content and amount with serial hemoglobin tests and vital signs evaluations are also essential.
- Inspect the abdominal wall and scrotum to look for hematomas that present in the first hours, which indicate acute and severe bleeding.
- A significantly distended abdomen should alert the surgeon to serious intraabdominal bleeding that usually requires open reexploration.

Chain of Actions for Laparoscopic Reexploration Due to Bleeding

- During the anesthesia process and moving forward, connect the gas insufflations tube to the previous drainage tube. This maneuver allows pneumoperitonium to be restored quickly, provides compression, and helps maintain hemostasis while the other trocars are reinserted.
- In deciding to reexplore a laparoscopic bleeding case, first consider if the patient is stable and continues to be stable after the anesthesia. Also take into account type of previous surgery and whether it will allow safe and useful laparoscopic exploration. A useful example would be partial nephrectomy, where the surgeon would need to reexplore the complete surgery bed. If the patient is stable, then a laparoscopic approach is permitted to explore the area of kidney resection and manage the bleeding accordingly. In the case of a previous laparoscopic cystectomy, it is difficult to laparoscopically reexplore the complete bed since the pouch is now connected to the urethra and the mesentery would interfere with a safe and efficient laparoscopic approach. In this case, if reexploration is necessary, then an open approach should be used.

References

1. Cadeddu J. Complications of laparoscopic procedures after concentrated training in urological laparocopy. *J Urol.* 2001;166(6):2109-2111.
2. Vallancien G, Cathelineau X, Baumert H, Doublet JD, Guillonneau B. Complications of transperitoneal laparoscopic surgery in urology: review of 1, 311 procedures at a single center. *J Urol.* 2002;168(1):23-26.
3. Abreu SC, Sharp DS, Ramani AP, et al. Thoracic complications during urological laparoscopy. *J Urol.* 2004;171(4):1451-1455.
4. Castillo O, Cortés O. Complicaciones en cirugía laparoscópica urológica. *Actas Urol Esp.* 2006;30(5):541-554.
5. Porter JR. Vascular complications during urologic laparoscopy. In: Gill IS, ed. *Textbook of Laparoscopic Urology.* New York, NY: Informa Healthcare; 2006:901-910.
6. Venkatesh R, Landman J. Laparoscopic complications: gastrointestinal. In: Gill IS, ed. *Textbook of Laparoscopic Urology.* New York, NY: Informa Healthcare; 2006:911-922.
7. French DB, Marcovich R. Laparoscopic complications: neuromuscular. In: Gill IS, ed. *Textbook of Laparoscopic Urology.* New York, NY: Informa Healthcare; 2006:923-932.
8. Abreu SC, Cerqueira JBG, Fonseca GN. Complications: Thoracic. In: Gill IS, ed. *Textbook of Laparoscopic Urology.* New York, NY: Informa Healthcare; 2006:933-938.
9. Chandler JC, Corson SL, Way WL. Three spectra of laparoscopic entry access injuries. *J Am Coll Surg.* 2001;192:478-491.
10. Fahlenkamp D, Rassweiler J, Fornara P, Free T, Loening SA. Complications of laparoscopic procedures in urology: experience with 2, 407 procedures at 4 german centers. *J Urol.* 1999;162:765-771.
11. Permpongkosol S, Link RE, Su LM, et al. Complications of 2, 775 urological laparoscopic procedures: 1993 to 2005. *J Urol.* 2007;177:580-585.
12. Soulié M, Salomon L, Seguin P, et al. Multi-institutional of complications in 1085 laparoscopic urologic procedures. *Urology.* 2001;58(6):899-903.

13. Wolf S Jr, Marcovich R, Gill IS, et al. Survey of neuromuscular injuries to the patient and surgeon during urologic laparoscopic surgery. *Urology*. 2000;55(6):831-836.

14. Santinelli F, Carracedo M. Trucos y secretos cirugia laparoscopica en urologia. In: Sotelo R, Castillo O, Mirandolino M, Santinelli F, eds. *Lumboscopia: tecnica y secretos para su realizacion*. Venezuela: La Galaxia; 2006:59-70.

15. Gill IS, Clayman RV, Albala DM, et al. Retroperitoneal and pelvic extraperitoneal laparoscopy: an international perspective. *Urology*. 1998;52:566-571.

16. Meraney A, Samee A, Gill IS. Vascular and bowel complications during retroperitoneal laparoscopic surgery. *J Urol*. 2002;168:1941-1944.

17. Demey A, de la Taille A, Vordos D, et al. Complications of retroperitoneal laparoscopy based on a series of 500 cases. *Prog Urol*. 2006;16(2):128-133.

18. Liapis D, de la Taille A, Ploussard G, et al. Analysis of complications from 600 retroperitoneoscopic procedures of the upper urinary tract during the last 10 years. *World J Urol*. 2008;26(6):523-530.

19. Kumar M, Kumar R, Hemal AK, Gupta NP. Complications of retroperitoneoscopic surgery at one centre. *BJU Int*. 2001;87:607-612.

20. Hemal AK, Gupta NP, Wadhwa SN, Goel A, Kumar R. Retroperitoneoscopic nephrectomy and nephroureterectomy for benign nonfunctioning kidneys: a single center experience. *Urology*. 2001;57(4):644-649.

21. Hemal AK, Goel A, Kumar M. Evaluation of laparoscopic retroperitoneal surgery in urinary stone disease. *J Endourol*. 2001;15(7):701-705.

22. Winfield HN, Hamilton BD, Bravo EL, Novick AC. Laparoscopic adrenalectomy: the preferred choice? A comparison to open adrenalectomy. *J Urol*. 1998;160(2):325-329.

23. Hazzan D, Shiloni E, Golijanin D, Jurim O, Reissman P. Laparoscopic vs. open adrenalectomy for benign adrenal neoplasm. *Surg Endosc*. 2001;15(11):1356-1358.

24. Gill IS. The case for laparoscopic adrenalectomy. *J Urol*. 2001;166:429-436.

25. Soulié M, Seguin P, Richeux L, et al. Urological complications of laparoscopic surgery: experience with 350 procedures at a single center. *J Urol*. 2001;165:1960-1963.

26. Terachi T, Yoshida O, Matsuda T, et al. Complications of laparoscopic and retroperitoneoscopic adrenalectomies in 370 cases in Japan: a multi-institutional study. *Biomed Pharmacother*. 2000;54(Suppl 1):211s-214s.

27. Castillo O, Cortés O, Kerkebe M, Arellano L, Russo M, Pinto I. Adrenalectomía laparoscópica: lecciones aprendidas en 110 procedimientos consecutivos. *Rev Chil Cir*. 2006;58(3):175-180.

28. Doumas K, Skrepetis K, Lykourinas M. Laparoscopic ablation of symptomatic peripelvic renal cysts. *J Endourol*. 2004;18(1):45-48.

29. Rané A. Laparoscopic management of symptomatic simple renal cysts. *Int Urol Nephrol*. 2004;36(1):5-9.

30. Rubinstein SC, Hulbert JC, Pharand D, Schuessler WW, Vancaille TG, Kavoussi LR. Laparoscopic ablation of symptomatic renal cysts. *J Urol*. 1993;150:1103-1106.

31. Kim IY, Clayman RV. Laparoscopic radical nephrectomy: current status. In: Gill IS, ed. *Textbook of Laparoscopic Urology*. New York, NY: Informa; 2006:493-498.

32. Siqueira TM Jr, Kuo RL, Gardner TH, et al. Major complications in 213 laparoscopic nephrectomy cases: the Indianapolis experience. *J Urol*. 2002;168:1361-1365.

33. Gill IS, Kavoussi LR, Clayman RV, et al. Complications of laparoscopic nephrectomy in 185 patients: a multi-institutional revew. *J Urol*. 1995;154:479-483.

34. Parsons JK, Varkarakis I, Rha KH, Jarrett TW, Pinto PA, Kavoussi LR. Complications of abdominal urologic laparoscopy: longitudinal five years analysis. *Urology*. 2004;63:27-32.

35. Spaliviero M, Gill IS. Laparoscopic partial nephrectomy: current status. In: Gill IS, ed. *Textbook of Laparoscopic Urology*. New York, NY: Informa Healthcare; 2006:519-542.

36. Ramani AP, Desai MM, Steinberg AP, et al. Complications of laparoscopic partial nephrectomy in 200 cases. *J Urol*. 2005;173(1):42-47.

37. Celia A, Zeccolini G, Guazzoni G, et al. Laparoscopic nephron sparing surgery: a multi-institutional European survey of 592 cases. *Arch Ital Urol Androl*. 2008;80(3):85-91.

38. Pyo P, Chen A, Grasso M. Retroperitoneal laparoscopic partial nephrectomy: surgical experience and outcomes. *J Urol*. 2008;180(4):1279-1283.

39. Eden C, Gianduzzo T, Chang C, Thiruchelvam N, Jones A. Extraperitoneal laparoscopic pyeloplasty for primary and secondary ureteropelvic junction obstruction. *J Urol*. 2004; 172:2308-2311.

40. Inagaki T, Rha KH, Ong AM, Kavoussi LR, Jarrett TW. Laparoscopic pyeloplasty: current status. *BJU Int*. 2005;95(2):102-105.

41. Mariano MB, Tefilli MV, Graziottin TM, Morales CM, Goldraich IH. Laparoscopic prostatectomy for benign prostatic hyperplasia – a six-year experience. *Eur Urol*. 2006;49:127-132.

42. Sotelo R, Spaliviero M, Garcia-Sergi A, et al. Laparoscopic retropubic simple prostatectomy. *J Urol*. 2005;173:757-760.

43. Rassweiler J, Seemann O, Schulze M, Teber D, Hatzinger M, Frede T. Laparoscopic versus open radical prostatectomy: a comparative study at a single institution. *J Urol*. 2003;169: 1689-1693.

44. Lepor H, Nieder AM, Ferrandino MN. Intraoperative and postoperative complications of radical retropubic prostatectomy in a consecutive series of 1, 000 cases. *J Urol*. 2001;166: 1729-1733.

45. Benoit RM, Naslund MJ, Cohen JK. Complications after radical retropubic prostatectomy in the Medicare population. *Urology*. 2000;56:116-120.

46. Augustin H, Hammerer P, Graefen M, et al. Intraoperative and perioperative morbidity of contemporary radical retropubic prostatectomy in a consecutive series of 1243 patients: results of a single center between 1999 and 2002. *Eur Urol*. 2003;43:113-118.

47. Moinzadeh A, Abouassaly R, Gill IS, Libertino JA. Continuous needle vented Foley catheter suction for urinary leak after radical prostatectomy. *J Urol*. 2004;171:2366-2367.

48. Hu JC, Nelson RA, Wilson TG, et al. Perioperative complications of laparoscopic and robotic assisted laparoscopic radical prostatectomy. *J Urol*. 2006;175:541-546.

49. Hemal AK, Kumar R, Seth A, Gupta NP. Complications of laparoscopic radical cystectomy during the initial experience. *Int J Urol*. 2004;11(7):483-488.

50. Hollenbeck BK, Miller DC, Taub D, et al. Identifying risk factors for potentially avoidable complications following radical cystectomy. *J Urol*. 2005;174:1231-1237.

51. Denewer A, Kotb S, Hussein O, El-Maadawy M. Laparoscopic assisted cystectomy and lymphadenectomy for bladder cancer: initial experience. *World J Surg*. 1999;23:608-611.

52. Chiong E, Hegarty PK, Davis JW, Kamat MW, Pisters LL, Matin SF. Port-site hernias occurring after the use of bladeless expanding trocars. *Urology*. 2010;75(3):574-580.

Difficulties in Laparoscopic Training, Mentoring, and Medico-Legal Issues

30

Ahmed M. Al-Kandari and Inderbir S. Gill

Laparoscopy is a surgical technique that requires special knowledge, training, and skills. With the introduction of more complex cases (both extirpative and reconstructive), training is essential to enable the surgeon to do these procedures efficiently. Worldwide spread of laparoscopic urologic surgery has occurred over the years with different efforts by surgeons and their institutions.

According to one study, laparoscopic urologic surgery (LUS) is one of the fastest growing subspecialties in the surgical world. The procedures require technical expertise and finesse; unlike their open counterparts, there is significant limitation in the margin of error. Various ethical, medicolegal, and health economy demands have made training in laparoscopic urologic surgery challenging: to date, no study has documented a global consensus on optimal LUS training programs. The authors' search identified several models, some of which were applied successfully in the form of mini-fellowships. There remain no clear guidelines on the optimum LUS training program. The optimal program may need to be tailored to individual units based on resources (this includes country-specific health economics), mentor availability, and caseload.[1] Furthermore, some Spanish urology units have been developing special experimental training programs on laparoscopic radical prostatectomy, partial nephrectomy, or laparoscopic dismembered pyeloplasty with the Anderson-Hynes technique. It has been previously described that laparoscopic modular learning constitutes a very useful concept to avoid problems related to an incomplete and incorrect learning process. Also, it seems clear that laparoscopic training reduces the learning curve in laparoscopic urologic techniques.[2] Laparoscopic surgery is well known as having a long and variable learning curve. In fact, successive generations of surgeons were able to reduce their operative times and plateau their learning curves. The preliminary data suggests that younger trainees are faster to acquire new laparoscopic skills than older persons. This finding suggests a potential benefit from earlier integration of laparoscopic skills in medical education.[3]

Significant variation in outcomes is explained by factors describing aspects of surgical expertise. Variability in the surgical skill set is likely greatest during the laparoscopic learning curve, which raises quality-of-care concerns during the initial implementation of

A.M. Al-Kandari (✉)

Department of Surgery (Urology), Faculty of Medicine, Kuwait University, Jabriyah, Kuwait
e-mail: drakandari@hotmail.com

A.M. Al-Kandari and I.S. Gill (eds.), *Difficult Conditions in Laparoscopic Urologic Surgery*, **433**
DOI: 10.1007/978-1-84882-105-7_30, © Springer-Verlag London Limited 2011

the technique. Policies attempting to smooth the laparoscopic learning curve, such as mentoring and skill measurement prior to attainment of credentials, could improve the quality of care.[4]

Laparoscopic Urologic Training

There are several different ways of learning laparoscopic urologic surgery, including the following scenarios outlined in the following section.

Training During Residency

More programs worldwide have adopted laparoscopic urologic procedures, so residents typically have opportunities to assist during these procedures. But it is important to examine the difficulties that can occur during in this scenario:

Problem:

Some staff, especially those who have recently completely their fellowships, prefer to oversee cases entirely by themselves, which leaves the residents with fewer chances to completely master laparoscopic procedures.

Solutions:

1. Program directors should get feedback from their residents and take action to establish training tasks for residents when they assist staff during laparoscopic urologic surgery.
2. Residents should have opportunities for dry laparoscopic training on specific cases.
3. Animal laboratory facilities can be very helpful as residents can practice different laparoscopic techniques and become familiar with the different disposables and instruments.

Problem:

Lack of strict follow-up of resident operative log books, especially in laparoscopic surgery.

Solutions:

1. The program director and chairman should examine training issues and residents' log books to ensure solid training in laparoscopy.

2. Careful follow-up of each resident's performance is required to ensure that the resident has completed enough training suitable to his or her level.
3. Careful operative work division between residents in their senior year and in their fellowships is important to ensure that everyone gets a chance.

Training During Fellowships

There are worldwide laparoscopic urologic fellowship training programs. Most of these programs are recognized by the Endourological Society. An example is the Memorial Sloan-Kettering Cancer Center Urologic Oncologic Laparoscopic Program. It lasts 2 years and trains fellows and faculty. For fellows, the program consists of a 6-month, high-volume laparoscopic oncology rotation, during which dry lab, animal lab, video review, and operating room experience are required. For faculty, the program consists of one accredited continuing medical education course, 20 h of dry lab, one session animal lab, observation of laparoscopic cases, first assistant in a minimum of 15 laparoscopic cases, and performing laparoscopic cases under mentorship. The goals of a surgical education program should be the standardization of the acquisition of surgical skills and assessment of the performance in a uniform setting to ensure the maintenance of the acquisition of skills and to develop programs to teach new skills.[5]

These programs are an excellent opportunity for training, and many programs have structured training plans and close mentoring that help fellows progress through their training. However, there are some difficulties encountered in this scenario that may affect the outcome of fellowship training:

Problem:

Staff who do not teach operative steps to fellows either because they are new or they prefer to do their cases by themselves.

Solutions:

1. A structured, detailed training program for fellows is important to ensure that they receive the necessary training.
2. Feedback from the fellows about their training progress in periodic intervals is important to ensure adequate assessment of their training.
3. Accurate operative work division between senior residents and fellows is important to ensure adequate training for all trainees.
4. Staff who do not teach the operative steps to trainees should be instructed to participate in training. If a staff member does not improve or resolve this issue, then he or she should be denied resident and fellow support as this is important in training programs. This should be applied for both for senior residents and fellows.

Self-training

In many instances, especially in age of post-residency, a urologist will decide to learn laparoscopy on his or her own. The several different methods to achieve this goal will be discussed in the following section, along with some of the difficulties that may be encountered.

Attending Laparoscopic Courses and Workshops

Basic Laparoscopic Courses

Before beginning laparoscopy, one should know the basics, including instruments, access, positioning, technique, etc. There are worldwide courses that discuss these issues for urologists (as well as for other specialties), which are very useful. Some commercial companies (e.g., Ethicon, Storz) provide support for these courses, which is very helpful.

Problem:

Some of the courses may not be very useful if practical issues are not involved.

Solutions:

1. Obtain disposable instruments and practice with them on dry objects.
2. An animal model can be used to practice the techniques that were learned.
3. Regular practice of some techniques, especially intracorporeal suturing, is helpful in obtain the benefits of taking a laparoscopic course and also helps to improve and master techniques.

Technical Operative Courses and Advanced Courses

More centers and universities are conducting occasional, and sometimes annual, specialized and advanced courses that are very useful in attracting interest in laparoscopic surgery. An example of such is the Institut de Recherche contre les Cancers de l'Appareil Digestif (IRCAD) courses offered in Strasbourg, France.

Problems:

1. These courses are very helpful, but may be costly and require travel.
2. Sometimes the animal laboratory part of the course does not allow for sufficient training, since a large number of candidates on one animal does not allow for adequate practice.

Solutions:

1. The industry should increase participation in propagating laparoscopic surgery by establishing training centers worldwide. Offering support for doctors to attend will reduce costs and encourage more people to participate.
2. The industry should also provide more animals with more trainers to improve the utilization of animal laboratory to the best possible level.

Visiting Experts in Laparoscopic Urologic Surgery

Visiting experts in laparoscopy and observing them operate is a very helpful tool in improving training experience. Nowadays worldwide distribution of centers for laparoscopic urology is available, so one should consider preference, budget, and travel issues (Figs. 30.1 and 30.2).

Problem:

1. Lack of benefits for the visiting program

Solutions:

To make the best of the visiting program, one should try to do the following:

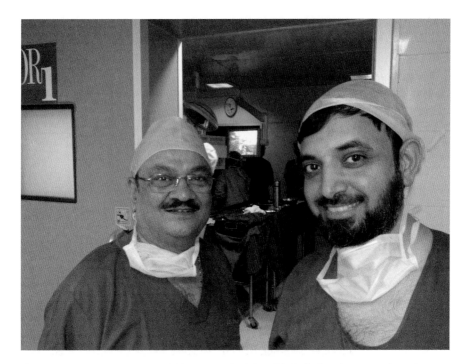

Fig. 30.1 Dr. Ahmed Al-Kandari visiting Dr. Mahesh Desai in India for a laparoscopic course

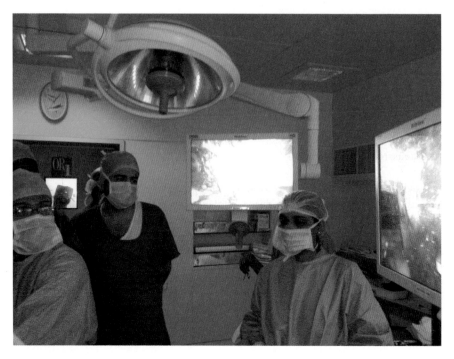

Fig. 30.2 International visitors observing laparoscopic surgery

1. Plan the visit with enough time for notification, and ask if it is possible for the center to line up more cases of your interest during your visit.
2. Avoid periods where there are many other visitors. Do this in order to take advantage of personal communication with the operating surgeon who can be more attentive and can answer questions easily.
3. Try to line up a visit before or after one of the annual meetings (i.e., the American Urological Association annual meeting), to help in time and cost management, especially when the meeting and the center are in the same country.
4. Extending a stay after a course or a workshop can be beneficial, especially when arrangements have been made for more opportunities to observe.

Inviting Experts to Your Center

One of the most important training opportunities is inviting world experts in laparoscopy to your center (Figs. 30.3–30.5). This leads to a tremendously valuable training opportunity, which allows one to be the first assistant during surgery, careful observation of the operative steps, and the ability to ask questions according to one's learning needs.

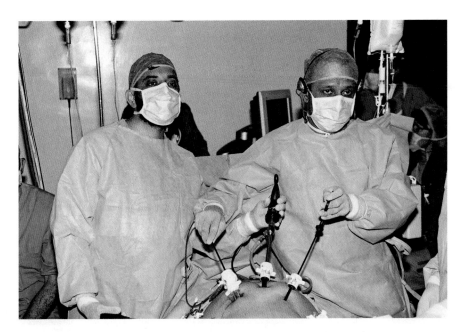

Fig. 30.3 Dr. Gill and Dr. Al-Kandari during a laparoscopic procedure in Kuwait

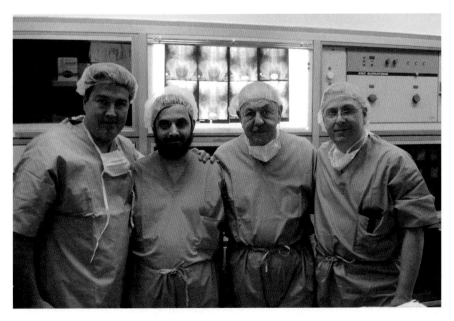

Fig. 30.4 Drs. Arthur Smith, Michael Grasso, Rene Sotello and Dr. Al-Kandari in the operating room during an Endourology and Laparoscopy Conference in Kuwait.

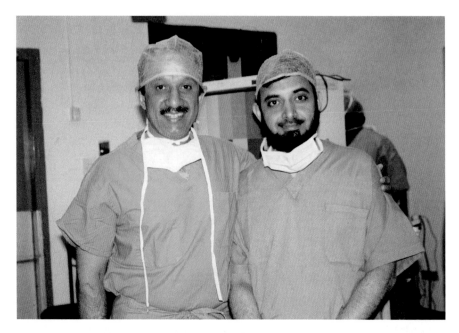

Fig. 30.5 Dr. Gill and Dr. Al-Kandari in the operating room during a laparoscopic workshop in Kuwait

Problem:

Conditions that make the visit less efficient occur, such as:

1. Suboptimal case types due to medical status, such as a patient with high-risk medical problems that are not well controlled before surgery and may lead to case cancelation.
2. Suboptimal laparoscopic cases, such as cases with multiple open surgeries or very large masses that may not be suitable for learning demonstrations.
3. Lack of adequate laparoscopic instruments may lead to technical difficulties or surgeon discomfort.
4. Lack of an experienced camera person, assistant, anesthetist, and scrub nurse, which may cause the procedure to be very difficult and uncomfortable.
5. Absence of audiovisual recording equipment, which leads to loss of a valuable educational material.

Solutions:

1. Proper case selection from all aspects is essential to ensure that the cases are done properly and a surgeon and his or her team can benefit from the visiting expert who will illustrate the steps properly.
2. Careful and detailed knowledge of all the important instruments and disposables that the visiting expert uses is essential ahead of time. If the instruments are not

available, or will take a long time to procure, then one can ask the expert to bring with as many instruments as possible to facilitate the procedure. One can also consider buying these instruments (if time allows) and keeping them for such cases after the visit.

3. It is essential for successful laparoscopic surgery that one has to have a complete, helpful, and experienced team that can support the laparoscopic experience and the learning process.

4. Recording the laparoscopic procedure performed by the visiting expert creates important educational material that helps (when reviewed accurately) teach the important surgical steps.

Using a Pelvic Trainer

Laparoscopic surgery is one of the surgical skills that requires adequate training and practice so that skills can be mastered when means of practice are utilized. One example is the pelvic trainer, where one can practice laparoscopic skills and improve technical skills. Repetitive practice of laparoscopic suturing and knot tying can facilitate surgeon proficiency in performing this reconstructive technique. There is no significant difference in proficiency between the students trained on a pelvic trainer and virtual reality trained medical students in performing laparoscopic cystorrhaphy in a pig model, although both groups require considerably more training before performing this procedure clinically. The pelvic trainer training may be more user-friendly for the novice surgeon to begin learning these challenging laparoscopic skills.[6]

The principle of a mechanical simulator (i.e., a box with the possibility of trocar insertion) has not changed during the last decade. However, the types of pelvic trainers and the models used inside of them have been improved significantly. For simulation purposes, various sophisticated models have been developed, including standardized phantoms, animal organs, and even perfused segments of porcine organs. For laparoscopic suturing, various step-by-step training concepts have been presented. These can be used for determination of the ability of a physician with an interest in laparoscopic surgery, but also to classify the training status of a laparoscopic surgeon. Training in laparoscopic surgery has become an important topic, not only in learning a procedure, but also in maintaining skills and preparing for the management of complications. For these purposes, mechanical simulators will definitely play an important role in the future.[7]

Different companies have produced different trainers (Fig. 30.6). To best utilize the pelvic trainer, some of difficulties in its use must be discussed:

Problems:

1. Some pelvic trainers are expensive.
2. The instruments that used for laparoscopic training can be expensive.
3. Some pelvic trainers require a camera person, which can be difficult to find and makes learning and practicing difficult.

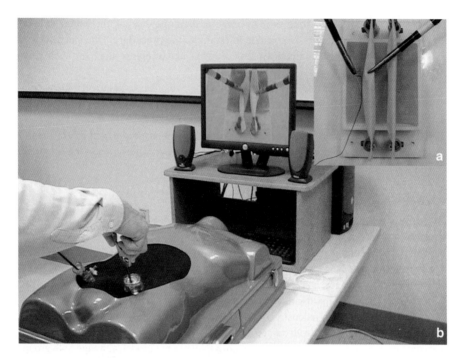

Fig. 30.6 A laparoscopic pelvic trainer (ProMIS computer-enhanced simulator, Haptica Ltd., Dublin, Ireland) (Reprinted from JSLS, Journal of the Society of Laparoendoscopic Surgeons. 2008;12(3):219–226)

Solutions:

1. If budget is an important limiting factor, some authors have described simpler home-made pelvic trainers that one may consider using.
2. In regard to the instruments needed for training and their cost, consider buying good quality used instruments that are often less costly. Also for suture practice, one may use only one needle holder – the other instrument can be any disposable forceps in good condition, which leads to cost reduction.
3. In regards to the need of a camera person (which may or may not be available), some companies have made pelvic trainers that do not require an assistant (Fig. 30.7). Others also have used special camera holder to obviate the need for an assistant.

Mentoring

Mentoring is one of the best ways to learn laparoscopic surgery. However, the availability of an experienced mentor to observe a surgeon who is operating and learning laparoscopy is limited. So if one has a chance to practice laparoscopy under mentor supervision then the following principles should be considered in order to reap the full benefits:

Fig. 30.7 Another type of pelvic trainer (Standard MITS with Joystick SimScope™, 3-Dmed®, Franklin, OH) used by Dr. Ahmed Al-Kandari

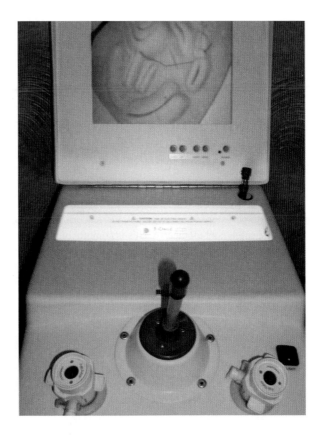

1. Select straightforward cases with minimal comorbid conditions.
2. Line up the largest possible number of cases to take full advantage of the opportunity to train.
3. Record these cases on video as they can can be a useful reference in future training.

Mutual Mentoring

Mutual mentoring allows for a greater output of cases, a high level of assistance, advice in intraoperative decisions, and the potential to "share" cases, reducing fatigue and increasing experience. It provides significant moral support in the difficult early days of starting the service. Its disadvantages are that it is time consuming and geographically restrictive. Mutual mentoring has allowed that authors to introduce a laparoscopic service at our respective hospitals with acceptable, high caseload complication rates.[8]

Video Mentoring

A number of studies have demonstrated that laparoscopic skills can be measured on a videotrainer and that ability improves with repetitive performance. Ultimately, preoperative images and data may be interfaced with robotic simulation software to allow practice of virtual operations with realistic tissue photo-representation prior to performing them on patients. Improvements in laparoscopic surgical simulation and application of these newly acquired skills on a simulated patient will ultimately eliminate the learning curve on actual patients and provide a useful means of establishing competence.[9]

Mentoring provides a useful adjunct to postgraduate urological training and the integration of laparoscopic techniques into the community based practice of urology.[10]

Telementoring

Telementoring is an interesting idea that facilitates mentoring through variable distances in which an experienced surgeon guides and teaches a less experienced surgeon how to do a procedure safely and efficiently. This is commonly done by the means of telecommunications, and lately through communication via the broadband Internet. Different centers have reported their experiences with such a teaching approach (Fig. 30.8).

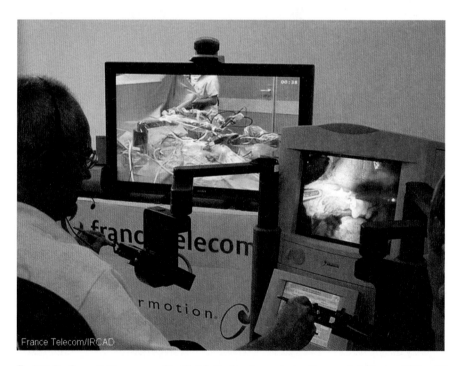

Fig. 30.8 Professor J. Marescaux of Institut de Recherche contre les Cancers de L'Appareil Digestif (IRCAD) performs the first transatlantic robotic assisted remote telepresence laparoscopic cholecystectomy (From Anvari M. Remote telepresence surgery: separation of surgeon from patient. http://www.laparoscopytoday.com/2005/01/remote_telepres.html. Accessed May 1, 2010. Reprinted with permission from the author)

To assess the feasibility of telementoring, a clinical telepresence system was developed. Telementoring was attempted in 14 advanced and 9 basic urologic laparoscopic procedures. The remote surgeon was located in a control room (>1,000 ft from operating room) while supervising an inexperienced surgeon. Mentoring was accomplished with real-time video images, two-way audio communication, a robotic arm used to control the videoendoscope, and a telestrator. The patient outcome, complications, and operative time were assessed and compared with patients undergoing matched procedures in which the experienced surgeon was working side by side with the primary surgeon. The overall telementoring success rate was 95.6% (22/23 cases) with no increase in complications. Telementoring of a laparoscopic radical nephrectomy failed secondary to improper positioning of the robotic arm. Operative times compared between telementored and traditionally mentored procedures were not statistically different for basic procedures, but were longer for advanced cases. Telementoring of laparoscopic procedures is safe and feasible. Further clinical studies are needed prior to implementing telementoring in surgical training.[11]

A laparoscopic adrenalectomy was telementored between Innsbruck, Austria, and Baltimore, Maryland (5,083 miles apart). A laparoscopic varicocelectomy was telementored between Bangkok, Thailand, and Baltimore, Maryland (10,880 miles apart) as well. Both procedures were performed over three integrated digital service network (ISDN) lines (384 kbps) with an approximate 1 s delay. Both procedures were successfully accomplished with an uneventful postoperative course. International telementoring is a viable method of instructing less experienced laparoscopic surgeons through potentially complex laparoscopic procedures, as well as potentially improving patient access to specialty care.[12]

Over a period of 3 months, two laparoscopic left spermatic vein ligations, one retroperitoneal renal biopsy, one laparoscopic nephrectomy, and one percutaneous access to the kidney were telementored. International telementoring is a feasible technique that can enhance surgeon education and decrease the likelihood of complications attributable to inexperience with new operative techniques.[13]

Medicolegal Issues with Laparoscopic Urologic Surgeries

Medicolegal issues in different surgical specialties have become a serious problem that may affect the outcome of different operations. To understand the important aspects in laparoscopy, the frequently possible scenarios will be listed and then the best ways of dealing with them will be discussed.

1. *Vascular injury during access performance*: Reports of major vascular accidents during access performance in laparoscopic urologic procedures have been reported and luckily are rare. This complication can lead to serious morbidity and even mortality; it can typically be a cause for litigation. The following are some important points to remember: The solution:

   - Be extremely careful, especially at the beginning of practice and in thin patients. Consider either an open approach to obtain access or carefully inserting a Visiport™ (Covidien, Mansfield, MA)

- Immediate conversion, with the request of vascular surgeon, can help salvage the situation and avoid the serious medical and legal issues

2. *Bowel injury*: Bowel injury during laparoscopic urologic surgery is possible and can be serious if unrecognized. If this occurs, the potential for litigation is high. Prevent bowel injury by doing the following:

   - Confirm the safety of all laparoscopic instruments, especially the ones attached to the monopolar cautery; if the insulation is broken (especially in reusable instruments) this can lead to bowel injury.
   - A safety margin of at least 2 cm from the bowel should be observed when dissecting adhesions or mobilizing the colon, especially with monopolar current since it has a widely spreading thermal effect.
   - Use other thermal energy dissecting instruments with less widespread effects such as ultrasound activated or bipolar activated sources.
   - Avoid cases with previous abdominal surgeries when beginning laparoscopy to avoid bowel injury.
   - Once the surgeon is comfortable with more cases, then he or she can try obtaining access either by the open technique or through an abdominal quadrant.

Prior reports of bowel injury during laparoscopic gynecologic surgery under litigation have illustrated important facts: The initial laparoscopic entry into the peritoneal cavity remains the major contributor to bowel injury in laparoscopic surgery. The open (Hasson) technique does not prevent bowel injuries. Delayed recognition was a major factor in assessment of liability.[14]

3. *Missed needles, gauze, or equipment*: It is very rare nowadays, with the strict responsibilities of operating theater nurses, that needles or broken instrument fragments are missed. It is essential that the count be correct when surgeons use intraperitoneal gauze since it can easily be missed, especially when bleeding occurs. These cases are definitely a cause for legal litigation that should be avoided.

General Points to Remember Regarding the Importance of Legal Issues in Laparoscopic Surgery

1. *Obtaining patient informed consent*: A full and detailed consent – which should be written and properly explained to the patient with emphasis related to potential complications tailored according to patient disease and surgical anatomy – is essential to avoid litigation when complications occur. Obtaining a detailed and clear informed consent is of key importance. In case of patient injury or death, the medicolegal aspects of the intraoperative complications and the liability of the surgical team are examined. However, it is always necessary to consider if the potential complications are predictable and/or preventable in accordance to the parameters of negligence, imprudence, and lack of knowledge. The same criteria have to be applied to assure compliance with preventive sanitary rules and that the conversion to laparotomy has been promptly carried out.[15]

   The requirement for patient informed consent has been confirmed by several decisions of the Appeals Court and is stated in the code of deontology. The value of classical oral information has been recently questioned in certain court cases. The authors have

analyzed the current legal situation in France and have tried to define the informational content required in the case of laparoscopic surgery, in addition to the way this information is provided and the means of obtaining informed consent:

- The information provided must be personalized.
- The patient must be informed that laparoscopy remains a surgical operation. It is licit to warn the patient of predictable risks according to statistical probabilities, of the team's experience, and of the patient's own status, including past history and psychological factors.
- A written statement may be prepared but must remain a document complementary to personalized oral information.
- The surgeon must obtain and assure good patient comprehension.
- The surgical community should publish risk rates in order for surgeons to have reliable references that can be used to define the notion of exceptional risk.[16]

2. *Obtaining consent for problem-solving laparoscopic surgery or open conversion*: In this situation, it is important to emphasize the risks to the patient. A good example would be a laparoscopic partial nephrectomy, especially for a larger mass (less than 7 cm), which is commonly performed nowadays. Since there is the possibility of s laparoscopic radical nephrectomy or an open conversion, this should be explained to the patient and included in the consent form to help in post operative patient satisfaction and to avoid medicolegal issues.

3. *Number requirement for proficiency in laparoscopic surgery (and avoiding legal problems when complications arise)*: There is no absolute number of cases that assures one competence in laparoscopic urologic surgery. The surgeon has to know his or her ability, recognize difficulties, deal with possible intraoperative complications, and consider all the options – even open conversion – to correct problems. It is well known that, before competence is achieved, a number of cases are needed to overcome the learning curve – a similar observation was made in a study by Dagash et al. on pediatric laparoscopic urologic procedures.[17]

4. *Use of reusable instruments*: Reusing instruments can be a source of medicolegal problems due to different factors, including:
   - Loss of insulation, which can lead to bowel injury during usage of the monopolar cautery.
   - Incomplete sterilization can be an issue, as reported by some authors. The use of such inadequately reprocessed single-use instruments increases the risk for the patient, and can lead to nosocomial infection and to legal consequences for the healthcare facility.[18]

5. *Robotic-assisted laparoscopic procedures*: It is recognized by world experts that robotic-assisted surgery requires basic training and teamwork to complete a procedure safely and efficiently. Subsequently proctoring, mentoring, and taking courses are essential aspects of being safe with the technique and avoiding medicolegal problems. A report has been published from the Society of Urologic Robotic Surgeons regarding the training, credentialing, proctoring, and medicolegal risks of robotic urological surgery; especially focusing on robotic-assisted radical prostatectomy.

   The implementation of guidelines and proctoring recommendations is necessary to protect surgeons, proctors, institutions and, above all, the patients who are associated with the institutional introduction of a robot-assisted radical prostatectomy program.[19]

Conclusion

Laparoscopic urologic surgery requires adequate training to facilitate surgery and to minimize or possibly avoid complications. The surgeon who plans to adopt laparoscopic surgery must spend the essential effort in training – including courses, mini-fellowships, inviting and learning from experts, and, occasionally, telementoring. It is always important to have all the adequate instruments and to utilize teamwork to accomplish procedures. Knowledge of the different complications and a careful, detailed consent will hopefully prevent medicolegal litigations related to laparoscopy.

References

1. Kommu SS, Dickinson AJ, Rané A. Optimizing outcomes in laparoscopic urologic training: toward a standardized global consensus. *J Endourol.* 2007;21(4):378-385.
2. Usón Gargallo J, Sánchez Margallo FM, Díaz-Güemes Martín-Portugués I, Loscertales Martín de Agar B, Soria Gálvez F, Pascual Sánchez-Gijón S. Animal models in urological laparoscopic training. *Actas Urol Esp.* 2006;30(5):443–450.
3. Salkini MW, Hamilton AJ. The effect of age on acquiring laparoscopic skills. *J Endourol.* 2010;24(3):377-379.
4. Hollenbeck BK, Roberts WW, Wolf JS. Importance of perioperative processes of care for length of hospital stay after laparoscopic surgery. *J Endourol.* 2006;20(10):776-781.
5. Touijer K, Guillonneau B. Teaching laparoscopic urologic oncology. The Memorial Sloan-Kettering Cancer Center experience. *Actas Urol Esp.* 2006;30(5):464-468.
6. McDougall EM, Kolla SB, Santos RT, et al. Preliminary study of virtual reality and model simulation for learning laparoscopic suturing skills. *J Urol.* 2009;182(3):1018-1025.
7. Rassweiler J, Klein J, Teber D, Schulze M, Frede T. Mechanical simulators for training for laparoscopic surgery in urology. *J Endourol.* 2007;21(3):252-262.
8. Jones A, Eden C, Sullivan ME. Mutual mentoring in laparoscopic urology - a natural progression from laparoscopic fellowship. *Ann R Coll Surg Engl.* 2007;89(4):422-425.
9. Hedican SP, Nakada SY. Videotape mentoring and surgical simulation in laparoscopic courses. *J Endourol.* 2007;21(3):288-293.
10. Marguet CG, Young MD, L'Esperance JO, et al. Hand assisted laparoscopic training for postgraduate urologists: the role of mentoring. *J Urol.* 2004;172(1):286-289.
11. Moore RG, Adams JB, Partin AW, Docimo SG, Kavoussi LR. Telementoring of laparoscopic procedures: initial clinical experience. *Surg Endosc.* 1996;10(2):107-110.
12. Lee BR, Caddedu JA, Janetschek G, Schulam P, Docimo SG. International surgical telementoring: our initial experience. *Stud Health Technol Inform.* 1998;50:41-47.
13. Micali S, Virgili G, Vannozzi E, et al. Feasibility of telementoring between Baltimore (USA) and Rome (Italy): the first five cases. *J Endourol.* 2000;14(6):493-496.
14. Vilos GA. Laparoscopic bowel injuries: forty litigated gynaecological cases in Canada. *J Obstet Gynaecol Can.* 2002;24(3):224-230.
15. Chisari MG, Finocchiaro A, Lo Menzo E, Rosato V, Basile G. Laparoscopic surgery: from clinic to legal medicine. *Minerva Chir.* 2004;59(6):589-596.
16. Rougé C, Tuesch JJ, Casa C, Ludes B, Arnaud JP. Patient information and obtaining informed consent in laparoscopic surgery. *J Chir (Paris).* 1997;134(7–8):340-344.
17. Dagash H, Chowdhury M, Pierro A. When can I be proficient in laparoscopic surgery? A systematic review of the evidence. *J Pediatr Surg.* 2003;38(5):720-724.

18. Roth K, Heeg P, Reichl R. Specific hygiene issues relating to reprocessing and reuse of single-use devices for laparoscopic surgery. *Surg Endosc*. 2002;16(7):1091-1097.

19. Zorn KC, Gautam G, Shalhav AL, et al. Training, credentialing, proctoring and medicolegal risks of robotic urological surgery: recommendations of the society of urologic robotic surgeons. *J Urol*. 2009;182(3):1126-1132.

Index

A.M. Al-Kandari and I.S. Gill (eds.), *Difficult Conditions in Laparoscopic Urologic Surgery*,   **451**
DOI: 10.1007/978-1-84882-105-7, © Springer-Verlag London Limited 2011